PHYSIOLOGY

OF

RESPIRATION

PHYSIOLOGY

JULIUS H. COMROE, JR., M.D., D.Sc.

Professor of Physiology

University of California, San Francisco

OF RESPIRATION

An

Introductory Text

SECOND EDITION

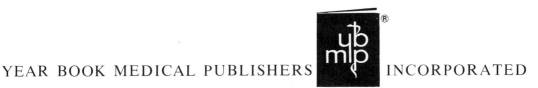

YEAR BOOK MEDICAL PUBLISHERS INCORPORATED

35 EAST WACKER DRIVE, CHICAGO

Reprinted, January 1966

Reprinted, September 1967

Reprinted, January 1968

Reprinted, April 1968

Reprinted, January 1969

Reprinted, February 1970

Reprinted, February 1971

Reprinted, October 1972

Second Edition, 1974

Library of Congress Catalog Card Number: 73-86837

Cloth: 0-8151-1826-0   Paper: 0-8151-1827-9

PRINTED IN U.S.A.

Preface to the Second Edition

THE LAST DECADE has seen rapid advances in knowledge of every aspect of respiratory and pulmonary disorders: early diagnosis of emphysema and diseases of small airways, management of respiratory distress syndrome of the newborn and "shock lung" of adults, regulation of breathing in patients with chronic hypoxia and those whose carotid bodies have been removed, the role of vagal reflexes from the lungs of unanesthetized man, the effect of gravity on airways and pulmonary circulation, new methods to detect nonmatching alveolar ventilation and pulmonary capillary blood flow, the effect of diphosphoglycerate (DPG) on the uptake and release of oxygen by hemoglobin, evaluation of acid-base disorders, defense mechanisms of the lung, new functions of the lungs and pulmonary circulation, biochemistry of the lungs, maturation of lungs from the fetus to the newborn to the adult and scanning electron microscopy to provide three-dimensional, detailed pictures of airway and lung surfaces. The last decade has also seen the general acceptance of the respiratory intensive care unit for newborn children and adults as a place where new knowledge is continuously applied to saving lives. In addition, it has seen the beginnings of the artificial lung and pulmonary transplantation, which to be clinically useful, still require intensive research on basic biological mechanisms.

The last decade has seen a revolution in pulmonary disease as a specialty: the emergence of strong research and teaching groups in pulmonary disease in American medical schools, the support of research and training in pulmonary disease by the National Heart Institute that in 1969 became the National Heart *and Lung* Institute and the recognition, at last, in 1973, by the old National Tuberculosis Association that it is, in fact, the American Lung Association. Of special significance has been the realization that, to a greater degree than in any other specialty, the finest clinical practice of pulmonary and respiratory disease requires a thorough knowlege of the sciences basic to this specialty. The medical student may continue to question the "relevance" of science in his medical education until he has become a physician responsible for a newborn or adult respiratory intensive care unit or a special pulmonary diagnostic laboratory, when he suddenly realizes the unity of basic sciences and clinical practice—that he cannot make complete diagnoses and correct decisions about treatment without knowing pulmonary and respiratory physiology, pharmacology and biochemistry. He also learns quickly that few of his patients oblige him by presenting an illness that can be managed by rote. He then realizes that his earlier philosophy of anti-intellectualism has "done him in" and that he needs something more than compassion to save the lives of his patients with pulmonary insufficiency and respiratory failure. He should also realize that the next decade will see another revolution in understanding, diagnosis and treatment and that he will need a good scientific base to understand and evaluate what is ahead.

The explosion of new knowledge and its application has resulted in revision of all chapters of the first edition of this volume, the extensive revision of ten of these, complete revision of two and addition of two new chapters (Defense Mechanisms of the Lung and Nonrespiratory Functions of the Lung). The first edition contained 111 figures. The second edition contains 140; of these, 65 are new and another 17 have been redrawn or revised.

I express my appreciation to Helen Gee Jeung who drew all of the original illustrations, to colleagues and publishers who permitted me to use their published illustrations, and to the following who provided unusually fine unpublished illustrations to use in this edition: John Clements, Gordon Gamsu, Alain Junod, Donald M. McDonald, Abraham Rudolph, John Severinghaus, Una Smith, Norman Staub and Judy Strum. I also acknowledge the generous advice and criticism of William Briscoe, John Clements, Robert Forster, Warren Gold and Abraham Rudolph with several parts of the text.

J. H. C.

Preface to the First Edition

SOME BOOKS for medical students seem to be written for their professors, for research specialists, for book reviewers—or for all three. This one is really intended for students of medicine—whether they are in medical school, in residency training or in the practice of medicine. Some parts of this book may seem to negate this statement, but not if the views that I and many others hold on the aims of medical education are accepted; these parts are included to show how physiological evidence is obtained, analyzed and evaluated; how conclusions are drawn; how hypotheses turn into concepts; how new concepts replace the previously accepted ones; how difficult and complex all of this is; how little we know "for sure" and how much remains to be learned.

Most of the text is a synthesis of what is currently known of the physiology of respiration that may be of direct help or interest to a physician on this planet. It is *not* a revision of *The Lung: Clinical Physiology and Pulmonary Function Tests* by Comroe, Forster, DuBois, Briscoe and Carlsen; its scope is far broader—from the regulation of ventilation to tissue gas exchange. It does, of course, include sections on pulmonary function, but these are placed in proper perspective in relation to a much larger subject.

There are few direct references in the text to the original publications of the many scientists who are responsible for modern respiratory physiology, and the bibliography contains only selected references. Further, because of the nature and size of this volume, some aspects of respiratory physiology have been omitted from it. I believe this is justified because of the publication in 1964 and 1965 of Section 3 of the monumental reference series, *The Handbook of Physiology;* in two of its many volumes are more than 100,000 square inches of text devoted to the Physiology of Respiration, compared to a mere 10,000 in this volume.

I express my appreciation to the many colleagues and publishers who permitted me to reproduce illustrations and to the following, who provided me with unusually fine unpublished illustrations to include in this volume: Robert Byck, Michel Campiche, John Clements, Abraham Guz, Julien Hoffman, Averill Liebow, Robert Mitchell, Lorraine Mortimer, Sergei Sorokin and William Tooley. I acknowledge also the generous assistance of Moran Campbell and Jack Howell with several parts of the text, and the artistry of Helen Gee, who drew all of the original illustrations.

I welcome suggestions for additional sections if accompanied by suggestions for deletions of an equal amount of material.

JULIUS H. COMROE, JR.

Table of Contents

1

Introduction

THE MAIN FUNCTION of respiration is to provide oxygen to the cells of the body and to remove excess carbon dioxide from them. Different species achieve this in different ways. Unicellular organisms get their O_2 by diffusion from the fluid surrounding them and eliminate CO_2 in the same way; larger organisms cannot. Krogh estimated that a spheri- cal creature with a radius of 1 cm that used 100 ml of O_2/kg/hour (about half of the O_2 consumption of resting man) would need an external O_2 pressure of 25 atmospheres, or 19,000 torr (mm Hg), to supply O_2 to its center by diffusion. He calculated that an organism cannot have a radius greater than 0.5 mm if it is to live by diffusion alone, assum-

Fig. 1-1.—Schema of the lungs and pulmonary circulation. The *rounded areas* represent alveoli; the *shaded tubes* leading to them represent all of the conducting airways. Mixed venous blood (*dark*) flows through vessels in intimate contact with ventilated alveoli and becomes arterial blood (*light*). The *thick arrows* represent inspired and expired tidal volume. The *fine arrows* represent the transfer of O_2 and CO_2 between gas and blood.

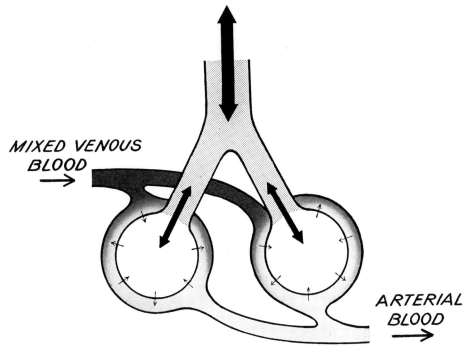

MIXED VENOUS
BLOOD
→

ARTERIAL
BLOOD
→

1

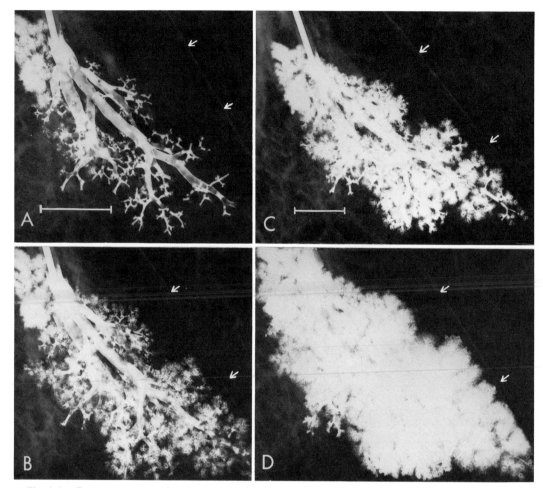

Fig. 1-2. — Roentgenograms showing progressive opacification by tantalum dust of a segment of a human bronchial tree distal to a wedged catheter. Initially, **A,** mainly nonrespiratory bronchioles are visible with some early filling of acini, producing stippling and rosettes. After further opacification, **B** to **D,** the mosaic of more spherical, superimposed but distinct acini is visible. *Arrows* indicate the pleural surface. Marker in **A** represents 2.2 cm in **A, B** and **D;** that in **C** represents 1.8 cm. (From Gamsu, G., *et al.*: Invest. Radiol. 6:171, 1971.)

ing that it lives in water almost completely saturated with air at 1 atmosphere of pressure.

Some larger organisms that live in air (certain insects) do get enough O_2 by diffusion alone, but they have a special system of air tubes (tracheae or spiracles) that pipe air directly to many regions of the body, so that the distances that O_2 must diffuse to reach tissue cells are short.

Large animals, including man, make use of two systems: (1) a blood circulatory system to carry whatever is necessary to and from the tissue cells, with the help of a remarkable chemical, hemoglobin, which insures the transport of large quantities of O_2 and CO_2, and (2) a respiratory system, a gas exchanger, to load the blood with O_2 and remove excess CO_2. In fish, blood flows through the gill vessels and extracts O_2 from water flowing around them. In man, the respiratory surfaces are folded within the body to prevent drying of the delicate membranes; air saturated with water vapor is drawn into intimate

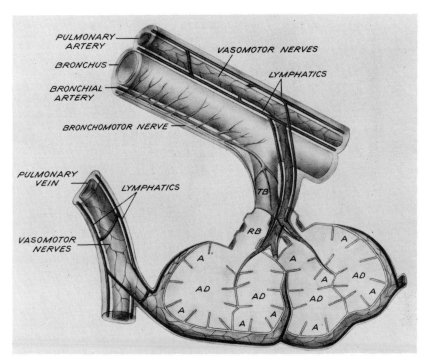

Fig. 1-3. — Lung model showing arrangement of blood and air tubes to terminal air units. Note the relations of the bronchial blood supply, lymphatics and motor innervation, insofar as they are known. Possibilities for selective interactions that regulate local ventilation to local blood flow become apparent in this model. A = anatomic alveolus; AD = alveolar ducts; RB = respiratory bronchiole; TB = terminal bronchiole. (From Staub, N. C., in Gray, T. C., and Nunn, J. F. [eds.]: *General Anesthesia* [3d ed.: London, Butterworth & Company, Ltd. 1971], vol. 1, chapter 5.)

contact with the blood flowing through the pulmonary capillaries, and gases are exchanged.

These two systems cooperate to supply the needs of the tissues. One system supplies air; the other supplies blood. Their ultimate purpose is the transfer of gases between air and all tissue cells. The respiratory system uses an air pump, which draws fresh air through air tubes to small air sacs (alveoli) that have very thin membranes. The circulatory system uses a blood pump, which drives the whole output of the heart through fine, thin-walled blood tubes (capillaries) surrounding the alveoli.

The respiratory system is sometimes oversimplified so that it looks like Figure 1-1, which shows that there are 2 main parts to the system: (1) a conducting airway, where practically no gas is exchanged, and (2) alveoli, where large amounts of O_2 and CO_2 are rapidly exchanged. But, in reality, the respiratory system is a very complex distributing system. It starts as 2 nasal tubes (sometimes a third tube, the mouth, is also used), and then becomes one, the trachea. The trachea subdivides into 2 main branches, the right and left bronchi, and each of these divides into 2 more, and each of these usually into 2 more. In all, there are $20-23$ subdivisions. A simple calculation shows that 20 divisions of this type produce about a million terminal tubes. At the end of each are numerous blind pouches, the alveoli; here gas exchange occurs (Fig. 1-2). There are about 300 million of these in the 2 lungs of man; their diameter varies from 75 to 300 μ. Some are very close to the center of the lung (the hilum) and some are at the apex or base of the lung, as much as $20-30$ cm away from

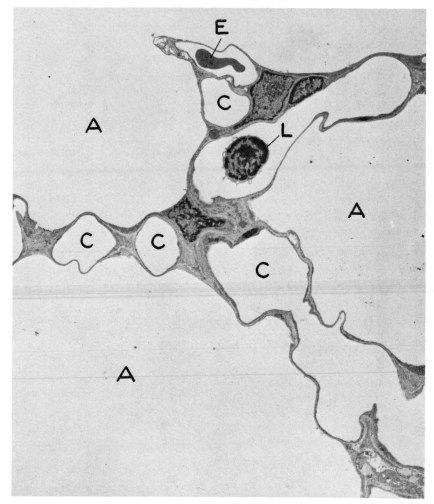

Fig. 1-4.—Electron micrograph of inflated lung that has been perfused with glutaraldehyde fixative. Most capillaries (*C*) are free of blood cells, but one of them contains an erythrocyte (*E*), and another contains a lymphocyte (*L*). Capillary endothelium, basement membrane and alveolar epithelium separate gas in alveoli (*A*) from blood in capillaries. Rat. ×2,000. (Courtesy of Dr. Judy Strum.)

the hilum. Figure 1-3 shows a terminal unit and its alveoli schematically; Figure 1-4 is an electron micrograph of alveoli and their capillaries. To distribute the proper amount of fresh air almost simultaneously to 300 million alveoli of varying sizes through 1 million tubes of varying lengths and diameters requires a remarkable engineering design. Further, since the air in the conducting tubes does not participate in gas exchange, the internal diameter of the tubes must be small (to minimize the volume of wasted air), but not so small that the respiratory pump must do excessive work against friction in moving air through them.

Another remarkable engineering feat provides a vast and extremely thin surface for the transfer of gases between air and blood (Fig. 1-4). Man at rest requires a transfer of only 200–250 ml of O_2/minute, but during maximal exercise he may need more than 20 times this amount—up to 5,500 ml. The surface area of the membrane available for this transfer is huge—about 70 m², or 40 times the surface area of the body; the membrane is less than 0.1 μ thick.

The system for supplying blood is often simplified so that it looks like Figure 1-5, but it is as remarkable and complex as the respiratory system. The pump—the right ventricle—drives venous blood into 1 large tube, the pulmonary trunk. This divides and subdivides (Figs. 1-6 and 1-7) until ultimately blood flows through millions of short, thin-walled capillaries surrounding the alveoli. The surface area of this capillary bed is about 70 m², the thickness of each capillary wall is less than 0.1 μ and the diameter of each vessel is about $10-14$ μ. Yet the resistance to flow through the whole bed is so low that $5-10$ L of blood can flow through it each minute with a driving pressure of less than 10 mm Hg. The pump has a wide range. It can push 4 L/minute through the capillaries in man at rest, but as much as $30-40$ L/minute when he exercises maximally.

The air and blood pumps are constructed

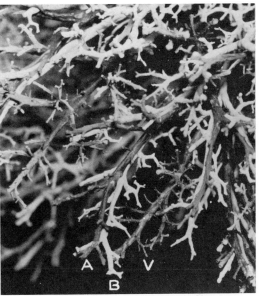

Fig. 1-6.—The blood and gas distributing and collecting systems. Arteries (A), bronchi (B), and veins (V) have been demonstrated by injecting them and digesting away all tissue. The artery and bronchus are close to each other. The vein is midway between the broncho-arterial rays. (Courtesy of Dr. Averill Liebow.)

Fig. 1-5.—Schematic representation of the pulmonary and systemic circulations. RA = right atrium; LA = left atrium, RV = right ventricle; LV = left ventricle.

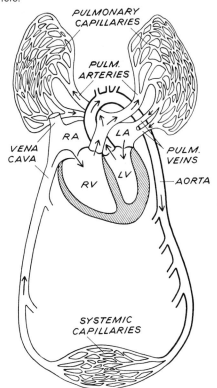

quite differently. The blood is driven by a muscular pump, the right ventricle, which pushes blood in one direction; the tricuspid valves prevent backflow into the right atrium during systole, and the pulmonic valves prevent backflow into the right ventricle during diastole. Blood flows through a conducting system (pulmonary arteries) to the exchange system (capillaries) and a collecting system (pulmonary veins) into a second pump (the left ventricle) for distribution to body cells.

The air pump differs by having no valves; it moves air back and forth (like the tides) through the same set of tubes; these tubes both conduct fresh air to the alveoli and collect alveolar gas from them. Little or no gas is exchanged in these tubes; they are "dead space." This dead space in the air pump is a disadvantage in one respect: it requires more ventilation and more pump work. It is an advantage in another: it permits more space in the lungs for diffusion of gases because it

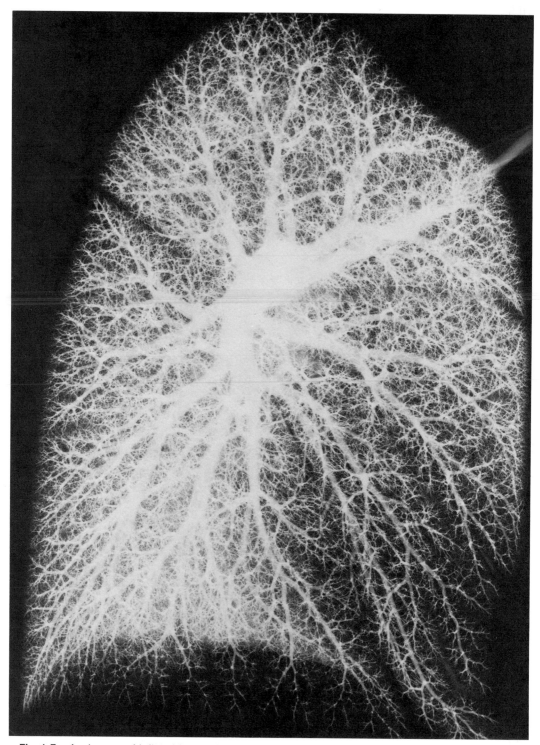

Fig. 1-7.—Angiogram of inflated human lung injected at autopsy with radiopaque material (Courtesy of Dr. Robert Wright; from Comroe, J. H.: Scient. Am. 214:56, 1966.)

eliminates the need for a different set of collecting tubes for expired gas. The air pump differs from the blood pump in another respect: it is a "negative" (subatmospheric), rather than a positive, pressure pump. A positive-pressure pump would *compress* the lungs, push alveolar gas out of the thorax and then allow fresh air to enter during recoil. The negative-pressure pump actively *enlarges* the thorax and lowers the pressure in the alveoli below atmospheric pressure so that air, at atmospheric pressure, flows in; it then recoils passively to its resting position to push air out.

To meet the varying needs of tissue cells, the heart and lungs must be variable pumps. Ideally, they should also be regulated with exquisite precision, so that they meet every need with the least cost in energy. Further, the supply of air and the supply of blood produced by the two pumps must be matched not only in overall amounts but also in every region of the lung. This requires responsive decision centers, supplied with necessary information and the power to enforce decisions.

Respiratory regulation, of course, involves more than maintaining a supply of air for gas exchange. For example, expired air is used for speaking, singing, blowing, coughing; respiratory muscles are involved in sighing, yawning, laughing, sobbing, hiccuping, sucking, sniffing, straining and vomiting. In some animals, expired air is an important means of eliminating heat. And there are special regulatory mechanisms to protect the lung from the entry of solids, liquids and irritant gases.

The pulmonary gas exchange system is not an end in itself. It exists to meet the needs of organs, tissues and cells. Physiologists usually think of respiration as the movement of the lungs, thorax and air. Biochemists think of respiration as the cellular processes in tissues that use O_2 and give off CO_2. Some call the first "external respiration" and the second "internal respiration" or "tissue respiration." In this volume we shall discuss all of the processes involving exchange of gases — between air and the alveoli, between the alveoli and pulmonary capillary blood, between tissue capillaries and tissue cells and between air-containing spaces and blood. We shall leave to the biochemists the actual cellular processes that use O_2.

2

Alveolar Ventilation

THE MOST IMPORTANT FUNCTION of the lung and of pulmonary ventilation is to supply tissue cells with enough O_2 and to remove excess CO_2. To accomplish this, pulmonary ventilation must increase the partial pressure of O_2 in the alveoli well above that in the venous blood flowing through the alveolar capillaries; this loads the blood destined for tissue cells with O_2. It must also lower the partial pressure of CO_2 in the alveoli below that in venous blood; this unloads excess CO_2 from the blood destined for tissue cells. Since gases move between alveoli and their capillary blood and between tissues and their capillary blood because of a difference in their partial pressures, it is well to define partial pressures of gases at this time.

PARTIAL PRESSURE OF OXYGEN (Po₂) AND OF CARBON DIOXIDE (Pco₂)

Partial Pressure of a Gas in a Mixture of Gases

P stands for pressure; Po_2 is the pressure of oxygen and Pco_2 the pressure of carbon dioxide (Table 2-1). A pure gas does not behave like a continuous fluid, but like an enormous number of tiny particles. At atmospheric pressure, 1 mole of a gas contains 6×10^{23} particles (Avogadro's number), and these occupy 22.4 L at 0 C. These particles (molecules) are separated by distances that are large in relation to their own dimensions. They are in a continuous state of random motion, but exert no forces on one another except when they collide. During collision with other molecules or with the walls of the containing vessels, there is no chemical reaction; the collisions may be regarded as perfectly elastic, and the pressure depends on the number of collisions.

In 1643 Torricelli found that the total pressure of atmospheric gases at sea level was sufficient to maintain a column of mercury 760 mm high. For more than 300 years thereafter, the total and partial pressures of gases have been expressed in mm Hg. A few years ago, some respiratory physiologists decided to replace the clumsy term "millimeters of mercury" with "torr." "Torr" specifically refers to the pressure required to support a column of mercury 1 mm high when the mercury is of standard density and subject to standard acceleration. (These conditions are met at 0 C and 45 latitude, where the acceleration of gravity is 980.6 cm/sec².) "Torr" has become a synonym for "mm Hg." In this book I use "torr" to refer to partial or total pressures of gases. I have

TABLE 2-1.—PARTIAL PRESSURE OF GASES: SYMBOLS AND DEFINITIONS

P	= Pressure
Po_2 or CO_2 or N_2 or H_2O	= Partial pressure of oxygen or carbon dioxide or nitrogen or water
PI_{O_2}	= Partial pressure of oxygen in inspired gas
PA_{O_2}	= Partial pressure of oxygen in alveolar gas
Pa_{O_2}	= Partial pressure of oxygen in arterial blood
$P\bar{v}_{O_2}$	= Partial pressure of oxygen in mixed venous blood

continued to use "mm Hg" for blood pressure because the term is still preferred by cardiovascular physiologists.

If we have a container of pure, dry O_2 at sea level, its Po_2 is the same as the total pressure, 760 torr, since all of the molecules are O_2. If instead we have a mixture of gases, the pressure exerted by each is the same as it would be if that gas alone occupied the whole volume (Dalton's law). For example, the gases in dry air are $O_2(20.93\%)$, $CO_2(0.04\%)$ and N_2 (79.03%). If the O_2 molecules were suddenly alone and the volume of the container remained the same, there would be only 20.93% as many collisions as before, and the pressure would be 20.93% of 760, or 159.1 torr. Likewise, if the CO_2 occupied the volume alone, the pressure would be 0.04% of 760, or 0.3 torr. Nitrogen in a similar situation would have a pressure of 79.03% of 760, or 600.6 torr. The sum of all the partial pressures, $159.1 + 0.3 + 600.6$, gives the total pressure, 760 torr.

In the lungs, the gases are O_2, CO_2, N_2 and H_2O (as water vapor); at 37 C their partial pressures are 104, 40, 569 and 47, respectively (Table 2-2). These are average values for healthy resting man at sea level; values of Po_2, Pco_2 and Pn_2 fluctuate from breath to breath and during a single breath. The partial pressure of a gas in a mixture of gases can be measured in many ways. Both O_2 and CO_2 have long been measured by chemical ab-sorption technics in the Haldane, Van Slyke or Scholander apparatus. Oxygen can now be measured by a rapid O_2 electrode or by a paramagnetic analyzer, CO_2 by a continuous infrared analyzer and N_2 by emission spectroscopy. These gases can also be measured by gas chromatography or mass spectrometry.

Partial Pressure of Water Vapor

The partial pressure of water vapor in air is a special problem. The molecules of a liquid, like those of a gas, are in constant motion; those at the liquid-air surface tend to escape into the gas above the liquid. The greater the temperature, the greater is the kinetic energy of the water molecules and the greater their tendency to escape. Therefore, water-vapor pressure depends directly on temperature. Water vapor at body temperature (37 C) maintains a partial pressure of 47 torr, regardless of changes in barometric pressure. Some water-vapor pressures covering the range encountered in physiologic conditions are given in Table 2-3.

Room air usually contains some water vapor. But, regardless of whether it contains water vapor or not, it becomes saturated with water vapor at body temperature as soon as it is drawn through the nose, mouth and pharynx. Therefore, inspired gas in the trachea has a Ph_2O of 47 torr. Since the total gas pressure in the trachea must equal atmospheric pressure (760 torr), only $760 - 47$, or 713, torr is available for the sum of the partial pressures of O_2, CO_2 and N_2.

TABLE 2-2.—TOTAL AND PARTIAL
PRESSURES OF GASES (TORR)*

	DRY AIR	MOIST TRACHEAL AIR (37 C)	ALVEOLAR GAS	ARTERIAL BLOOD	MIXED VENOUS BLOOD
Po_2	159.1†	149.2†	104†	100	40
Pco_2	0.3	0.3	40	40	46
Ph_2O	0.0	47.0	47	47	47
Pn_2‡	600.6	563.5	569	573	573
P total	760.0	760.0	760	760	706

*Usual values in a resting, healthy man at sea level (barometric pressure = 760 torr).
†This is an approximate value and holds approximately only for man breathing air at sea level (760 torr). The total atmospheric pressure at Denver or Salt Lake City is about 640 torr, and the partial pressure of O_2 in inspired and alveolar gas is well below values for man at lea level.
‡Includes small amounts of rare gases.

TABLE 2-3.—WATER VAPOR PRESSURES (Ph_2O)
AT DIFFERENT TEMPERATURES

TEMP. (C)	Ph_2O (TORR)	TEMP. (C)	Ph_2O (TORR)
20	17.5	29	30.0
21	18.7	30	31.8
22	19.8	31	33.7
23	21.1	32	35.7
24	22.4	33	37.7
25	23.8	34	39.9
26	25.2	35	42.2
27	26.7	36	44.6
28	28.3	37	47.0

O₂ ELECTRODE

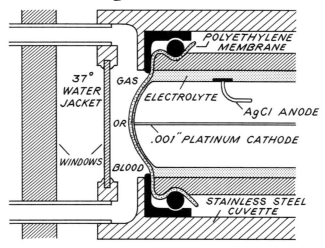

CO₂ ELECTRODE

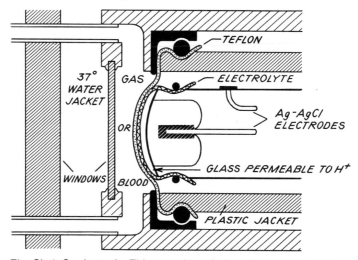

Fig. 2-1 (top). — The Clark O_2 electrode. This uses the polarigraphic method, which is essentially careful electrolysis of dilute solutions containing reducible or oxidizable substances, including O_2. When a suitable voltage is applied to an electrode immersed in a solution containing O_2, O_2 is reduced (takes up electrons). This transfer of electrons is measured by a galvanometer; the current flowing is a function of O_2 tension. For measurement of the partial pressure of O_2 in a mixture of gases, a bare platinum wire can be used. For measurement of Po_2 of blood, the platinum wire (bare only at its tip) must be protected from contamination by a polyethylene or polypropylene membrane that is permeable to O_2 molecules.

Fig. 2-2 (bottom). — The Severinghaus CO_2 electrode. This consists of a glass electrode (permeable to H^+) covered with a thin film of electrolyte (0.01M $NaHCO_3$ and 0.1M NaCl) in a "spacer." This film is separated from the gas or blood sample by a thin Teflon membrane (25 μ thick) that is permeable to CO_2 but not to H^+ Carbon dioxide molecules diffuse from the sample through the Teflon membrane and react with water in the electrolyte to form H^+ and HCO_3^-. The H ions pass through the special glass and are measured as in a pH meter. (Δ pH $= 0.95\Delta$ log Pco_2.) A water jacket keeps the sample at 37 C. (Redrawn from Severinghaus, J. W. in Handbook of Physiology. Respiration, Vol. II. Ed. by Fenn, W. O. and Rahn, H. [Washington: American Physiological Society, 1965], pp. 1475–87.)

The P_{O_2} of moist inspired gas *in the trachea* is, therefore, 20.93% of *713*, or 149 torr, and not 20.93% of 760, or 159, as in dry air.

Partial Pressure of a Gas in a Liquid

The concept of a partial pressure, or tension, of a gas in a liquid such as saline, plasma or blood is harder to grasp. ("Partial pressure" and "tension" of a gas are often used interchangeably.) One can remove all gases from a liquid (by chemical absorption, boiling or exposure to a vacuum); the pressure of gases in the liquid is then zero. However, when this liquid is exposed to air, the O_2, CO_2 and N_2 molecules in the air move by diffusion into the liquid until the gas pressures in the liquid and air are equal. When the partial pressure of a particular gas tending to come out of solution is equal to the partial pressure of the same gas tending to go back into solution, the system is in equilibrium for that particular gas.

One can prepare blood or other perfusion fluids by equilibrating them with gases of known partial pressure; this is done regularly during cardiopulmonary bypass, using an artificial heart and lung (or pump-oxygenator) in patients undergoing open heart surgery. Equilibration is hastened by using small volumes of liquid, large volumes of gas and a large contact surface.

When the tension of O_2 or CO_2 in blood is unknown (as in a sample of arterial blood), one can measure it in a few minutes using O_2 or CO_2 electrodes; Figures 2-1 and 2-2 show schematically the principles of operation of these electrodes.

The partial pressure (torr) of a gas in a liquid may be low, but the content (ml) may be very high. This is because different gases have different solubilities in various liquids. Large *amounts* of very soluble gases (such as acetone) may be dissolved at very low *partial pressures;* very small amounts of insoluble gases dissolve in the same liquid, even when partial pressure is quite high. It is possible, therefore, to have more milliliters of a very soluble gas in 1 L of liquid than in

1 L of a gas mixture on top of it at equilibrium (equal partial pressures).

ALVEOLAR GAS

Because tissues engaged in aerobic metabolism use O_2 and form CO_2, they remove O_2 from capillary blood and add CO_2 to it. This lowers the P_{O_2} of venous blood below that of arterial blood and raises the P_{CO_2} of venous blood (see Table 2-2). The more active the tissues, the lower will be the P_{O_2} and the higher the P_{CO_2} of mixed venous blood. To keep arterial blood at steady levels of P_{O_2} and P_{CO_2}, the lungs – by the process of alveolar ventilation – must supply to alveoli the amount of O_2 removed from blood by tissues and must remove from alveoli an amount of CO_2 added to blood by tissues.

The main purpose of ventilation, then, is to maintain an optimal composition of alveolar gas. We can think of alveolar gas as a compartment of gas lying between atmospheric air and alveolar capillary blood. Oxygen is continuously removed from the alveolar gas and CO_2 continuously added to it by blood flowing through alveolar capillaries. Oxygen is supplied to the alveolar gas and CO_2 removed from it by the cyclic process of ventilation – the inspiration of fresh air followed by the expiration of some alveolar gas.

Alveolar P_{O_2} varies during a breath (Fig. 2-3), from one breath to another and in different alveoli. A *mean* alveolar P_{O_2} can be calculated if one estimates mean alveolar P_{CO_2} (from measured P_{CO_2} of arterial blood) and measures R, the respiratory exchange ratio (ml CO_2 excreted/ml O_2 absorbed). At sea level, the equation is

$$P_{A_{O_2}} = F_{I_{O_2}}(713) - P_{A_{CO_2}}\left[F_{I_{O_2}} + \frac{1 - F_{I_{O_2}}}{R}\right],$$

where $F_{I_{O_2}}$ = fraction of O_2 in inspired air; $P_{A_{CO_2}}$ = mean alveolar P_{CO_2}, and R = respiratory exchange ratio. Note that if R = 1.0 (CO_2 added to alveolar gas/minute = O_2 absorbed/minute), the values in the brackets equal 1.0 and alveolar P_{O_2} is simply the P_{O_2} of moist inspired gas (tracheal gas) minus

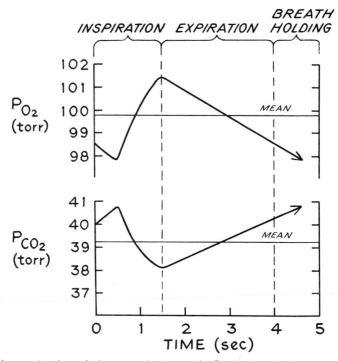

Fig. 2-3. — Alveolar gas tensions during a respiratory cycle. During *inspiration*, one would expect that alveolar Po_2 would rise because fresh air ($Po_2 = 149$ torr when saturated with water vapor at 37 C) is added to the alveolar gas ($Po_2 = 98.5$ torr at end-expiration). During *expiration*, one would expect that alveolar Po_2 would decrease and alveolar Pco_2 would increase; this is because expiration is essentially breath-holding (with lung volume decreasing throughout the expiration), during which blood continues to flow through pulmonary capillaries and continues to remove O_2 and add CO_2.

Note, however, that at the beginning of inspiration, alveolar Po_2 continues to fall (instead of rising) and alveolar Pco_2 continues to rise (instead of falling). This is because the first gas to enter alveoli during inspiration is alveolar gas that filled the anatomic dead space at the end of the previous expiration; it does not alter the composition of gas in alveoli, and exchange of O_2 and CO_2 continues as it did during expiration. After the dead-space gas is drawn in, alveolar Po_2 rises sharply because *fresh inspired air* now adds O_2 to alveoli far more rapidly than it is absorbed. (Redrawn from Comroe, J. H., Jr., *et al.*: *The Lung* [2d ed.; Chicago: Year Book Medical Publishers, Inc., 1962].)

alveolar Pco_2. This means that the equation, though it appears to be formidable, is a simple one. All it states is that the total pressure of alveolar gases (O_2, CO_2, N_2 and H_2O) at sea level equals 760 torr. Since inspired tracheal gas is moist, the total pressure for O_2, CO_2 and N_2 is $760 - 47$, or 713. If $FI_{O_2} = 0.2093$, the Po_2 of tracheal gas is 149 torr. If pulmonary capillary blood adds 5.6% CO_2 to this gas and simultaneously absorbs O_2 equal to 5.6% of the total, the alveolar $Fo_2 = (0.2093 - 0.0560)$, or 0.1533, and the Po_2 is now 0.1533×713, or 109, and the Pco_2 is 0.056×713, or 40 torr; Po_2 decreases by 40 torr, Pco_2 increases by 40 torr and PN_2 does not change. Usually, the O_2 absorbed is greater than the CO_2 excreted, and the equation corrects for the resulting increase in PN_2.

ALVEOLAR VENTILATION VERSUS TOTAL VENTILATION

Total ventilation is the volume of air entering or leaving the nose and mouth during each breath (tidal volume) or each minute (minute ventilation or minute volume). It can be measured breath by breath by volume recorders (spirometers) or by using flowmeters (pneumotachographs) and then obtaining volume by integration of flow records. The volume of gas in the lungs at body temperature, saturated with water vapor, may be 10% greater than the volume measured in a spirometer at room temperature. To correct gas volumes in a spirometer to those in the lungs, use the equation

Volume in lungs = Volume in spirometer
   (BTPS)   (ATPS)

where P_B = barometric pressure, P_{H_2O} = water vapor pressure at room temperature, BTPS = body temperature and pressure saturated with water vapor and ATPS = ambient temperature and pressure saturated with water vapor.

Alveolar ventilation is the volume of *fresh* air entering the alveoli each breath (or each minute). Alveolar ventilation is always less than total ventilation—how much less depends on the anatomic dead space, tidal volume and frequency of breathing.

Anatomic Dead Space and Tidal Volume

Fresh air does not go directly to alveoli. It goes first through the conducting airway (nose, mouth, pharynx, larynx, trachea, bronchi and bronchioles). Because there is no significant exchange of O_2 and CO_2 between gas and blood in the conducting airway, the internal volume of the airway is called the *anatomic dead space.*

Values for anatomic dead space in healthy men and women are given in Table 2-4. Anatomic dead space can be measured (see Fig. 13-1, p. 170), but most physicians estimate it from standard tables, taking into account

TABLE 2-4.— ANATOMIC DEAD SPACE (ML) IN HEALTHY SUBJECTS
(mean value)

Young women (semirecumbent)	104
Young men (semirecumbent)	156
Young men (supine)	115
Young men (during maximal expiration)	110
Young men (during maximal inspiration)	230
Older men (semirecumbent)	180

factors such as age, sex, lung volume and tidal volume. Radford has noted that an adult's anatomic dead space in milliliters is about equal to his ideal weight in pounds; physicians often use this as an approximate value.

At the end of a normal expiration (pre-in-

$$\left(\frac{273+37}{273+\text{room temp.}} \times \frac{P_B - P_{H_2O}}{P_B - 47}\right),$$

spiration), the conducting airway is filled with *alveolar* gas, which has a P_{O_2} of 100 rather than 149 torr and a P_{CO_2} of 40 rather than 0.3 torr (Fig. 2-4). Let us say that its volume is 150 ml and that the volume of the next inspiration (tidal volume) will be 450 ml. The alveoli receive a volume of 450 ml, but the composition of this 450 ml differs from that entering the nose or mouth. The alveoli first receive 150 ml of gas from the conducting airway (this gas does not raise alveolar P_{O_2} or lower alveolar P_{CO_2}, since it has the same composition as alveolar gas) and then 300 ml of fresh air. The remaining 150 ml of fresh air remains in the conducting airway at end-inspiration.

[A special case of alveolar ventilation by dead space (or alveolar) gas exists when a segmental bronchus in one lobe is obstructed but gas enters the alveoli beyond the obstruction through collateral channels; these may be channels in the alveolar walls (pores of Kohn) or communications between the bronchioles and alveoli (Lambert's canals). If the alveoli with obstructed airways receive their gas through pores connected to ventilated alveoli, the former receive alveolar gas and not fresh air; this gas does little to arterialize mixed venous blood flowing past it.]

It is obvious that the volume of the dead space and the tidal volume are important factors in determining the amount of alveolar ventilation. The total volume of each breath is called the *tidal volume* because, like the tides, it moves back and forth over the same path. Tidal volume is usually about 400–500 ml, but can be very much larger. The greatest

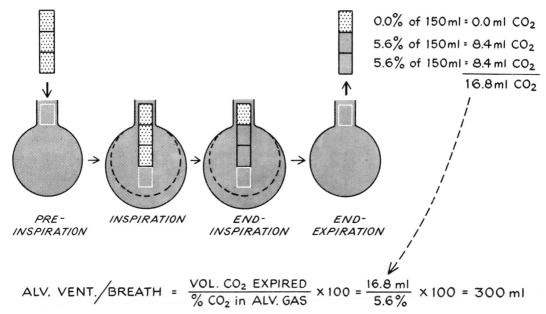

$$\text{ALV. VENT.} / \text{BREATH} = \frac{\text{VOL. } CO_2 \text{ EXPIRED}}{\% \ CO_2 \text{ in ALV. GAS}} \times 100 = \frac{16.8 \text{ ml}}{5.6\%} \times 100 = 300 \text{ ml}$$

Fig. 2-4.—Alveolar ventilation and anatomic dead space. Each block represents 150 ml of gas. *Dotted blocks* represent inspired air; *shaded blocks*, alveolar gas. During inspiration, 150 ml of dead space gas plus 300 ml of inspired air enter the alveoli; by end-inspiration this has mixed with and become alveolar gas. One block of inspired gas fills the anatomic dead space at end-inspiration and is washed out by alveolar gas during expiration. *Dashed lines* show preinspiratory lung volume. The Bohr equation is used to calculate alveolar ventilation per breath. Total ventilation minus alveolar ventilation = dead space.

Note: Drawing is schematic. Air does not flow with a square front but in spike or cone form. (Redrawn from Comroe, J. H., Jr., *et al.*: *The Lung* [2d ed.; Chicago: Year Book Medical Publishers, Inc., 1962].)

volume that a healthy man can inspire, beginning at the end of a quiet expiration, is about 3,600 ml; this is called the *inspiratory capacity* (Fig. 2-5 and Tables 2-5 and 2-6). After a maximal expiration, he can inspire about 4,800 ml. If tidal volume is 1,000 and anatomic dead space is 150 ml, then 850/1,000, or 85%, of the gas entering the alveoli is fresh air. If tidal volume is 200 and dead space is 150 ml, only 50/200, or 25%, of the gas entering the alveoli is fresh air.[1]

---

[1]The anatomic dead space is decreased by pneumonectomy and by tracheotomy because of the removal or bypass of some of the conducting airway. Tracheotomy has occasionally been performed as a therapeutic measure to improve alveolar ventilation in patients who have a very low, fixed tidal volume, such as may occur in advanced emphysema; the advisability of tracheotomy has been questioned because it decreases the efficacy of coughing. Anatomic dead space may be reduced in asthma (as a result of bronchial narrowing) or enlarged by diseases such as bronchiectasis, which widens the air ducts, or emphysema, in which the whole lung volume, including the anatomic dead space, is enlarged.

Alveolar Ventilation, Lung Volume and $P_{A_{O_2}}$

Lungs do not collapse to the airless state (Fig. 2-6) with each expiration. Indeed, they cannot be emptied of gas by the most forceful expiration possible; some gas still remains—the *residual volume* (Fig. 2-5). At the end of a normal expiration, much more air remains in the lungs; this is the *functioning* residual volume and is called the *functional residual capacity (FRC)* (Fig. 2-5). The FRC acts as a buffer against extreme changes in alveolar P_{O_2} with each breath. If there were no FRC, alveolar P_{O_2} would decrease to that of venous blood in the pulmonary capillaries at end-expiration and rise to near 149 with deep inspiration; blood P_{O_2} and content would also fluctuate widely with each breath.

All of the lung volumes except the residual volume can be measured by volume recorders. The residual volume may be calculated

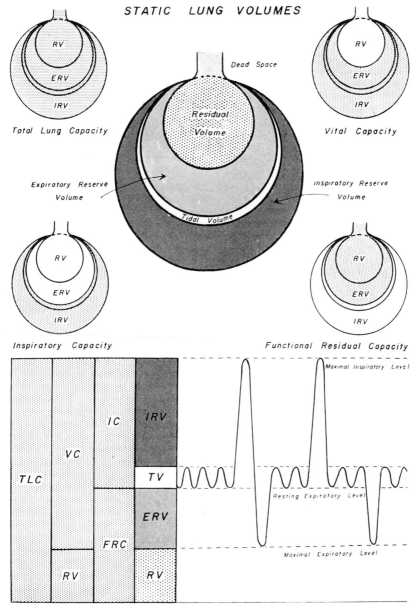

Fig. 2-5.—Lung volumes and capacities. **Top,** the large central diagram illustrates the 4 primary lung volumes and their relative magnitude. The 4 satellite diagrams show the 4 lung capacities (*shaded areas*). Note that the lung *volumes* do not overlap but that the *capacities* include 2 or more of the primary volumes. **Bottom,** lung volumes as they appear in a spirogram; *shadings* in the first vertical bar to the left of the tracing correspond to those in the central diagram above. For definitions, see Table 2-5. (From Comroe, J. H., Jr., *et al.: The Lung* [2d ed.; Chicago: Year Book Medical Publishers, Inc., 1962].)

by gas dilution methods, using either O_2 or He to dilute alveolar N_2; actually FRC is usually measured and expiratory reserve volume subtracted to obtain residual volume. The FRC (and hence RV) is more often measured using a body plethysmograph (Fig. 2-7).

The alveolar Po_2 is an important determinant of diffusion of O_2 from gas to blood. The amount of alveolar ventilation is more impor-

TABLE 2-5.—THE LUNG VOLUMES AND
CAPACITIES
(see Fig. 2-5)

LUNG VOLUMES

Tidal volume, or the depth of breathing—the volume of gas inspired or expired during each respiratory cycle

Inspiratory reserve volume—the maximal amount of gas that can be inspired from the end tidal-inspiratory position

Expiratory reserve volume—the maximal volume of gas that can be expired from the resting end-expiratory level

Residual volume—the volume of gas remaining in the lungs at the end of a maximal expiration

LUNG CAPACITIES

Total lung capacity—the amount of gas contained in the lung at the end of a maximal inspiration

Vital capacity—the maximal volume of gas that can be expelled from the lungs by forceful effort following a maximal inspiration

Inspiratory capacity—the maximal volume of gas that can be inspired from the resting expiratory level

Functional residual capacity—the volume of gas remaining in the lungs at the resting expiratory level

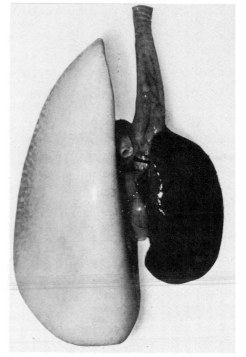

Fig. 2-6.—Fully inflated and airless lungs (rat). The fully inflated lung is actually pink; the completely airless lung is actually deep red. The airless lung, outside the body, is considerably smaller than the space in the closed hemithorax that at full expiration normally contained the lung and its residual gas volume. When a lung becomes completely airless *within the thorax*, the space previously occupied by its residual gas volume is filled by an elevation of that hemidiaphragm or a shift of the mediastinum and other lung into that hemithorax. (Courtesy of Dr. Norman Staub.)

TABLE 2-6.—LUNG VOLUMES IN HEALTHY
RECUMBENT SUBJECTS
(Approximate values, in ml)*

	MALES AGED 20–30 1.7 M²	MALES AGED 50–60 1.7 M²	FEMALES AGED 20–30 1.6 M²
Inspiratory capacity	3,600	2,600	2,400
Expiratory reserve capacity	1,200	1,000	800
Vital capacity	4,800	3,600	3,200
Residual volume (RV)	1,200	2,400	1,000
Functional residual capacity	2,400	3,400	1,800
Total lung capacity (TLC)	6,000	6,000	4,200
(RV/TLC) × 100	20%	40%	24%

*From Comroe, J. H., Jr., *et al.*: *The Lung* (2d ed.; Chicago: Year Book Medical Publishers, Inc., 1962).

tant in determining alveolar P_{O_2} than the size of the FRC. If the pulmonary capillary blood removes 250 ml of O_2/minute, only 250 ml of O_2 must be added to alveolar gas by the process of ventilation to maintain alveolar P_{O_2}; this is true whether the FRC is 2,000 ml or 4,000 ml. An analogy may be helpful here. If 250 ml of O_2 were absorbed chemically each minute in a *small* airtight box containing air, and simultaneously 250 ml of O_2 were piped into the box each minute, the O_2 concentration in the box would remain constant; if 250 ml of O_2 were absorbed chemically each minute in a *large* airtight room containing air, and simultaneously 250 ml of O_2 were piped into the room, the O_2 concentration of the large room would also remain constant. If there is rapid and uniform distribution in both the small box and the large room, the volume of the container is unimportant in determining the O_2 concentration and partial pressure *in a steady state*.

On the other hand, the size of the FRC is important when a rapid *change* in alveolar gas *composition* is necessary. For example, if a patient breathes 100% O_2 instead of air, he will achieve a high alveolar O_2 concentra-

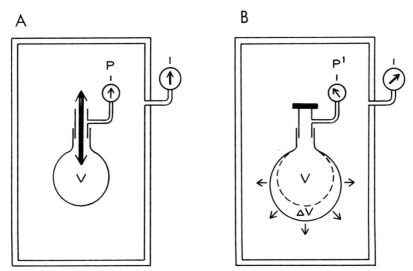

Fig. 2-7.—Measurement of thoracic gas volume; body plethysmograph technic. The rectangle is an air-tight body box. The patient (represented by his alveoli and conducting airway) breathes air about him. The two circles with pointers represent pressure gauges; one measures pressure in the box and the other measures airway pressure, which equals alveolar pressure when there is no air flow. **A,** at end-expiration alveolar pressure equals atmospheric pressure; V is unknown. The airway is then occluded, **B,** and the patient inspires; this creates a new gas volume $(V+\Delta V)$ and a new pressure, P'. Knowing P, P' and ΔV, V (initial, unknown thoracic gas volume) can be calculated using Boyle's law. $PV = P'V'$.

tion more slowly if his FRC is large than if it is small (Fig. 2-8). Again, when inducing anesthesia with gases such as N_2O or halothane or inducing hyperpnea by $10\% \, CO_2$ in air, it will take longer to achieve the desired alveolar concentration of the gas if the FRC is large (other things being equal). Again, an analogy using small and large closed spaces may be helpful. If a man were to smoke in an airtight phone booth, the smoke concentration would rise much more rapidly than if he were to smoke in a large room.

Consider the simple case of a man given O_2 to breathe (Fig. 2-9). Let us say that his FRC is 3,000 ml, dead space is 150 and alveolar ventilation per breath is 350. Each inspiration first enlarges the alveolar gas volume from 3,000 to 3,150 ml by the flow into the alveoli of alveolar gas in the anatomic dead space; the further inspiration of 350 ml of O_2 then dilutes the N_2 in alveolar gas by 350/3,500, or 10%. The alveolar N_2, as a result, decreases from 80 to 72%. On the next inspiration, the FRC is again diluted

Fig. 2-8.—N_2 washout at 2 lung volumes. Breathing either 250 or 500 ml of O_2 15 times/minute washes out alveolar N_2 more slowly when FRC is 4,500 than when it is 2,500 ml. $T.V. =$ tidal volume; $FRC =$ functional residual capacity; $N_2 =$ concentration of N_2 in alveolar gas after 1 minute or 15 breaths (initial concentration = 80% N_2).

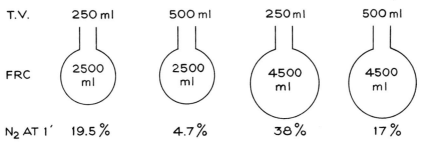

T.V.	250 ml	500 ml	250 ml	500 ml
FRC	2500 ml	2500 ml	4500 ml	4500 ml
N_2 AT 1′	19.5%	4.7%	38%	17%

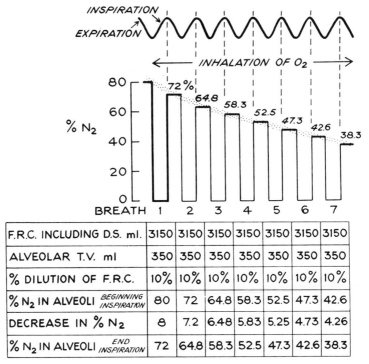

Fig. 2-9. — Pulmonary N_2 washout curve. A man with uniform distribution of inspired gas breathes O_2 at a constant alveolar tidal volume of 350 ml; the N_2 concentration of inspired and expired gas is recorded continuously by a N_2 meter. The plateaus represent expired *alveolar* gas (after washout of anatomic dead space). This N_2 washout curve is a single exponential curve. The alveolar N_2 concentrations at the beginning and end of each inspiration show a 10% dilution with each breath. (Redrawn from Comroe, J. H., Jr., *et al.*: *The Lung* [2d ed.; Chicago: Year Book Medical Publishers, Inc., 1962].)

10%, and at the end of the second inspiration, the alveolar N_2 is 64.8%. This continues until alveolar N_2 is washed out[2] and the lung contains only O_2, CO_2 and H_2O. The rate of this washout of N_2 and replacement by O_2 (or by another gas such as helium or N_2O) is increased by a small FRC, rapid breathing, large tidal volume and small dead space; it is decreased by a large FRC, slow breathing, small tidal volume and large dead space. We shall learn later that the rates of washout may be different in different parts of abnormal lungs if some regions are poorly ventilated and some well ventilated.

---

[2]The N_2 initially in the lungs may be washed out in a few minutes, but N_2 in blood and tissues is eliminated more slowly. Further, some N_2 may enter capillary blood through skin, and this can be prevented only if the patient is surrounded by O_2

How Much Alveolar Ventilation Is Enough?

Because the main purpose of ventilation is to maintain an optimal concentration of alveolar gases, alveolar ventilation is "enough" for O_2 when it matches O_2 use with O_2 supply. Assume that the tidal volume is 250 ml, dead space 150 and alveolar ventilation per breath 100; if the patient breathes 20 times/minute, he supplies the alveoli with 20×100, or 2,000 ml, of air/minute. If 20.93% of this is O_2, the O_2 supplied per minute is 418 ml. Some make the mistake of saying that 418 ml is far more than the average amount of O_2 used by resting man per minute (240 ml), and therefore that such a patient is *hyper*ventilating. Their error lies in a failure to realize that inspiration is fol-

TABLE 2-7.—EFFECTS OF HYPOVENTILATION
(Patient breathing air or O_2)*

Let us assume that the frequency of breathing is 20/minute and that hypoventilation is so extreme that alveolar ventilation is only 100 ml instead of 350 ml/breath. During the first of these small tidal volumes the following exchange of O_2 would occur.

BREATHING AIR

O_2 *added to alveoli / breath (O_2 inspired minus O_2 expired)*
  100 ml inspired air (20.93% O_2) contains   20.93 ml O_2
  100 ml expired alveolar gas (14% O_2) contains   14.00 ml O_2
                     = 6.93 ml O_2/breath
O_2 *removed from alveoli / breath (O_2 consumption, 240 ml / minute)* = 12.00 ml O_2/breath
  Volume of O_2 removed exceeds volume of O_2 added;
   alveolar and arterial O_2 tensions must fall.

BREATHING OXYGEN

O_2 *added to alveoli / breath (O_2 inspired minus O_2 expired)*
  100 ml inspired O_2 (100% O_2) contains   100 ml O_2
  100 ml expired alveolar gas (18% O_2†) contains   18 ml O_2
                     = 82 ml O_2/breath
O_2 *removed from alveoli / breath (O_2 consumption, 240 ml / minute)* = 12 ml O_2/breath
  Volume of O_2 added exceeds volume of O_2 removed;
   alveolar and arterial O_2 tensions must rise.

 However, *no matter whether air or O_2 is breathed, hypoventilation always leads to an accumulation of CO_2.* The following calculations make this clear.

BREATHING AIR OR OXYGEN

CO_2 *eliminated from alveoli / breath (CO_2 expired minus CO_2 inspired)*
  100 ml expired alveolar gas (5.6% CO_2) contains   5.6 ml CO_2
  100 ml inspired air (0.04% CO_2) contains   0.0 ml CO_2
                     = 5.6 ml CO_2/breath
CO_2 *added to alveoli / breath (CO_2 production, 200 ml / minute)* = 10.0 ml CO_2/breath
  Volume of CO_2 added exceeds volume of CO_2 eliminated;
   alveolar and arterial tensions must rise.

---

*From Comroe, J. H., Jr., *et al.*: *The Lung* (2d ed.; Chicago: Year Book Medical Publishers, Inc., 1962).

†A single breath of 100 ml O_2 will instantaneously raise the O_2 concentration of alveolar gas from 14 to about 18%.

lowed by expiration and that O_2 supplied to alveoli per breath is the *difference* between that inspired and that expired. This is made clear in Table 2-7. When this *difference* is less than the O_2 removed by the pulmonary capillary blood, the patient is *hypoventilating* and his alveolar and arterial Po_2 must fall.

The "wisdom of the body" has decided that an alveolar Po_2 of about 100 torr and a Pco_2 of about 40 torr best meet the needs of the body for O_2 supply, CO_2 removal and

regulation of blood acidity (see Chapter 16), and remarkable mechanisms regulate ventilation to keep alveolar Po_2 and Pco_2 at or near these levels (see following chapters). *Alveolar hyperventilation* occurs when more O_2 is supplied and more CO_2 removed than the metabolic rate requires; alveolar and arterial O_2 pressures rise and those of CO_2 fall. If the supply of fresh air is very large and the metabolic rate very low, the alveolar Po_2 and Pco_2 approach those of moist tracheal air (149 and 0.3 torr, respectively).

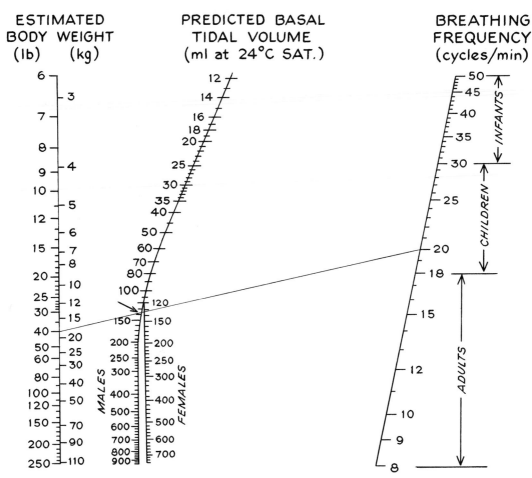

Fig. 2-10. — Radford nomogram for predicting basal tidal volume. To determine the minimal tidal volume required for a patient breathing (or being ventilated mechanically) at various rates, connect the estimated body weight and breathing frequency with a straight line and note where this line crosses the basal tidal volume line. The following corrections may be required: for fever, add 5% for each degree above 99 F.; for activity, add 10%; for altitude, add 5% for each 2,000 ft above sea level; for breathing equipment, add internal volume of mask and apparatus dead space; for tracheotomy, subtract volume equal to $1/2$ body weight in pounds.

In patients with abnormal lungs, larger tidal volumes are necessary. (Redrawn from Radford, E. P., Jr.: J. Appl. Physiol. 7:451, 1955, and N. Engl. J. Med. 251:877, 1954.)

They do not *reach* these values because some O_2 is always removed from, and some CO_2 is always added to, the alveolar gas unless the heart has stopped (see Fig. 13-3). *Alveolar hypoventilation* occurs when less O_2 is supplied and less CO_2 removed than the metabolic rate requires; alveolar and arterial O_2 pressures decrease and those of CO_2 rise.

The amount of air per minute that a healthy man at sea level should breathe (minute volume or minute ventilation) is determined by his anatomic dead space, tidal volume and frequency of breathing on the one hand and his metabolic requirements on the other. Radford has constructed a nomogram to predict how much ventilation is "enough" in healthy persons (Fig. 2-10). When a patient has abnormal lungs, a normal alveolar Po_2 is not enough to oxygenate his blood (because of impaired diffusion, poor matching of blood and gas or shunts; see Chapters 12 and 13), and his alveolar or arterial Po_2 is no longer a satisfactory guide to the amount of alveolar ventilation that he needs. Under these circumstances, alveolar or arterial Pco_2 is a good guide and for this reason is measured routinely in intensive-care units to determine the adequacy of ventilation. *Over*ventilation with air to correct hypoxemia (decreased O_2 in arterial blood) will lower PA_{CO_2} and Pa_{CO_2}, possibly exces-

sively, and produce harmful effects (see p. 258); underventilation with 100% O_2 may correct hypoxemia but allow PA_{CO_2} and Pa_{CO_2} to rise excessively and produce a different set of harmful effects (see p. 257). In this situation, sufficient alveolar ventilation to keep Pa_{CO_2} near 40 torr prevents the harmful effects of too high or too low Pa_{CO_2}, and enrichment of the inspired gas with O_2 can relieve or reduce hypoxemia. Because it is easy to measure alveolar Pco_2 with an infrared analyzer or arterial Pco_2 with a CO_2 electrode, physicians can judge whether a patient's ventilation is "enough" by measuring his Pco_2.

The "rule" that *in*creased Pa_{CO_2} is a certain indication of *hypo*ventilation and *de*creased Pa_{CO_2} is a sure indication of *hyper*ventilation has at least one exception. Anesthetists sometimes hyperventilate a patient mechanically during surgical operations for long enough periods to deplete his blood and tissue stores of CO_2. At the end of the mechanical hyperventilation, a long time is required for enough CO_2 to be formed metabolically to bring tissue and blood Pco_2 back to 40 torr, and during this period the patient hypoventilates and becomes hypoxemic. His CO_2 stores can be filled only by hypoventilation relative to his metabolic rate, and during this repletion period hypoventilation occurs with low Pa_{CO_2}.

3

Regulation of Respiration – The Respiratory Centers

WHEN WE THINK OF RESPIRATION, we think of an automatic, involuntary activity that, without any thought or concern on our part, manages to bring enough air into pulmonary alveoli just often enough to maintain the O_2 and CO_2 tensions of alveolar gas or arterial blood at optimal levels—whether we are resting, engaged in vigorous physical activity or at any intermediate stage. This remarkable activity must depend on systems that feed information on need to a decision center that has the authority to increase or decrease contractions of the respiratory muscles continuously, appropriately and economically.

But respiration, unlike other involuntary, automatic activities, is also under our voluntary control. We can order that breathing stop (at least to the breaking point of breath holding), and we can order that breathing increase (at least till hyperventilation reduces the Pco_2 of arterial blood to such low levels that cerebral vessels constrict and cerebral ischemia causes us to faint). And we can use our expired air for speaking, singing, blowing or coughing and our inspired air for sucking or sniffing. Respiratory muscles are also commandeered for involuntary acts other than breathing, such as sighing, yawning, laughing, hiccuping and vomiting. All of these voluntary and involuntary acts temporarily suspend the otherwise continuous, involuntary regulation of breathing. All are complex acts requiring fine coordination of respiratory, and sometimes nonrespiratory, muscles in a precise sequence: contraction or relaxation of pectoral, thoracic and abdominal muscles, the diaphragm, facial, glottic, pharyngeal and laryngeal muscles and the bronchiolar smooth muscle. Further, to achieve optimal effects, respiratory changes are often coordinated with complex cardiovascular changes.

It is logical to believe that one system regulates *automatic* respiratory activity and another is responsible for *voluntary* respiratory acts. Good evidence now points to the existence of separate neurologic structures for automatic and for voluntary control, although the two systems can interact. The cerebral hemispheres are in charge of voluntary breathing and can be effective even when automatic centers no longer function; the automatic centers can be effective in patients who, because of anesthesia or lesions in the brain, can no longer influence breathing voluntarily. The more primitive automatic control system is in the brain stem and probably sends its messages to respiratory muscles over ventral reticulospinal tracts. The voluntary control system is in the somatic motor cortex and limbic forebrain structures and transmits its impulses partly to the medullary reticulum and partly directly to respiratory muscles over direct corticobullar and corticospinal paths. Almost all experimental work on respiratory centers has been done on anesthetized animals in which the voluntary control system is inoperative. Therefore, most of what follows in this chapter concerns the automatic centers and most of what follows in Chapters 4 and 9 concerns the information required by the automatic centers to serve the needs of the body.

FUNCTION OF THE AUTOMATIC RESPIRATORY CENTERS

A heart may continue to beat rhythmically for many hours after it has been removed from the body if its coronary arteries are supplied with nutrient fluids, because it has an *inherent property* of rhythmic impulse formation. This normally is a function of the sinoatrial node, but if this node is destroyed, other parts of the heart display their own rhythmic contraction.

The muscles of respiration possess no in-herent rhythm. They do not contract if they are separated from the central nervous system by cutting the motor nerves innervating them. Therefore, the rhythmic sequence of inspiration, expiration, inspiration must originate in the spinal cord or brain. In 1812 Legallois found that breathing is still rhythmic if the cerebrum and part of the upper brain stem and cerebellum are removed. He concluded that rhythmic breathing depends on a small portion of the medulla near the level where the vagus nerves emerge. Flourens (1851) described a "vital node"—a pinpoint area at the level of the calamus scriptorius of the medulla—whose destruction was sufficient to cause death. Later (1859) he redefined this as a larger area—a bilateral structure about 2.5 mm in diameter at the midline, close to the level of the obex (Fig. 3-1)—and stated that rhythmic respiration could not continue unless this area was intact and connected to the spinal cord. The concept of a small, bilateral, inherently rhythmic *center* (*the* center of respiratory events) has been an attractive one ever since.

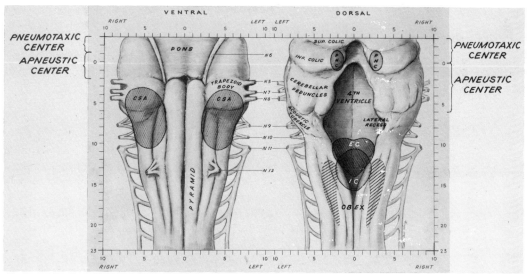

Fig. 3-1.—Medullary and pontine respiratory centers in the cat. *Shaded areas* in *dorsal* diagram show level of inspiratory center (*IC*), expiratory center (*EC*) (IC and EC lie 2–8 mm beneath the floor of the fourth ventricle) and pneumotaxic center (*PNC*); *hatched areas* represent regions of inspiratory and expiratory activity recorded from microelectrodes. *Shaded areas* in *ventral* diagram show surface chemosensitive areas (*CSA*); the apneustic and pneumotaxic centers lie above these in the pons. *Numbers* on border represent stereotaxic coordinates in millimeters. *N6 to N12* represent cranial nerves. (From Mitchell, R. A., in Brooks, C. M., Kao, F. F., and Lloyd, B. B. (eds.): *Cerebrospinal Fluid and the Regulation of Ventilation* [Oxford: Blackwell Scientific Publications, 1965].)

However, as stated earlier, respiratory centers must do much more than generate rhythmic sequences of inspiration and expiration; they must also have connections with many other parts of the brain, so that complex patterns of muscular activity can be carried out in smooth sequence.

The respiratory centers must now be redefined as a group of neurons and synapses capable of receiving, evaluating and sending information so that simple or complex patterns of breathing or other acts that increase or decrease respiration result. The location of the respiratory centers, in the medulla and pons, is a strategic one for interaction with other systems, because the reticular formation, consisting of many groups of richly interconnecting neurons, is also here (Fig. 3-2).

We know little about how respiratory centers make decisions. Sometimes information received from one part of the body calls for the same action as that received from another part of the body—e.g., both call for apnea or both call for hyperpnea; here the decision is easy. Sometimes requests coming from the cerebral cortex conflict with requests from chemoreceptors—e.g., one calls for breath holding and the other for deep breathing; now decision centers must decide which request shall take precedence (be prepotent) and which shall be suppressed (be impotent). We are especially ignorant about the working of decision centers in unanesthetized animals or man. We do know, however, that apnea, so easy to produce reflexly in anesthetized animals (by activating reflexes from the upper respiratory tract, lungs or carotid sinus), is rarely permitted by the decision centers of awake, unanesthetized man; possibly this is because alerting centers in the reticular activating system are important in decision making, and these are readily suppressed by general anesthesia or possibly by deep sleep.

LOCATION OF THE AUTOMATIC RESPIRATORY CENTERS

Physiologists have tried to locate the respiratory centers in many ways:

1. By watching for changes in respiratory patterns while cutting away various parts of the brain, starting with the cerebral cortex and working down toward the spinal cord. This classic technic is far from ideal, because a slice across the whole brain or brain stem interrupts every ascending and descending fiber, whether it serves respiration or not. Further, it causes bleeding and edema and, for an uncertain period, injures every cell or fiber at the level of the section. The immediate effect of such a traumatic procedure may be quite different from the chronic effect. The use of fine, precisely placed lesions avoids some of these problems, but not all. Byck's new technic of producing a reversible cold "section" may prove to be the best of these methods.

The failure of respiration to change appreciably after one part of the brain stem is elim-

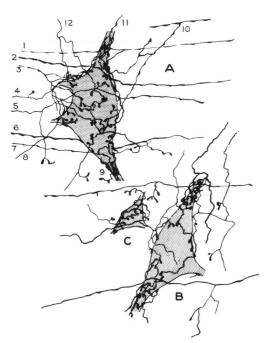

Fig. 3-2.—Synaptic relations of neurons in medial medullary reticular formation in a kitten. This drawing illustrates 3 neurons (A, B, C) and the many fibers terminating on each; 1–12 terminate on A. (From Scheibel, M. E., and Scheibel, A. B.: *Reticular Formation of Brain* [Boston: Little, Brown & Company, 1958].)

inated does not mean that the cells destroyed have no influence on respiration under any conditions. For example, if one destroys the hypothalamus in an animal that is panting because its body temperature is increased, the change in respiration will be different than if this same lesion is made in an animal with a normal or low body temperature. One would also anticipate that the response would be totally different if this were done in man, who does not pant as a means of eliminating excess body heat.

2. By electrically stimulating small regions of the brain or brain stem and determining the respiratory response. This technic has identified areas in the cerebral cortex, hypothalamus, pons or medulla that can affect respiration. The responsive area may be a true center (a group of interacting cells) or a bundle of nearby descending motor fibers or, because of spread of current, both. Some physiologists have also injected small

amounts of chemical stimulants to map regions capable of initiating coordinated respiratory responses.

3. By electrically recording the spontaneous activity of small regions of the brain with microelectrodes and correlating electrical activity with changes in respiration.

4. By evoking activity in small groups of cells by stimulating afferent vagal or other fibers that influence respiration.

There is now general agreement on a few facts, though not on their interpretation. These facts are:

1. Removal of the cerebrum and cerebellum has no important effect on respiration of animals. (This does not mean that there is no cortical influence on the respiratory muscles; see pp. 22 and 29.)

2. Removal of the midbrain has no effect on respiration (Section *1*, Fig. 3-3).

3. Separation of the upper third of the pons from the lower brain stem (Section *2*,

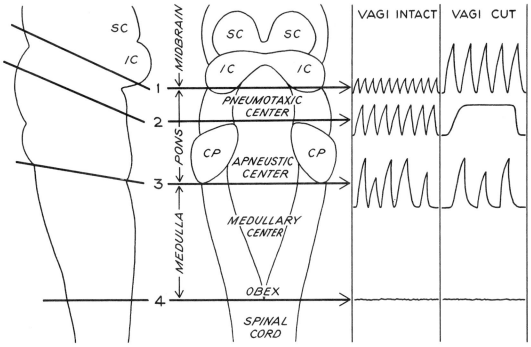

Fig. 3-3.–Patterns of respiration after four brain stem sections. The diagram in the *center* is a dorsal view of the brain stem; that to the *left* is a lateral view. The four patterns on the *right* are representative of those that follow complete sections at each level. Section below the medulla results in complete apnea. *SC* = superior colliculus; *IC* = inferior colliculus; *CP* = cerebellar peduncles.

Fig. 3-3) leads to slight respiratory slowing and increase in tidal volume, but as a rule, to no remarkable change in rate or rhythm; if both vagus nerves are then cut, breathing stops in full inspiration (apneusis) or becomes apneustic (inspiratory spasms interrupted regularly or irregularly by expiration; Table 3-1).

4. Section *3* across the lower border of the pons leads to gasping breathing, which may be regular or irregular.

5. Section *4* across the lower medulla leads to complete apnea.

These facts have led to the conclusion that there are at least 3 major parts of the respiratory center:

TABLE 3-1.— NORMAL AND ABNORMAL PATTERNS OF BREATHING

EUPNEA: normal breathing—repeated rhythmic inspiratory-expiratory cycles without inspiratory or expiratory pause; inspiration is active and expiration passive.

HYPERPNEA: increased breathing; usually refers to increased tidal volume with or without increased frequency. May or may not be related to increased metabolism.

POLYPNEA, TACHYPNEA: increased frequency of breathing.

HYPERVENTILATION: increased alveolar ventilation in relation to metabolic rate (i.e., decreases alveolar P_{CO_2} to less than 37 torr).

HYPOVENTILATION: decreased alveolar ventilation in relation to metabolic rate (i.e., permits alveolar P_{CO_2} to rise above 43 torr).

APNEA: cessation of respiration in the resting expiratory position.

APNEUSIS: cessation of respiration in the inspiratory position.

APNEUSTIC BREATHING: apneusis interrupted periodically by expiration; may be rhythmic.

GASPING: spasmodic inspiratory effort, usually maximal, brief and terminating abruptly; may be rhythmic or irregular.

CHEYNE-STOKES RESPIRATION: cycles of gradually increasing tidal volume followed by gradually decreasing tidal volume (see Fig. 3-6).

BIOT'S RESPIRATION: originally described in patients with meningitis by Biot (Lyon Med. 23:571, 561, 1876) as irregular respiration with pauses; today, it refers to sequences of uniformly deep gasps, apnea, then deep gasps.

---

1. A *medullary center* capable of initiating and maintaining sequences of inspiration, expiration and inspiration, though these are not normal in character.

2. An *apneustic center* in the middle and lower pons that, if uncontrolled, may produce prolonged, uninterrupted inspiratory spasm or apneustic breathing.

3. A *pneumotaxic center* in the upper third of the pons that, along with the dominant vagal impulses, restrains the apneustic center periodically.

THE MEDULLARY CENTER

This contains the minimal number of neurons necessary for the basic coordinated sequence of inspiration, expiration, inspiration. This neuronal activity is inherent and persists when all known afferent stimuli have been cut off.[1] Respiration is not eupneic in an animal whose brain stem is sectioned between the pons and medulla, but is usually gasping and arrhythmic. (Some use the word "rhythmic" to mean sequences of inspiration, expiration, inspiration as opposed to apneusis or apnea. I use the word to mean *regular spacing* between respiratory cycles, just as the cardiologist uses it to mean regular spacing between cardiac contractions.)

The medullary center is sometimes separated into an inspiratory and an expiratory center, because maximal sustained inspiration follows electrical stimulation of some regions and maximal expiration follows stimulation of adjacent regions (Fig. 3-4). Appropriate alternate stimulation of these 2 areas can cause regular sequences of inspiration and expiration. The existence of predominantly inspiratory and predominantly expira-

---

[1]Pitts found that isolation of the medulla from the pons led to prolonged apneusis, persisting sometimes to death, and concluded that some inhibitory impulses from outside the medulla were needed periodically to inhibit inspiration and permit expiration. His transections might have been a little high, so that a millimeter or two of the pons remained connected to the medulla; this could allow parts of the apneustic center to dominate medullary respiration.

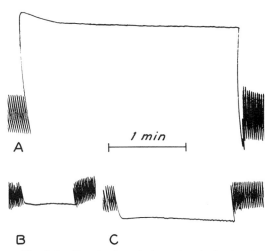

Fig. 3-4.—Respiration during electrical stimulation of medulla of the cat. *A,* maximal inspiratory response; *B,* expiratory response; *C,* maximal expiratory response. Inspiration, up. Responses were obtained from areas *IC* and *EC* shown on Figure 3-1, *dorsal.* (From Pitts, R. F., Magoun, H. W., and Ranson, S. W.: Am. J. Physiol. 126:673, 1939.)

tory regions has been confirmed by recording electrical activity from the medulla, though these regions are somewhat more lateral and caudal. It is unlikely that there is a clear separation of all inspiratory from all expiratory neurons, and at least some of each must be intermingled. Indeed, chemical stimuli injected into this area *can* cause a smooth hyperventilation. It is likely that inspiratory and expiratory neurons are linked closely and that inspiratory activity probably inhibits the expiratory neurons, and vice versa, to produce coordinated responses. Normal, quiet breathing is characterized by active contraction of only the inspiratory muscles; expiration occurs passively by cessation of contraction of the muscles of inspiration. The expiratory muscles, however, become active when there is obstruction to expiration or when minute ventilation increases greatly. Vigorous expiratory contractions represent an unaccustomed type of muscular effort.

The medullary center receives information from many receptors, directly or indirectly; it has connections with the higher respiratory centers in the pons and with areas in the hypothalamus, cortex and the reticular activating system (RAS).

The medullary center was originally thought to be the area in the brain that responded to an increase in arterial Pco_2 and produced the classic CO_2 hyperpnea. It is now believed that the central action of CO_2 is largely on special receptors located on the lateral surfaces of the upper part of the medulla (see Fig. 3-1). These receptors are believed to respond to changes in hydrogen ion concentration (H^+) rather than to Pco_2 itself. They are called central H^+ receptors; they respond to changes in the Pco_2 of their environment because this changes their (H^+) (see Chapter 6). We do not know whether increased Pco_2, acting on the medulla, can cause hyperpnea after specific inactivation of the H^+ receptors.

THE APNEUSTIC CENTER

The role of this center is revealed when both the pneumotaxic center and the vagi are inactivated; prolonged apneusis then results (Fig. 3-5). Apneusis does not occur if one vagus nerve or one part of the bilateral pneumotaxic center is intact. This suggests that the unrestrained apneustic center causes prolonged activity of the inspiratory neurons in the medulla. It is closely associated with neurons of the RAS in the medulla and pons, presumably with neurons that have the specific respiratory function of facilitating inspiration. The apneustic center appears to be restrained periodically by (1) impulses generated in the pneumotaxic center or passing through it or (2) afferent impulses of the inflation reflex that travel up the vagi and impinge directly on the apneustic center, without first ascending to the pneumotaxic center. Functionally, the apneustic center seems to be a central station for the vagal inflation reflex, although, anatomically, vagal afferents have not been traced to it.

The activity of the apneustic center is influenced by other factors—the height of the inspiratory spasm may increase if arterial

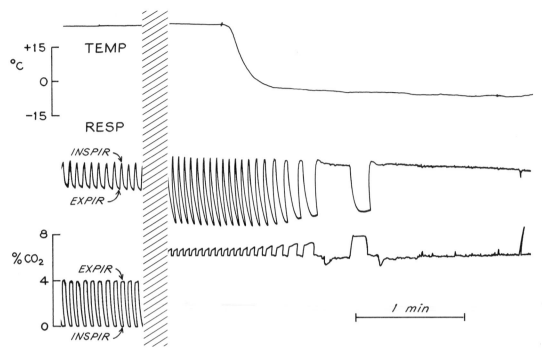

Fig. 3-5.—Apneusis resulting from inactivation of pneumotaxic center and vagi; thermode inserted into mid pons. *Left,* cat breathing air; *right,* cat given 6% CO_2 in air to breathe (note hyperpnea and high alveolar CO_2). When cold fluid was pumped through the thermode, breathing slowed and then stopped in inspiration. Recovery occurred when the pons was rewarmed. The inspiratory apnea was produced repeatedly by repeated cooling. *TEMP* = temperature of cold fluid in thermode just outside brain; temperature of the pons was about 15 degrees higher. % CO_2 = % in inspired and expired gas, measured continuously. (Courtesy of Dr. Robert Byck.)

P_{CO_2} is elevated (Fig. 3-5), or if certain sensory nerves are stimulated. The apneustic center does not require afferent impulses from sensory receptors in the carotid bodies (p. 36) for its function; denervation of the carotid sinuses and carotid bodies does not abolish apneusis once it is established.

THE PNEUMOTAXIC CENTER

Lumsden, using ablation, concluded that this center in the cat lies bilaterally in the upper few millimeters of the pons, at least 10 mm above the medullary inspiratory and expiratory centers (see Fig. 3-3). More precise studies have located the pneumotaxic center in the nucleus parabrachialis medialis.

The pneumotaxic center is probably not an inherently rhythmic pacemaker; it seems to depend on impulses from elsewhere. These might come over ascending pathways from the inspiratory center. Pitts postulated that inspiration sets up impulses that ascend from the medullary inspiratory center to the pneumotaxic center, where they generate impulses that descend to excite the expiratory center and inhibit the inspiratory—a negative feedback mechanism. The function of the pneumotaxic center appears to be somewhat equivalent to that of the inflation reflex (p. 74): it does not facilitate inspiration but encourages rhythmic respiration. The pneumotaxic center is not necessary to mediate the respiratory effects of somatic pain, vagal reflexes, increased arterial blood P_{CO_2} or decreased P_{O_2}.

It is obvious that we can no longer refer to *a* respiratory center, because we know of two such centers in the pons and one in the medulla, plus one special chemoreceptor area. In the *upper pons* is the pneumotaxic center. In the *lower pons* is the apneustic center. In the *upper and lateral medulla* are the chemoreceptors for H^+. In the *lower medulla* are the reflex integrative inspiratory-expiratory centers. Since only one true *center* has been identified in the medulla, we shall call the inspiratory-expiratory centers there simply the *medullary respiratory center.*

EFFECTS OF CENTRAL NERVOUS SYSTEM DISEASE ON RESPIRATION IN MAN

If the respiratory centers in man correspond in location and function to those of the cat and dog, physicians should occasionally see patterns of breathing in patients that result from increase or decrease in the function of each specific respiratory center. However, disorders of the brain in man are rarely the result of single, small lesions of the type produced experimentally; usually they result from decrease or lack of blood flow (by block of large or small arteries), compression (by tumors) or irritation or destruction (by hemorrhage, infectious agents or injury).

Neurologists have described several distinct patterns of abnormal breathing that are associated with the use of depressant drugs or with structural disease of the central nervous system. These are (1) hypoventilation or apnea; (2) hyperventilation; (3) periodic respiration (Cheyne-Stokes); (4) posthyperventilation apnea; (5) diminished maximal voluntary ventilation, and (6) apneusis.

Hypoventilation or Apnea

This may be caused by (1) an overdose of depressants, such as general anesthetic agents, morphine or barbiturates; (2) specific diseases, such as tumors of the medulla, bulbar poliomyelitis and some types of meningitis; (3) general increase in intracranial pressure, and (4) cerebral thrombosis or embolism, often seen in polycythemia. In experimental embolism, Netsky has shown that the vertebral arteries must be blocked to affect respiration; the circulation to the cerebral cortex and the hypothalamus through the carotid arteries can be completely shut off without bringing about a change in respiration. Experimental embolization of the vertebral arteries in animals leads either to apnea or to polypnea, which is soon followed by slow breathing and apnea; the respiratory reaction is accompanied by a marked rise in systemic arterial blood pressure (by as much as 150 mm Hg), bradycardia and an increased pulse pressure.

In most patients with hypoventilation due to central lesions or to depressant drugs, breathing becomes slow and, often, intermittent. The breaths may be irregularly spaced and the tidal volume irregular. Respiration responds poorly to inhalation of air enriched with CO_2, but the response to low O_2 concentrations persists fairly well. If the patients are conscious, the hypoventilation becomes more severe during sleep. It may be partly overcome by commands or other abrupt increase in sensory input. These observations suggest that the hypoventilation may be due to depression of the reticular activating system (or of the sensory input to it), to depression of medullary chemoreceptors, or both. Narcotics and anesthetic agents depress or inactivate the medullary or pontile centers or the RAS; ischemia due to vascular obstruction or compression may depress centers that facilitate breathing or excite those that inhibit it; infectious agents may alter the blood-CSF (cerebrospinal fluid) barrier and permit protein buffers to enter the CSF and increase its pH, which depresses the medullary chemoreceptors (p. 61).

Rarely, a patient is apneic unless commanded to breathe. As long as he receives orders to breathe, he does; when orders stop, breathing stops. This syndrome has been called, quite incorrectly, "Ondine's curse." Ondine, a water nymph, took a mortal lover, who subsequently became unfaithful. Thereupon the king of the water nymphs, using his supernatural powers, suppressed all of the automatic functions of her lover so that if he relaxed his vigilance, he no longer saw, heard, moved or breathed. Ondine placed no curse and indeed was heartbroken when she could not dissuade her king from executing his sentence. (See *Ondine* by Jean Giraudoux.)

SLEEP APNEA. Recent studies on dogs and man during sleep have shown that (1) apnea is much easier to produce and more prolonged in sleeping than in awake dogs, (2) periods of apnea are the rule in sleeping babies (and may play a role in sudden infant death that all too frequently occurs between 1 and 3 months of age and (3) apnea lasting as long as 150 seconds can occur in sleeping adults who have no known neurologic disorder, and may lead to asphyxia, cardiovascular changes and abrupt awakening; these episodes may be a factor in chronic insomnia or even in cardiovascular disasters that sometimes occur during sleep. The influence of sensory stimuli and of wakefulness on respiration is discussed further in Chapter 9.

Hyperventilation

This may be due to (1) some types of meningitis or encephalitis, which cause chemical irritation of receptors or centers, or (2) pontile lesions. Plum, a neurologist, has noted that patients with certain pontile lesions are usually stuporous or comatose and have metronomically regular, moderately deep, rapid and labored breathing lasting for hours or days. The breathing pattern is very much like that in man during muscular exercise or severe acidosis. Inspiration and expiration are about equal in length; expiration is active. When alveolar ventilation is increased and there is no impaired diffusion or uneven matching of ventilation and blood flow in the lungs, there is no hypoxemia, and inhalation of O_2 does not depress breathing significantly. Inhalation of CO_2 does increase ventilation further, but not more than in healthy men. The CO_2 threshold (see p. 64) is markedly reduced.

Histologic studies show necrosis of the central part of the pons; the lower part and medulla are usually intact. The necrosis is caused by thrombosis or embolism of the midpontile portion of the basilar artery. The hyperventilation could be due to destruction of regions normally restraining breathing or to irritation of excitatory centers by accumulation of metabolic products (continued metabolism without blood flow) or by substances liberated during destruction of cells.

Cheyne-Stokes Respiration

This is a regularly recurring series of cycles of gradually increasing and decreasing tidal volumes (Fig. 3-6). Plum has proposed that it is due to brain damage and states that patients with this abnormal pattern usually have bilateral interruption of the descending motor paths, as a rule at the midbrain level. A cardiologist, Hecht, has proposed that Cheyne-Stokes respiration is due to heart failure, with a prolonged circulation time between lungs and brain. Probably both are correct. The neurologic and circulatory disturbances may well be interrelated, because marked slowing of circulation predisposes to thrombosis and damage of the central nervous system.

NEUROLOGIC FACTOR. Patients with Cheyne-Stokes respiration hyperventilate; even during the phase of diminishing ventilation, arterial P_{CO_2} is below normal (< 40 torr). Therefore, something other than P_{CO_2} is driving respiration. It is not hypoxia, because the hyperventilation persists even when the arterial P_{O_2} is increased to normal. The CO_2 threshold is normal, but the CO_2 response curve (p. 57) shows that the sensitivity to CO_2 is almost 3 times that of normal subjects. Since some patients with Cheyne-Stokes respiration have no detectable heart disease and no slowing of circulation to the brain, a neurologic disorder is a likely cause of their respiratory arrhythmia.

CIRCULATORY FACTOR. To understand the mechanism involved, we must first explain regulation in a closed system with negative feedback. The simplest example is that of a

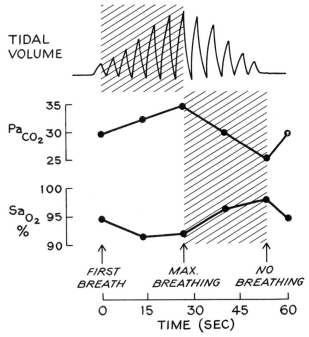

TIDAL VOLUME

Pa_{CO_2}

35
30
25

Sa_{O_2} %

100
95
90

FIRST BREATH   MAX. BREATHING   NO BREATHING

TIME (SEC)
0   15   30   45   60

Fig. 3-6.—Cheyne-Stokes respiration in man. Pattern of increasing, followed by decreasing, tidal volume related to arterial CO_2 tension (Pa_{CO_2}) and arterial O_2 saturation (Sa_{O_2}). *Hatched areas* illustrate lag between increasing breathing (*left*) and decreasing Pco_2 and increasing Po_2 in systemic arterial blood (*right*). (Drawn from the data for patient A. K., Brown, H. W., and Plum, F.: Am. J. Med. 30:849, 1961.)

heating system consisting of a central hot-air furnace, ducts, a room and a thermometer; the furnace can be turned on or off, but the fan continues to circulate air through the ducts and the room. The thermometer sends information about the room temperature back to the furnace; if the room temperature is too low, the furnace continues to supply heat to the room; if it is too high, the furnace shuts down. However, the process of regulation must involve slight increase and decrease above the desired room temperature; feedback control can never operate without some error, because an error is required to bring about the correction. The error will be small if the furnace is immediately adjacent to the room, so that there are no ducts (no dead space), if the thermometer responds and signals quickly and if the furnace increases or decreases its output promptly. The error will be large if the furnace is far away or the fan is inadequate and a long time is required for hot air to reach the room, and if the thermometer is at the far end of the room.

If sensory receptors sensitive to decreased Po_2 and increased Pco_2 control breathing; if these are all located in the lungs at the end of the pulmonary capillaries; and if nerve impulses speed to and from the respiratory centers infinitely fast, the error in regulation of arterial blood O_2 and CO_2 will be extremely small. However, if receptors reporting arterial Po_2 and Pco_2 are in peripheral arteries and the circulation time from the lung to the receptors is so long that they cannot sample arterial blood until 30 seconds or more after it leaves the pulmonary capillaries, the error will be large. Suppose that the arterial chemoreceptors signal for increased ventilation; this occurs at once and promptly decreases the Pco_2 and increases the Po_2 of blood in the pulmonary capillaries. However, if this blood does not reach systemic arterial chemoreceptors for 30 seconds, the increased ventilation continues, and in the arterial blood, Pco_2 decreases and Po_2 increases further (Fig. 3-6). At the end of 30 seconds, chemoreceptor drive diminishes and respiration slows or stops, but blood with little or no chemical stimulation continues to reach chemoreceptors for 30 seconds, and hypoventilation continues. When blood of high P_{CO_2} and low P_{O_2} (due to hypoventilation) reaches the chemoreceptors, hyperpnea begins again. Thus, we have sequences of overventilation, underventilation, overventilation. This over- and undercorrection can cause the system to "oscillate" permanently. The "input" (the arterial blood gases) oscillates, and the "output" that it produces (pulmonary ventilation) must also oscillate and at the same frequency. However, the input and output cycles are not synchronous; when one cycle is a half cycle behind the other, the feedback maintains the oscillation — in this case, hyperpneic and apneic phases of breathing.

Guyton has produced or maintained Cheyne-Stokes respiration by greatly increasing the time for circulation of the blood between lung and brain from 10 to as much as 300 seconds. Hecht, studying patients who had Cheyne-Stokes respiration, found that the lung-to-brain circulation time was prolonged and was approximately one-half the length of the Cheyne-Stokes respiration cycle. These two observations support the theory that oscillation is due to a long circulation time between lungs and chemoreceptors.

But many patients with congestive heart failure and long circulation times do not have Cheyne-Stokes respiration. It is likely that a neurologic disorder often initiates the respiratory arrhythmia and that circulatory slowing aggravates or maintains it. However, the matter is complex, because there are at least 2 types of chemoreceptors — those in the carotid and aortic bodies (sensitive to P_{CO_2} and P_{O_2}), which respond almost instantly, and those in the medulla (sensitive to $[H^+]$), which respond more slowly (p. 59).

Posthyperventilation Apnea

This is usually associated with lesions of the reticular activating system. Since apnea usually does not follow hyperventilation in healthy, alert man, its occurrence may be a diagnostic sign of damage to the pons.

Diminished Maximal Voluntary Ventilation

Cerebellar lesions produce ataxia of limb muscles and may produce a disturbance of respiratory muscles that decreases both vital capacity and maximal voluntary hyperventilation (MVV). Patients with rigidity, spasticity or weakness because of strokes or parkinsonism (with lesions in the basal ganglia) may also have decreased MVV. Patients with destruction of their motor pathways may have spasticity, weakness or paralysis and decreased MVV.

Apneusis

Lateral, bilateral pontine lesions in man at or below the level of the trigeminal nucleus (an area corresponding to the pneumotaxic center in animals) result in a pattern of irregular breathing in which tonic inspiratory cramps (apneusis) alternate with periods of apnea, with totally irregular breathing in between. Patients may live for days with such lesions. Their responsiveness to inhalation of CO_2 is quite low; this suggests that this area, when intact, may be CO_2-sensitive in man.

4

The Response to Oxygen and Oxygen Lack

ONE MIGHT GUESS that respiration would increase whenever cells of the body use more O_2 and form more CO_2 and would decrease whenever they need less O_2 and form less CO_2. This, indeed, is the case. Respiration does increase as body metabolism increases, and usually in proportion to it. This obviously requires very fine regulation, and to achieve it, the body should be able to sense or measure levels of certain materials used or formed by cell activity, such as O_2, CO_2 or H^+, and report these levels to the respiratory centers so that they can increase or decrease ventilation.

It is logical to ask first whether respiration is regulated primarily to maintain a proper supply of O_2. The answer is an unexpected one: the body's mechanisms for detecting O_2 lack, and it alone, are relatively insensitive. Figure 4-1 and Table 4-1 show how little respiration increases in healthy men when, instead of breathing 20.93% O_2 (air), they breathe 18, 16, 14 or 12%. But there *is* a powerful response when the O_2 concentration in inspired air is decreased further, to 8, 6 or 4%.[1] This leaves no doubt that there are O_2 detectors somewhere, but they are rela-

tively unresponsive when the O_2 concentration of inspired gas decreases a little or even moderately and are aroused fully only when life is threatened by a serious decrease in O_2 supply.

TABLE 4-1.—EFFECT OF BRIEF HYPOXEMIA (8–10 MIN) ON PULMONARY VENTILATION*

CONCENTRATION OF O₂ IN INSPIRED AIR (%)	TIDAL VOL. (ML)	FREQUENCY (BREATHS/MIN)	RESPIRATORY MIN VOL. (L/MIN)	ALVEOLA VENTILATI (L/MIN)
20.93	500	14	7.0	4.9
18.0	500	14	7.0	4.9
16.0	536	14	7.5	5.4
12.0	536	14	7.5	5.4
10.0	593	14	8.3	6.2
8.0	812	16	13.0	10.4
6.0			18.0	
5.2			22.0	
4.2	933	30	28.0	23.2

*From Dripps, R. D., and Comroe, J. H., Jr.: Am. J. Physiol. 149:277, 1947. All data are mean values and the same as those in Figure 4-1; predicted anatomic dead space was used to calculate alveolar ventilation, and increases in tidal volume were taken into account. Note that the first response is an increase in tidal volume. This increases *alveolar* ventilation and alveolar Po₂ (brings it closer to inspired Po₂) and so helps to counteract the low inspired Po₂.

THE OXYGEN RECEPTORS

Receptors sensitive to the level of O_2 were unknown until the discovery of the carotid and aortic chemoreceptors (1927–30). So deeply entrenched was the concept of central regulation of breathing by CO_2 (p. 55) and so skeptical were respiratory physiologists

---

[1] The first real demonstration that the decreased Po₂ of inspired air was responsible for the increased breathing of men at high altitude was made by Paul Bert and recorded in *La Pression barométrique* (Paris: Masson, 1878, p. 744; M. A. and F. A. Hitchcock [tr.] [Columbus, Ohio: College Book Company, 1943], p. 692).

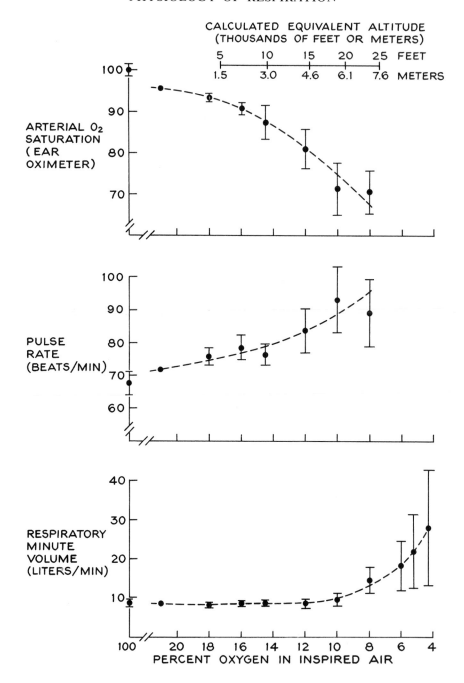

Fig. 4-1.—Effect of brief hypoxia in man. Healthy men breathed gas mixtures low or high in O_2 for 8 min. Measurements are average values of arterial O_2 saturation, pulse rate and respiratory minute volume for the last 3 min. Cross lines represent 1 standard deviation from the mean. Note the wide variation in individual responses to inhalation of the same gas mixtures; this is an index of the wide range of sensitivity of chemoreceptor response to hypoxia in man. The men who increased their ventilation most in response to low O_2 had the highest arterial O_2 saturation. Some men show *no* respiratory stimulation even when breathing 10% O_2. (Data from Dripps, R. D., and Comroe, J. H., Jr.: Am. J. Physiol. 149:277, 1947.)

(they still are—regarding discoveries made by others!) that Haldane and Priestley, in 1935, wrote, "On the whole it seems that the reflex control of breathing by chemical stimulation of the carotid nerve endings (by O_2 lack) has not been established." However, there is now general agreement that most of the useful respiratory (and probably circulatory) response to a decrease in arterial Po_2 originates in special chemosensitive cells in the aortic bodies attached to the arch of the aorta and in the carotid bodies near the division of the common carotid into the internal and external carotids (Fig. 4-2).

Specific organs and tissues other than these bodies do not seem to have special receptors to warn the respiratory center of local tissue hypoxia, though they do have local mechanisms to increase local blood flow. For example, when limbs are made hypoxic either by lowering the Po_2 of arterial blood supplying them or by injecting cyanide into

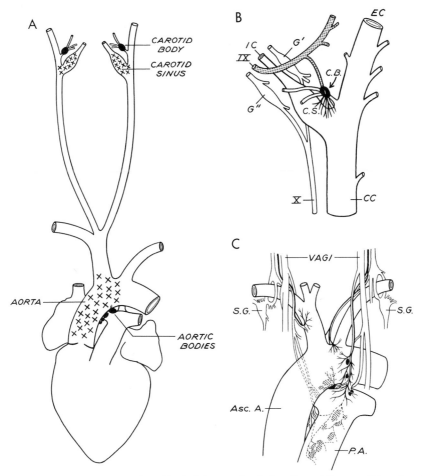

Fig. 4-2.—The carotid and aortic bodies (dog). **A,** approximate location of the carotid and aortic chemoreceptors (*black ovals*) and stretch receptors (*crosses*). **B,** the carotid body (*C.B.*) receives its arterial blood from the occipital artery, which is the first branch of the external carotid (*EC*). Its afferent fibers run in the carotid branch of the ninth cranial nerve (*IX*). *X* = vagus nerve, *CC* = common carotid artery, *C.S.* = carotid sinus, *IC* = internal carotid, *G'* = superior cervical sympathetic ganglion, and *G"* = nodose ganglion of the vagus. (Redrawn from Adams, W. E.: *The Comparative Morphology of the Carotid Body and Carotid Sinus* [Springfield, Ill.: Charles C Thomas, Publisher, 1958].) **C,** aortic chemoreceptor cells lie on the anterior (*black ovals*) and posterior (*hatched ovals*) surfaces of the aortic arch and pulmonary artery (*P.A.*); in the dog they receive their blood from a small branch of the aortic arch. *S.G.* = stellate ganglion; *Asc.A.* = ascending aorta. (Redrawn from Nonidez, J. F.: Anat. Rec. 69:299, 1937.)

this blood, respiration is not stimulated, but local blood flow increases. Even complete cessation of blood flow to the limbs, which increases the P_{CO_2} and (H^+) of these tissues, besides lowering their P_{O_2}, does not increase respiration unless nerve endings for pain are stimulated. The same is true for the pulmonary circulation: marked lowering of P_{O_2} of blood flowing through it does not increase respiratory minute volume.

The main exception is the brain. Cutting off its blood supply by clamping all arteries to it or by increasing the external pressure around it does increase breathing temporarily. Stopping blood flow produces complex effects because it permits CO_2 and H^+ to accumulate in the brain, besides causing O_2 lack; in addition, hypoxia depresses many neurons and activities of the brain.

CAROTID AND AORTIC BODIES

The carotid bodies have been known to anatomists since 1743, but their neurovascular nature and probable chemoreceptor function were not suggested until about 200 years later by a histologist, de Castro, in 1926. At about the same time, Heymans and Heymans found that blood low in O_2 or high in CO_2, limited to the left ventricle and first part of the aorta, caused stimulation of breathing, but only when the vagus nerves were intact. Shortly thereafter, Heymans found that the carotid arteries had similar chemosensitive zones; these were located in the carotid bodies. In 1938 Heymans was awarded the Nobel prize in medicine and physiology for this discovery.

I shall use the word *chemoreceptors* to mean sensory nerve endings that normally respond to changes in their *natural* chemical environment. For example, receptors in the tongue and nose have as their prime function the detection of chemical changes in their environment (taste and smell) and are therefore chemoreceptors. The carotid and aortic receptors sense changes in blood P_{O_2}, P_{CO_2} or (H^+) and are likewise chemoreceptors. On the other hand, a large number of recep-

tors respond (often powerfully) to chemical agents (often in minute amounts) that are not present in the normal or even in the diseased body, and presumably are not physiologic stimuli to the receptors; stretch receptors of the Hering-Breuer inflation reflex, pressoreceptors of the aortic arch and carotid sinuses and pacinian corpuscles may be stimulated by chemical agents (such as veratridine or nicotine) that are not the natural stimuli to these receptors. They are true mechanoreceptors which, for some reason, can be stimulated by low concentrations of certain chemicals. All reflexes initiated by the action of chemical substances on nerve endings are called *chemoreflexes*, but not all result from excitation of true *chemoreceptors*.

Where Are the Carotid and Aortic Bodies?

The carotid bodies are small, pinkish nodules located just beyond the division of each common carotid artery into the external and internal carotids (see Fig. 4-2); in man, each is about 3 – 5 mm in diameter. Each receives its arterial blood from a branch of the external or internal carotid artery. In some species the bodies are so closely associated with nerve fibers coming from the carotid sinus pressoreceptors that they were long thought to be part of the carotid sinuses. Afferent nerve fibers from both the carotid sinus and carotid body do run in the same carotid sinus nerve to join the glossopharyngeal nerve. The carotid bodies, however, are completely different from the carotid sinuses in structure and function. The carotid sinuses contain mechanoreceptors that respond to changes in stretch or deformation of the vessel wall; the carotid bodies contain chemoreceptors that respond to certain changes in their chemical environment.

The aortic bodies contain chemoreceptors that function separately from the aortic pressoreceptors in the wall of the ascending arch of the aorta. Most of the aortic chemoreceptors are scattered between the arch of the aorta and the pulmonary artery or lie on the dorsal aspect of the pulmonary artery (see Fig. 4-2). In some species chemoreceptor tissue is attached to major arterial trunks just above the arch of the aorta, but this tissue seems to be insensitive to known chemical stimulants and is presumably unimportant in the regulation of respiration and circulation.

The afferent nerve fibers from the aortic bodies enter the vagosympathetic trunks, usually along with the recurrent laryngeal nerves. Their cell bodies are in the nodose ganglia of the vagus nerves; in some animals there is a separate aortic nerve or aortic depressor nerve, and the aortic body fibers run with it.

The arterial blood supply of the aortic chemoreceptors of adult animals comes from small branches of either the coronary artery or the aortic arch. In the fetus these chemoreceptors may receive blood from the pulmonary artery as well; in the human embryo, there is a pulmonary arterial branch to the aortic body that persists until birth. In late fetal stages, this is supplemented by branches from the coronary arteries, usually the left; after birth, the pulmonary artery branch retrogresses completely, just as does the ductus arteriosus.

The embryology of these chemoreceptors is of physiologic interest. Koch developed the concept that each of the branchial (aortic) arches of primitive organisms (which also appear at different stages of development of mammalian embryos) is provided with receptors and nerves for pressure reception. In the mammalian embryo (Fig. 4-3), the first two arches disappear; the third aortic arch becomes the internal carotid artery and the carotid sinus, innervated by the glossopharyngeal nerve; the fourth becomes the right subclavian (right side) and the aortic arch (left side), innervated by the laryngeal branch of the vagus and the aortic nerves; the fifth disappears, and the sixth develops into the pulmonary artery (right side) and the ductus arteriosus (left side).

Schmidt suggested that chemo- as well as

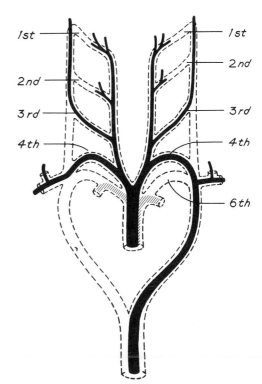

Fig. 4-3.—Aortic arches of the embryo. The dashed channels are the embryonic arches, the solid black are the main arteries of the adult systemic circulation and the shaded tubes are the main arteries of the adult pulmonary circulation. See text. (Adapted from Licata, R., in Abramson, D. I.: *Blood Vessels and Lymphatics* [New York: Academic Press, 1962].)

pressoreceptors might be associated with each of the persisting branchial arch structures. Chemoreceptor-like cells have been found in association with the first (mandibular) arch, innervated by the fifth nerve; the second (hyoid) arch, innervated by the seventh cranial nerve; the third (the carotid body); the fourth (aortic body), and the sixth arch (Liebow's cells associated with pulmonary venules). Schmidt also suggested that the strong stimulant effects of hypoxia and the relatively weak effects of increasing CO_2 on these tissues might represent survival in the air-breathing adult mammal of a reflex essential to the gill system in the fish. Fish take up O_2 from water as it flows through the branchial (gill) system. This branchial respiration in aquatic animals is regulated by the tension of O_2 in the water, decreased tension stimulating respiration. Krogh observed that gill movements of fishes are far more sensitive to decreased O_2 tension than to increased CO_2 tension in the water. It seems probable, therefore, that the carotid and aortic bodies in higher forms of life represent the survival of structures of great importance in the control of respiration in water-breathing animals.

What Stimulates the Carotid and Aortic Bodies?

1. DECREASE IN O_2 SUPPLY RELATIVE TO O_2 USE. First let me define hypoxia and hypoxemia. *Hypoxia* is a general term that signifies a decrease in O_2 below normal levels—in inspired gas, alveolar air, blood or tissues; see page 277 for a classification of types of hypoxia. *Hypoxemia* signifies a decrease in O_2 saturation of hemoglobin or a decrease in O_2 tension or both to below normal levels in blood; in this book it always refers to *systemic arterial* blood. The *amount* of O_2 in systemic arterial blood is also decreased in anemia (decrease in number of erythrocytes or amount of hemoglobin or both), but the arterial Po_2 and saturation of hemoglobin with O_2 are normal in patients with uncomplicated anemia. Anemia is really a type of hypoxemia (since the ml of O_2/100 ml of blood are less than normal), but we shall use "hypoxemia" to mean a decrease in O_2 in arterial blood *not* due to anemia.

The amount of O_2 available to tissues is discussed in Chapters 14 and 15; it depends on the amount of blood flow through tissues, as well as on the amount of O_2 contained in blood and the willingness of Hb to release it. For cells (including sensory receptors) to be hypoxic, the supply of O_2 must have decreased relative to their use of O_2; this lowers extra- and intracellular Po_2.

It is known that perfusion of isolated carotid bodies (connected to the body only by their nerves) with blood low in O_2 leads to increased ventilation. It was once believed that the carotid body cells simply acted as a meter sitting in the arterial blood flowing past them, that they sensed the amount of O_2 in it and flashed a message to the brain. This belief was strengthened by finding that, normally, the total O_2 in blood leaving the carotid body was almost as great as the total O_2 in blood entering it. But we know now that chemoreceptors do use O_2—about 0.09 ml/gm of tissue per minute—and not merely sample it. The reason for the high venous O_2 content is that the carotid body is an unusually vascular organ (Fig. 4-4) and has a tremendous blood flow (20 ml/gm/minute) in relation to its size; because of this, the carotid body removes only about 2% of the O_2 in arterial blood flowing through it.

Certain conclusions can be drawn from these relationships:

1. If blood flow is normal, the supply of O_2 is huge, the carotid body cells draw off little O_2 from each unit of blood and the Po_2 of arterial blood, chemoreceptor cell and carotid body end-capillary blood are almost equal (100 and 88; see row 1, Table 4-2), the cells are not stimulated.

2. If the Po_2 of inspired gas and arterial blood is decreased (row 2, Table 4-2) to 27 torr, the Po_2 of cells in the carotid body must be less than this, despite a huge blood flow, and the cells are stimulated.

3. If the arterial Po_2 is kept normal at 100 torr and blood flow to the carotid body is reduced to one fourth of normal (as in hypotension due to hemorrhage), O_2 uptake from each unit of blood increases 4-fold, the Po_2 of carotid body tissues decreases to 60 torr and some receptors are stimulated by low Po_2 alone (row 3, Table 4-2). However, when blood flow decreases and cell metabolism continues, metabolites such as H^+ and CO_2 accumulate locally, and these not only stimulate the carotid body but potentiate the effects of low O_2. In this case, the arterial blood Po_2 gives no clue to the actual Po_2 of the receptors, and even if one knew their Po_2, it would not indicate their activity, because ischemia has permitted the accumulation of CO_2 and H^+ to stimulant levels. This

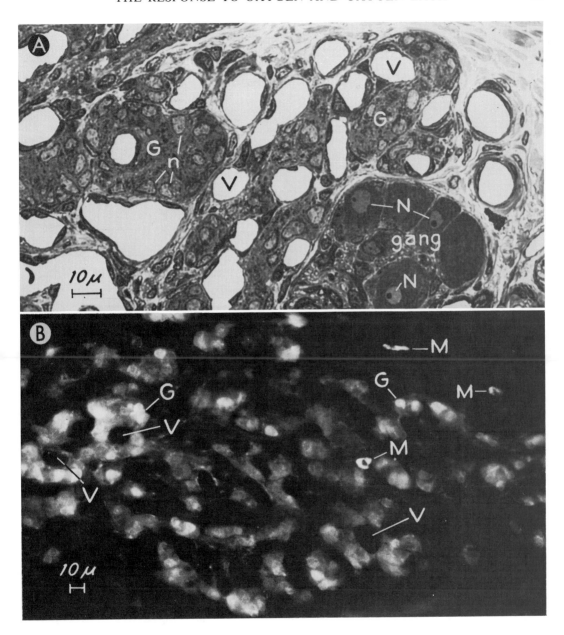

Fig. 4-4.—Structure of the carotid body (rat). **A,** note the large number of vascular channels surrounded by clumps of carotid body (glomus) cells. *V* = thin-walled blood vessel emptied of blood by perfused fixative; *G* = groups of glomus cells, the nuclei of which (*n*) are stained less than their cytoplasm; *gang* = a group of autonomic ganglion cells, probably parasympathetic to blood vessels in the carotid body; the nuclei (*N*) of these cells have prominent nucleoli. Light micrograph, ×750, stained with toluidine blue.

B, histochemical method of Falck and Hillarp used to demonstrate catecholamines in tissues by fluorescence microscopy. *G* = groups of glomus cells containing catecholamines that have been converted to intensely fluorescent compounds. The intensity of the fluorescence varies and is probably related to the concentration of catecholamines in glomus cells; *V* = blood vessels containing no fluorescent material appear black; *M* = mast cells contain material which is autofluorescent; the histochemical reaction is not required to induce fluorescence in mast cells. Light micrograph, × 350. (Courtesy of Dr. Donald M. McDonald.)

TABLE 4-2.—O₂ TENSION OF ARTERIAL AND CAROTID BODY (END-CAPILLARY) BLOOD

	ARTERIAL BLOOD			BLOOD FLOW/MIN TO CAROTID BODY	O_2 REMOVED† (ml O_2/100 ml)	CAROTID BODY END-CAPILLARY BLOOD			INCREASED RESPIRATION CAUSED BY CAROTID BODY REFLEXES
	O_2 Saturation (%)	Po_2 (torr)	O_2 Content* (ml O_2/100 ml)			O_2 Content (ml O_2/100 ml)	O_2 Saturation (%)	Po_2 (torr)	
1. Normal‡ (15 gm Hb)	98.5	100	19.7 + 0.3 = 20.0	normal	0.5	19.5	96.0	88	No
2. Hypoxemia (15 gm Hb)	50.0	27	10.0 + 0.08 = 10.08	normal	0.5	9.58	47.5	25	Yes
3. Hypotension	98.5	100+	19.7 + 0.3 = 20.0	¼ normal	2.0	18.0	89.0	60	Slight
4. Anemia (50%) (7.5 gm Hb)	98.5	100	9.85 + 0.3 = 10.15	normal	0.5	9.65	94.5	80	No
5. Anemia (20%) (3 gm Hb)	98.5	100	3.94 + 0.3 = 4.24	normal	0.5	3.74	87.5	55	Slight
6. Saline (no Hb)		150	0.45	2 × normal	0.25	0.2		66	No
7. HbCO (7.5 gm active Hb)	98.5 (50%)§	99+	9.85 + 0.3 = 10.15	normal	0.5	9.65	94.5	80–50	No

*The O_2 content is calculated as the sum of O_2 combined with Hb and O_2 dissolved in the blood. This calculation is explained in Chapter 14 and Figure 14-1.

†There is no measurable difference between O_2 in arterial blood entering the carotid body and venous blood leaving it, when blood flow is rapid. The value in this column is computed from the measured difference of 2 ml O_2/100 ml blood when blood flow is deliberately reduced to ¼ normal. This may be a high value because of increased chemoreceptor activity during ischemia.

‡Normal blood is assumed to contain 15 gm Hb/100 ml. Each gm can combine with 1.34 ml O_2; the O_2 capacity of Hb of 100 ml of this blood is 20 ml (Fig. 14-1).

§Fifty percent of total Hb is active and is 98.5% saturated with O_2.

is also true if the receptors' own metabolism is increased.

This relationship between O_2 supply and O_2 demand explains several clinical and experimental observations:

1. Patients with severe anemia do not have increased respiration at rest, even though their hemoglobin may be very low. If their lungs, alveolar and arterial Po_2 and blood pressure and blood flow through chemoreceptors are normal, the Po_2 of the chemoreceptors will not fall to critical levels. Moderate anemia (row 4, Table 4-2) results in a chemoreceptor Po_2 of 80 torr and no stimulation; severe anemia will lower carotid body Po_2 to 55, and this is just borderline for effective excitation of the chemoreceptors (row 5). In the case of anemia, blood flow is rapid, and CO_2 and H^+ do not accumulate.

Experimentally, perfusion of the carotid bodies with hemoglobin-free saline (Po_2 150 torr) does not cause stimulation; the fluid flow through the vessels more than doubles because of the low viscosity of saline, and this supplies enough dissolved O_2 to maintain a high tissue Po_2 (row 6, Table 4-2).

2. Patients with CO poisoning do not have increased breathing. This is because of the greater affinity of hemoglobin for CO than for O_2 (210:1). This means that only 1/210 as much CO as O_2 is needed in alveolar gas for CO to compete on even terms with O_2 for hemoglobin. Thus, the continued presence of a Pco of less than 0.5 torr in alveolar gas (Po_2 100 torr) will produce 50% HbCO and 50% HbO_2 at equilibrium. Although hypoxemia is severe, the O_2 in inspired air will be reduced only from 20.93% to 20.91% (a reduction of only 0.15 torr Po_2—from 159.0 to 158.85 torr). Thus CO poisoning creates the special situation of an infinitesimal reduction in alveolar and arterial O_2 *tension* with a marked reduction in arterial O_2 *content*. Calculations (based on removal of 0.5 ml O_2 from Hb that still combines with O_2) show that the Po_2 of carotid body cells should be 80 torr (row 7, Table 4-2). However, CO has a second effect on O_2 transport; it hinders the release of O_2 from HbO_2 (see p.

192). In this case, the 0.5 ml of O_2 is not released until carotid body tissue Po_2 falls to about 50 torr; this is borderline for stimulation of a significant number of chemoreceptors.

Chiodi and associates exposed 4 unanesthetized men to 0.15–0.35% CO for several hours. In 13 experiments the HbCO was 30–40%, in nine experiments 40–50% and in one experiment, 52%. Nevertheless, in none did minute volume of respiration increase. Mills and Edwards explain this paradox by suggesting that chemoreceptors in man are excited by this tissue Po_2 but that medullary centers are depressed at the same time because their Po_2 is much lower (the brain has a high metabolic rate relative to its blood flow). It is easy to see why inhalation of CO can be very dangerous: there is no hyperpnea, no dyspnea and not even cyanosis, since HbCO is cherry red.

3. Methemoglobin poisoning represents another condition in which some hemoglobin is converted into an inactive form (does not carry O_2) at a time when the Po_2 of arterial blood is still normal. Men or animals with large quantities of circulating methemoglobin do not increase their breathing.

4. If blood flow is markedly decreased, the chemoreceptor cells can become hypoxic even though arterial Po_2 and content are normal. Blood flow may be reduced either because the pressure in the systemic arteries is low as a result of severe hemorrhage, or because the arterioles supplying the chemoreceptors have constricted, even though arterial blood pressure is reasonably high.

It seems best to define the hypoxic stimulus to the carotid and aortic bodies as a decrease in the O_2 supply to the chemoreceptors below the amount they use, rather than as a decrease in arterial Po_2. The latter *is* a specific stimulus *when blood flow to the carotid body is normal*, but low blood flow can result in stimulation even though arterial Po_2 is normal.

A word of caution here. Some physiologists believe that the carotid body blood flow decreases to zero when both common carotid arteries are occluded. In most species, the central arterial anastomoses through the circle of Willis are so abundant that carotid occlusion does not drastically reduce arterial blood flow to carotid bodies (Fig. 4-5). Arterial blood simply flows backward from the vertebral arteries into and through the carotid and occipital arteries. For this reason, occlusion of the common carotid arteries, either experimentally or by arterio-

Fig. 4-5.—Effects of carotid occlusion on carotid sinus blood pressure. Occlusion of both common carotid arteries in midneck can lead to little decrease in blood pressure in the artery above the clamp (A) or to marked decrease (B). In both, mean pressure decreased above the clamp.

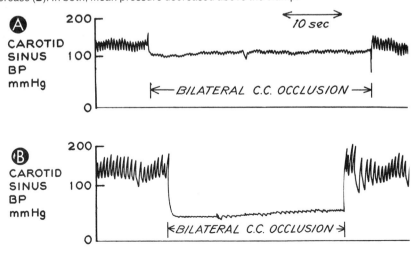

sclerosis, rarely produces marked ischemia of the carotid bodies.

2. INCREASE IN ARTERIAL P_{CO_2} AND (H^+). The role of the carotid and aortic bodies in the total response to increased CO_2 and H^+ is discussed in Chapters 5 and 6. As with O_2, the actual stimulus is the P_{CO_2} or (H^+) of the immediate environment of the chemoreceptors, rather than the concentration of these in arterial blood.

Perfusion of the carotid bodies of anesthetized animals with blood or solutions of varying P_{CO_2} or (H^+) has shown that reflex stimulation of ventilation does not occur until P_{CO_2} is increased by 10 torr or pH is decreased by $0.1 - 0.2$ pH units, even though action potentials in carotid nerve fibers may increase with less change.

However, there is interaction between stimulation of carotid bodies by low P_{O_2} and high P_{CO_2} or (H^+); this means that the effect of two (or three) acting together is greater than the sum of their individual actions. Therefore the two most serious threats to life (cardiac arrest or severe hypotension; respiratory failure or severe hypoventilation) excite the chemoreceptors more strongly than hypoxia alone because of the potentiation of the hypoxic stimulus by high P_{CO_2} during ischemia or asphyxia.

Is all chemoreceptor response, no matter what the apparent stimulus may be, initiated by an increase in local (H^+)? Certainly the response to increased P_{CO_2} and injection of acid could be so explained. Carbon dioxide is readily soluble in tissue fluids and passes through cell membranes rapidly. Inside cells it forms H_2CO_3, and this dissociates into H^+ and HCO_3^-. What about the response initiated by low O_2? Oxygen lack can cause intracellular accumulation of acids because of incomplete (anaerobic) metabolism of glucose. However, drugs such as nicotine (see next paragraph) do not seem to act by the same mechanism; they stimulate chemoreceptors powerfully, and their action can be blocked completely without any reduction in the response either to hypoxia or to cyanide.

Further, agents such as monoiodoacetic acid, which block glycolytic pathways and therefore prevent the accumulation of H^+, block the response to low O_2 — which fits the theory — but they also block the response to increased P_{CO_2} — which does not fit the theory, because CO_2 should still be able to diffuse into the cell, form H_2CO_3 and increase (H^+). Finally, low O_2 stimulates the carotid bodies at times when excess CO_2 does not (p. 59).

3. PHARMACOLOGIC STIMULI TO THE CAROTID BODIES. Many chemicals stimulate carotid and aortic chemoreceptors. Most of these fall into two classes: (1) chemicals known to interfere with tissue use of O_2 by an effect on cytochrome oxidase; a good example is sodium cyanide. Presumably, these chemicals act in the same way as low P_{O_2}. (2) Chemicals known to stimulate sympathetic ganglion cells; a good example is nicotine. Every substance known to stimulate sympathetic ganglion cells by a nicotine-like action also stimulates the carotid and, presumably, the aortic bodies. The clinical importance of drugs acting on the carotid bodies is discussed on page 53.

Mechanism of Stimulation of the Carotid Body

De Castro, who in 1926 was impressed by seeing clumps of special cells almost sitting in lakes of blood, was the first to propose that the carotid body had a sensory function. His concept was a simple one: the cells "tasted" the blood and reported to the brain on its chemical composition. He called these "chemoreceptor cells" and thought that an axon originating in each cell carried messages directly to the brain. With the advent of the electron microscope, it became apparent that the clumps of "chemoreceptor cells" have no axons, and de Castro's concept required revision.

What do we know of the fine structure of the carotid body, and how does this help us understand how chemical changes in the ar-

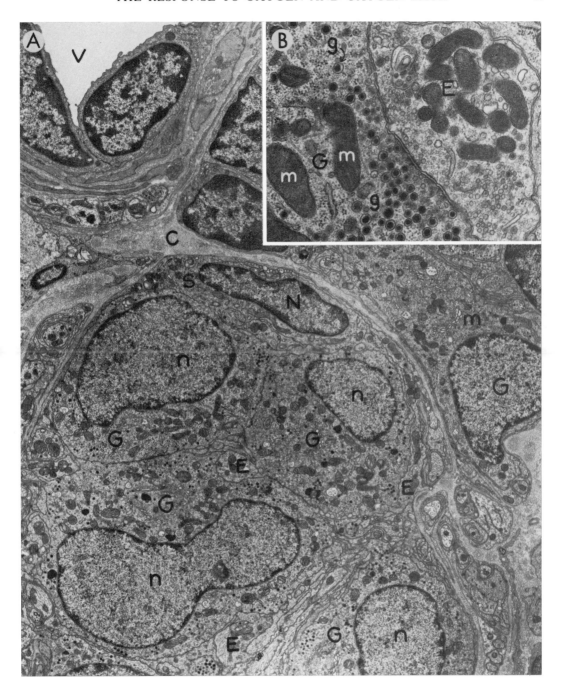

Fig. 4-6.—Fine structure of carotid body cells and nerve endings. **A,** rat carotid body, electron micrograph, × 7100. *V* = small arteriole; *G* = glomus cells having electron-dense cytoplasmic vesicles and nucleus (*n*); *N* = nucleus of satellite cell; *S* = cytoplasm of the satellite cell, processes of which surround glomus cells. Satellite cells do not have cytoplasmic granules similar to those of glomus cells; *E* = endings of sensory nerves near the glomus cells; *C* = collagen in extracellular space.

B, rat carotid body, electron micrograph, × 24,000. *G* = cytoplasm of a glomus cell containing: *m* = mitochondria; *g* = vesicles (800–1500 A in diameter) with electron-dense cores. *E* = ending of a sensory nerve, the cell body of which is in the petrosal ganglion. (Courtesy of Dr. Donald M. McDonald.)

terial blood are translated into sensory nerve impulses? A striking feature of the carotid body, easily visible with the light microscope, is the large number of blood channels (see Fig. 4-4), larger than capillaries and lined with fenestrated endothelial cells. These are surrounded by groups, clumps or cords of two types of special cells. Fluorescent microscopy shows that the type I, or glomus, cells (formerly called "chemoreceptor cells") contain most of the carotid body's catecholamines (epinephrine, norepinephrine and dopamine) and 5-hydroxytryptamine — shown by chemical determination to be present in the carotid body (see Fig. 4-4).

Electron micrographs show that type I cells are complex in shape, with many finger-like extensions. Their most striking feature is the presence of electron-dense, cored vesicles scattered throughout the cytoplasm (Fig. 4-6). Type I cells are almost completely enveloped by octopus-like tentacles of type II cells (also called satellite, sustentacular or supporting cells). Type II cells also have a

close relationship to nerve endings and nerve fibers in the carotid body and may have a function similar to that of Schwann cells or of glial cells in the central nervous system. The carotid body also contains nonspecific acetylcholinesterase; there is no agreement on its intracellular location.

There are numerous nerves and nerve endings in the carotid body and occasional ganglion cells (see Fig. 4-4), probably parasympathetic, whose postganglionic fibers may run to blood vessels. There are also postganglionic sympathetic fibers that originate in the superior cervical ganglion and end on vessels and a few preganglionic fibers that end in close relation to type I cells. Most of the fibers in the glossopharyngeal and carotid nerves appear to be afferents that have their cell bodies in the petrosal ganglion and their endings on type I cells; some are efferents that also end on type I cells. This means that stimuli to the carotid body might act directly on afferent nerve endings or act on type I or II cells to release chemical transmitters

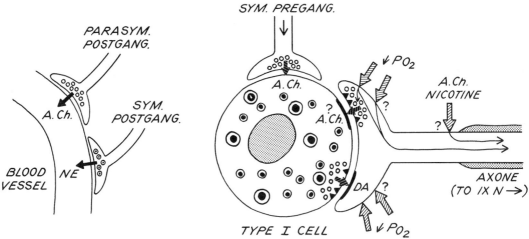

Fig. 4-7.—Schema of innervation of carotid body. The type I cell has at least 2 types of nerve endings—efferent sympathetic preganglionic nerve endings and afferent endings whose fibers run centrally in the carotid sinus nerve to the ninth cranial nerve. Low P_{O_2} may act on the sensory nerve ending rather than on the type I cell; simultaneously, however, low P_{O_2} may cause release of a chemical substance (acetylcholine?) which acts on the type I cell. The type I cell may in turn release dopamine (DA), which acts on the sensory nerve ending to modulate its activity. Stimulation of sympathetic preganglionic fibers to the type I cell may activate it (via A.Ch.) to release dopamine or other catecholamines. The schema pictures chemicals such as nicotine and acetylcholine activating afferent fibers central to the nerve ending. Autonomic nerves also end on blood vessels in the carotid body and can regulate their diameter and so influence blood flow. ? = site of action or nature of transmitter is speculative. (Schema based on electron microscopic and neurophysiologic observations of Dr. Donald M. McDonald).

which, in turn, stimulate afferent endings (Fig. 4-7).

Biscoe proposes that fine nonmyelinated nerve endings, enclosed almost to their terminal by type II cells, are the true chemoreceptors. He believes that type II cells perform the function of glial cells elsewhere in the nervous system and, in addition, may influence the nerve ending by altering its local environment. And he proposes that type I cells, rather than being receptors, influence true receptors by releasing chemical substances that alter their responsiveness; the release of materials from them may be regulated in part by efferent fibers whose endings make close contact with type I cells. Sympathetic and parasympathetic fibers may play a role by increasing or decreasing blood flow to the carotid body and so influencing the local concentration of stimulant materials. The true receptor (the nerve ending), according to Biscoe's concept, has a high O_2 consumption and is activated by a decreased Po_2, which slows the sodium pump in the nerve membrane; this in turn affects the potassium gradient and the membrane potential. Loss of potassium causes depolarization and initiates action potentials in the afferent fiber. He believes that the membrane potential of these very small fibers may be extremely sensitive to changes in Po_2 (and also to Pco_2 and $[H^+]$) because of their high surface-to-volume ratio.

Eyzaguirre, on the other hand, assigns to acetylcholine a critical role as a transmitter substance. He bases his concept on several observations: (1) Acetylcholine and cholinesterase are both present in the carotid body. (2) Acetylcholine, injected into arterial blood flowing through the carotid body, stimulates it. (3) When the perfusion of one carotid body is stopped (ischemic stimulation) and then begun again, the collected effluent contains a substance, thought to be acetylcholine, that can stimulate a second carotid body. Anticholinesterases (which prevent the destruction of acetylcholine) increase this effect. He believes that acetylcholine is released from type I cells by the action of hypoxia and then acts on nerve endings. The concept is interesting and ingenious. Not all agree with it, because some contend that agents that completely block the effect of acetylcholine on the carotid body do not reduce excitation by hypoxia.

A complete theory should also explain the role of catecholamines. Are they simply part of a system of catecholamine-containing cells scattered throughout the body, or do they have a specific role in initiating or modifying chemoreceptor impulses? The answer is not simple. Electron microscopic studies by McDonald show specialized regions of type I cells that are characteristic of a chemical synapse in which the transmitter would pass from type I cell to afferent nerve ending. But they also demonstrate chemical synapses in which the transmitter would pass from nerve ending (even the same ending) to the type I cell. The first transmitter could be acetylcholine, and its role could be to discharge material from the type I cell. The second transmitter could be a catecholamine such as dopamine (see Fig. 4-7). Dopamine depresses chemoreceptor activity in the cat, and its release locally, in minute amounts, might modulate chemoreceptor function and be responsible for the characteristic relationship between decrease in Po_2 and frequency of action potentials. But although the physiologic stimulus, hypoxia, produces similar effects in cats and dogs, dopamine *stimulates* chemoreceptors in dogs; perhaps dopamine has a physiologic action (to depress and modulate) in very low concentrations in the dog (as in the cat) but has an additional pharmacologic effect (stimulation) in the dog. We may be on the verge of learning the mechanism of action, but at the moment there is no general agreement on one concept.

What Does Stimulation of the Carotid and Aortic Bodies Do?

Chemoreceptor stimulation is usually thought to affect only respiration; however, it may lead to more widespread responses.

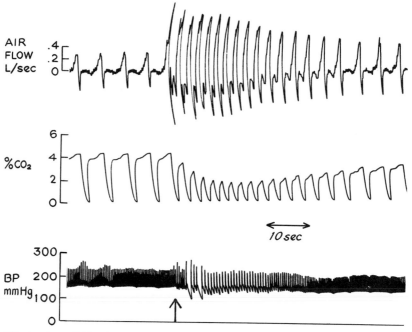

Fig. 4-8.—Effects of carotid body stimulation. A small amount of nicotine (5 μg) injected into the common carotid artery at the arrow causes increase in tidal volume, frequency and minute volume of breathing, decrease in Pco$_2$ of alveolar gas and bradycardia (anesthetized dog).

The known reflex effects are:

1. Increase in tidal volume, frequency and minute volume of breathing (Fig. 4-8).

2. Constriction of most of the peripheral vessels (except for cutaneous vessels).

3. Changes in heart rate. Bradycardia is characteristic of carotid body stimulation in laboratory experiments in which hyperpnea is prevented (Fig. 4-9); however, it is masked by a pulmonary reflex that causes tachycardia. The pulmonary reflex is activated by increased inflation of the lungs that occurs whenever tidal volume of breathing increases breathing, as it does during carotid body stimulation. The tachycardia is therefore an indirect result of carotid body stimulation. Tachycardia, however, appears to be a *direct* result of aortic body stimulation because it occurs even when there is no increase in tidal volume (see Fig. 4-9). Whenever something prevents lung inflation, such as neuromuscular block, immersion (the fetus is continuously immersed) or controlled ventilation, hypoxia is more apt

to produce bradycardia than tachycardia.

4. Increase in left ventricular performance.

5. Systemic arterial hypertension (Fig. 4-10).

6. Increase in bronchiolar tone.

7. Increase in functional residual capacity of the lungs.

8. Increase in pulmonary vascular resistance (in the dog, initiated by aortic, not carotid, body stimulation).

9. Increase in the secretion of the adrenal medulla and cortex and of the posterior pituitary.

10. Increase in the activity of the cerebral cortex, which may cause insomnia or, in experimental animals, convulsions.

Many physiologists consider that the aortic bodies are "weak" carotid bodies. This is not true, at least in the dog. Stimulation of carotid bodies results in reflex hyperpnea and vasoconstriction of limb vessels, and so does stimulation of the aortic bodies. But aortic body stimulation in the dog produces

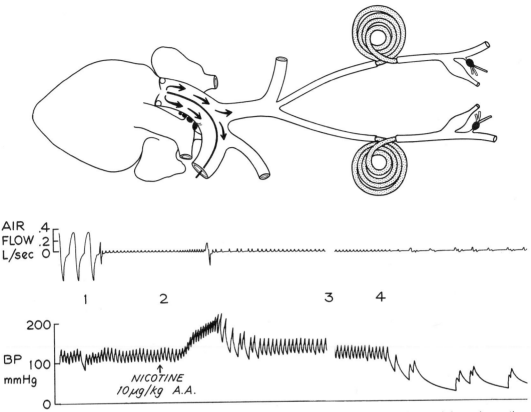

Fig. 4-9.—Temporal separation of aortic and carotid body stimulation. Nicotine injected through a catheter placed in the aorta of a dog just beyond the aortic valves reaches the aortic bodies within 1 second, but because it must pass through long delay paths (coils of plastic tubing) inserted in the common carotids, does not reach the carotid bodies until 75 seconds later. *Below,* nicotine, injected at *2,* stimulates aortic bodies and causes tachycardia and hypertension; later (at *4*) it reaches carotid bodies and causes bradycardia and hypotension. A neuromuscular blocking agent (succinylcholine) was injected at *1* to produce apnea and eliminate any effects of hyperventilation. Top tracing is respiratory air flow, bottom is carotid blood pressure. A portion of the record (45 seconds) was deleted at *3* to save space. *A.A.* = ascending aorta. (From Comroe, J. H., Jr., and Mortimer, L.: J. Pharmacol. Exp. Ther. 146:33, 1964.)

pulmonary vasoconstriction, and carotid body stimulation does not. Further, aortic body stimulation usually causes reflex tachycardia and systemic hypertension, whereas carotid body stimulation usually provokes reflex bradycardia.

Not every change that occurs in the acutely or chronically hypoxic patient results from stimulation of the chemoreceptors. The polycythemia (increased number of red blood cells, increased hematocrit and large blood volume) that characteristically occurs in chronically hypoxic animals does so even when the chemoreceptors have been denervated; indeed, it is even more severe, be-

cause arterial P_{O_2} is lower for a given inspired P_{O_2} when compensatory hyperpnea is no longer present. Increased formation of red blood cells is initiated by low O_2, but the stimulus to blood-forming organs is generally believed to be erythropoietin, a hormone released by the juxtaglomerular cells of the kidneys in response to local tissue hypoxia. Although the main source of erythropoietin is the kidneys, some must be produced elsewhere, since it is still present in patients who have no kidneys and who are kept alive by hemodialysis. Recently Tramezzani and his associates have reported experiments indicating that the carotid body, in addition to

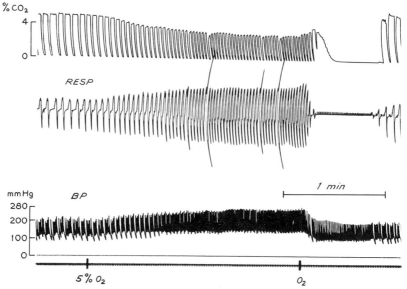

Fig. 4-10.—Effects of inhalation of 5% O_2 followed by 100% O_2. Inhalation of low O_2 causes increase in tidal volume and then in frequency of breathing (anesthetized dog). Alveolar ventilation increases and alveolar CO_2 decreases. Heart rate and systemic arterial blood pressure increase. Note the abrupt and prolonged apnea after the inhalation of O_2 which removes the hypoxic stimulus; breathing resumes when alveolar (and arterial) CO_2 has risen to previous levels.

other functions, is an endocrine organ secreting erythropoietin; they claim that removal of carotid bodies causes anemia and that extracts of carotid body stimulate the bone marrow to increase red cell production and release. These claims have not been confirmed; Wasserman found neither immediate nor delayed anemia in 40 patients after bilateral carotid body removal.

PHYSIOLOGIC IMPORTANCE OF THE OXYGEN RECEPTORS IN REGULATION OF BREATHING

ROLE WHEN THERE IS NO HYPOXEMIA. Is the carotid body important in the regulation of respiration when arterial Po_2 is in the normal range? Let us separate this into two questions:

1. Are the carotid and aortic bodies stimulated by the normal arterial Po_2 (100 torr) when man breathes air at sea level? Are they sending messages to the respiratory center because the Po_2 is 100 instead of, let us say, 600 torr? One way of determining this is to raise the arterial Po_2 of a normal man suddenly from 100 to more than 600 torr by giving him O_2 to inhale. This maneuver results in an immediate, though slight, depression of breathing. Assuming that it does nothing but raise arterial Po_2, we can conclude that the high Po_2 has physiologically "denervated" the O_2 receptors and that they must have been more active at the normal arterial Po_2 of 100 than at 600.

If persons first breathe 33% O_2 instead of air and then breathe pure O_2, there is usually little or no immediate depression of breathing. Experiments of this type suggest that some O_2-sensitive cells are firing messages to the respiratory center when arterial Po_2 is 100 torr (man breathing 20.93% O_2), but not when it has been raised to 170 or 180 (man breathing 33% O_2).

2. Do these cells respond to *small* changes in arterial Po_2, say from 100 to 95 torr, which might occur during a shallow breath or with a change from slight hyper- to slight hypoventilation? Figure 4-1 gives the best evidence on this point in una-

nesthetized men. They breathed first air and then 18, 16, 14.5, 12, 10 or 8% O_2. Neither tidal volume nor frequency of breathing changed in most men breathing 18% O_2. Inhalation of 16% O_2 increased the breathing in 17 of 20 men, but only by 6%. Not until they breathed 10% or even 8% O_2 was there significant hyperpnea in most men. Possibly a few men have chemoreceptors so sensitive and so powerful that they can increase breathing when 18% O_2 is breathed (and arterial Po_2 is decreased by 20 torr), but most do not develop hyperpnea until arterial Po_2 has decreased by 40–50 torr.

Figure 4-11 shows the number of impulses/second recorded in nerve fibers from the carotid body of a cat when the Po_2 of blood flowing through it varied from 550 to 30 torr. Note that there are a few impulses between 100 and 550, more between 100 and 50 and many more when Po_2 fell below 50 torr.

However, this is not the whole story. An increase in respiration caused by one stimulus, such as hypoxia, is always modified by changes in the intensity of other stimuli. For example, increased alveolar ventilation lowers arterial blood Pco_2 and reduces the response of both peripheral and central chemoreceptors even when the hypoxic stimulus remains constant. Again, increase in tidal volume increases lung inflation and increases the number of inhibitory nerve messages from the lung to the respiratory centers.

Physiologists like to know how much a specific respiratory stimulant or depressant affects ventilation of the whole person; this is easy to measure. They also like to know what a specific stimulus would do to respiration if uninfluenced and unchecked by any secondary effects; this is harder to measure. However, when subjects breathe low O_2 mixtures, enough CO_2 can be added to inspired air to keep arterial Pco_2 constant at a desired level; this is called the iso-Pco_2 technic. When alveolar Pco_2 is kept at normal or slightly subnormal levels by this technic, inhalation of low O_2 mixtures produces little significant change in ventilation until the alveolar Po_2 is 60 torr or less (Fig. 4-12). However, if the arterial Pco_2 is kept at a level greater than normal (43–44 torr), a reduction in Po_2 that previously produced no increase in ventilation may now do so. If the arterial Pco_2 is raised even higher (to 48–49 torr), and maintained at this level, there is still more stimulation, and respiration may now increase from changes in the Po_2 range between 140 and 60 torr, which normally produce little effect.

This means either that: (1) chemoreceptor cells *do* send messages to the medullary centers when the Po_2 decreases only a few millimeters, but these are ineffective unless the Pco_2 of the central cells is above normal; or (2) some potentiation occurs within chemoreceptor cells so that a simultaneous increase in Pco_2 and decrease in Po_2 produce nerve impulses not previously generated by decreased Po_2 alone.

A compromise point of view that seems to fit all evidence is that some chemoreceptor cells are tonically active at the normal Po_2 of arterial blood, and these can be inactivated by inhalation of 33% O_2, which produces a rise of 70–80 torr Po_2. However, most chemoreceptors are not stimulated effective-

Fig. 4-11.—Rate of chemoreceptor afferent discharges (impulses/sec) in a single fiber plotted against arterial blood oxygen tension (Pa_{O_2}). Note that there is little increase in rate when Pa_{O_2} decreases from 550 to 100 torr, more between 100 and 50 torr and a very sharp increase below 50 torr. The points of inflection vary in different fibers, but the shape of the curve is about the same. (Courtesy of Dr. Sanford Sampson.)

IMPULSES/SEC

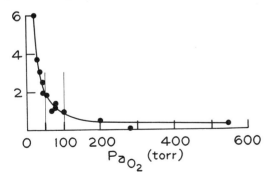

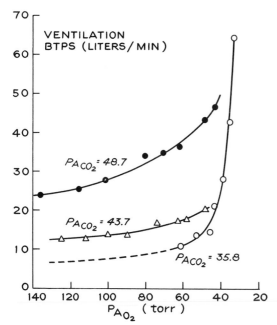

Fig. 4-12.—Increase in ventilation due to hypoxia associated with low and high levels of CO_2. Alveolar Pco_2 was maintained close to 35.8 torr (*bottom curve*), 43.7 torr (*middle curve*) and 48.7 torr (*top curve*) in a subject given low O_2 mixtures to breathe. Each curve starts at a higher level because of the effect of higher CO_2 tensions. Between 80 and 120 torr, the slope of the upper curve is steeper than that of the lower ones because of interaction between the low O_2 and high CO_2 stimuli. Volume of ventilation corrected to BTPS (body temperature, ambient pressure, saturated with water vapor). (Redrawn from Loeschke, H. H., and Gertz, K. H.: Arch. ges. Physiol. 267:460, 1958.)

ly or maximally until the Po_2 has fallen to 40 or 50 torr. Either the peripheral or central mechanism reacts more vigorously to small changes when arterial Pco_2 is above normal levels.

The role of the carotid and aortic bodies in the regulation of blood pressure in response to small changes in Po_2 has not been explored. When men inhale 18% or 16% O_2, slight tachycardia results, even though there is no significant increase in ventilation (see Fig. 4-1). If this is due to stimulation of peripheral chemoreceptors, then the carotid or, more likely, the aortic body must have more sensitive mechanisms for affecting circulation than for affecting respiration. It is not known whether changes in blood flow and O_2

supply of the carotid and aortic bodies that occur with small changes in systemic blood pressure activate receptors capable of influencing vasomotor centers; if they do, this could be an important mechanism for regulating the circulation.

Guazzi and Zanchetti believe that the carotid and aortic bodies play an important role in maintaining blood pressure during deep sleep. Blood pressure often falls moderately in cats during desynchronized sleep (a state characterized by a desynchronized EEG and rapid eye movements, associated with dreaming in man) but falls alarmingly after selective denervation of peripheral chemoreceptors. This suggests that chemoreceptors, when present, counter the initial fall in blood pressure by causing reflex vasoconstriction and so prevent periods of transient cerebral ischemia.

ROLE IN THE REGULATION OF RESPIRATION AND CIRCULATION IN ACUTE HYPOXEMIA. Is the hyperpnea of acute hypoxemia entirely reflex in origin? Before 1930, it was generally agreed that hypoxemia stimulated the medullary respiratory and vasomotor centers *directly*. The discovery of the carotid and aortic bodies and subsequent investigation of their function led to the belief that both the hyperpnea and the hypertension of hypoxemia were entirely *reflex* in origin and that hypoxemia led to pure depression of breathing and fall in blood pressure in animals deprived of their chemoreceptors. Actually, this is not true for either respiration or circulation. If lightly anesthetized or unanesthetized dogs whose carotid and aortic bodies have been denervated are given low O_2 to breathe, there is an initial period of reduced breathing. This is usually thought to be due to a simple depression of the respiratory center by hypoxia. Following this, respiratory minute volume increases above normal. The increase is not the typical hyperpnea of the intact, hypoxemic animal: it is delayed in onset, is characterized largely by an increase in rate and a decrease in tidal volume and persists for some minutes when the low O_2 mixture is replaced by air or O_2.

Studies on patients who have had both carotid bodies removed surgically have demonstrated that the respiratory response to moderate degrees of acute hypoxia is no longer present; the response to extreme hypoxia has, of course, not been tested as in animals.

What about the cardiovascular response? Denervated animals given O_2 to breathe also have an initial period of hypotension, but when hypoxia is sustained or very severe, the blood pressure may rise above normal. This rise may be due to stimulation of medullary, or even spinal, vasomotor centers by hypoxia, either because of metabolic acidosis or reduced cerebral blood flow. The late rise may also be due to release of catecholamines (epinephrine and norepinephrine) from the adrenal medulla as a direct effect of hypoxia on this gland or an indirect effect by stimulation of the vasomotor centers.

In patients in whom both carotid bodies were removed surgically, Lugliani and associates found that hypoxia (breathing 12% O_2) invariably led to a decrease in systolic and diastolic systemic blood pressure, even though the aortic bodies were still intact; the response to more severe hypoxia has not been tested. When these patients breathed 12% O_2, their heart rates increased as much as those of control patients with carotid bodies. The tachycardia could be due to aortic body reflexes, to hypoxia of the central nervous system or to reflexes associated with the fall in systemic blood pressure; it could not be attributed to reflexes initiated by lung inflation, since tidal volume of breathing did not increase.

In summary, the carotid and aortic bodies together seem to account for the hyperpnea and hypertension that result from slight, moderate or severe, acute hypoxemia. When hypoxemia is severe or prolonged, an additional, probably central, mechanism may augment breathing, particularly if the animal is unanesthetized. The tachycardia, vasoconstriction and hypertension that result from inhalation of low O_2 mixtures can be ac-counted for by carotid and aortic body reflexes—largely by the latter in the dog. Tachycardia may also occur as a result of pulmonary reflexes due to the associated hyperventilation. Severe hypoxemia, however, can cause a delayed increase in blood pressure without any of these reflexes.

Central chemoreceptors are, as a rule, easily depressed (by anesthesia, for example), but peripheral chemoreceptors, their afferent pathways, central connections and efferent components are not. It is clinically important that respiration of hypoxemic patients is relatively unresponsive to CO_2 at a time when it can still be "driven" by hypoxia acting through peripheral chemoreceptor reflexes. A sudden withdrawal of these—by giving the patient O_2 to inhale—may cause serious hypoventilation, CO_2 retention and coma, unless ventilation is maintained by some mechanical means. Thus, when a patient with emphysema and pulmonary insufficiency inhaled O_2, his arterial O_2 saturation increased from 69 to 95%, but this was accompanied by a decrease in minute volume of ventilation (from 4.6 to 2.2 L/minute), a rise in arterial P_{CO_2} (to 150 torr) and a decrease in arterial pH (to 7.06) (Table 4-3). This type of reaction is rare during O_2 therapy; however, it is important to recognize that it *can* occur and to be prepared to combat the hypoventilation with mechanical aids.

Chemoreceptor reflexes may also drive respiration in normal men who breathe very low O_2 mixtures, and inhalation of O_2 may be followed by complete apnea for a minute or more; this response has been termed "oxygen apnea" or "oxygen blackout" and is due to sudden withdrawal of the stimulant factor

TABLE 4-3.—EFFECT OF INHALATION OF O_2 IN PATIENT WITH PULMONARY INSUFFICIENCY*

	AIR	O_2
Art. O_2 sat., %	69	100
Art. P_{CO_2}, torr	125	150
Art. pH	7.12	7.06
Resp. MV, L/min	4.6	2.2
Resp. TV, ml	191	120

*From Comroe, J. H., Jr., *et al.*: *The Lung* (2d ed.; Chicago: Year Book Medical Publishers, Inc., 1962).

(peripheral chemoreceptor reflexes) by the abrupt rise in arterial Po_2 when the medullary centers are relatively unresponsive because of (1) severe hypoxia and (2) decrease in arterial Pco_2 below threshold levels by the preceding hypoxemic hyperventilation. In such cases, respiratory depression continues until the arterial Pco_2 rises to a level that can stimulate the depressed center or until the central depressant effects of hypoxia wear off (see Fig. 4-10).

Certain anesthetic agents (pentothal, cyclopropane, halothane) depress or abolish the response of the medullary chemoreceptors to CO_2, and the patient's ventilation may be maintained only by peripheral chemoreceptor reflexes excited by hypoxemia. Anesthetists prefer to prevent the hypoxemia by providing high concentrations of O_2 in the inspired gas mixture; this, of course, removes the reflex drive to respiration and may even lead to apnea. The anesthetist uses mechanical devices in such cases to provide adequate ventilation to keep arterial Pco_2 from rising during the operation.

ROLE IN THE REGULATION OF RESPIRATION IN CHRONIC HYPOXEMIA. Do the peripheral chemoreceptors continue to stimulate breathing indefinitely when hypoxemia becomes chronic — as in patients with cardiopulmonary disease or in man living at high altitude? Studies in both animals and man lead to the conclusion that the chemoreceptors respond for long periods; in neurophysiologic terms, they do not adapt readily. However, the response to hypoxia is blunted in men who live at high altitudes for many years and in children with congenital cyanotic heart disease (p. 252).

One can readily determine the extent to which hypoxemia is responsible for increasing or maintaining ventilation in a patient with chronic hypoxemia by measuring ventilation when he is breathing air and again *immediately after* O_2 is substituted for air. In a healthy man with normal arterial Po_2 and O_2 saturation, inhalation of O_2 decreases minute ventilation only slightly (3%) and only for a few minutes; after this, if inhalation of O_2 is continued, ventilation becomes about 10% greater than normal. If inhalation of O_2 leads to a greater *immediate* depression of breathing or to a sustained hypoventilation, the O_2 receptors must have been driving ventilation more than normally.

What does "physiologic denervation" accomplish in persons known to be hypoxemic? In some, inhalation of O_2 depresses ventilation no more than in healthy men; in some, as mentioned previously (p. 51), there may be serious and prolonged depression. How can we account for these varying responses?

1. Some men have little or no response to mild or moderate acute or chronic hypoxemia; their receptors are not excited until arterial Po_2 is very low.

2. Hypoxemia of patients is due to different disorders. Inhalation of O_2 "denervates" the O_2 receptors only when it relieves the hypoxemia. Inhalation of O_2 corrects hypoxemia in patients with hypoventilation, uneven ventilation in relation to pulmonary capillary blood flow and impairment of diffusion, but not in patients with right-to-left shunts (usually due to congenital heart disease), atelectasis or pulmonary artery-to-vein shunts, because the shunted blood does not come in contact with the high alveolar Po_2.

3. Some hypoxemic patients also have fever, pulmonary congestion, pleural effusion, hypotension and other disorders that increase respiration. Relief of hypoxemia does not depress breathing in them, because multiple factors are driving their respiration and the removal of one of these factors may effect little change.

4. In some chronically hypoxemic patients, O_2 inhalation does remove the hypoxemic drive, and respiration *is* markedly depressed, but this is unnoticed because the observer did not measure ventilation immediately after substitution of O_2 for air. If the measurement is made 20 minutes after the substitution, breathing may again be greater than normal and may appear not to have

been depressed by O_2 inhalation. Most men who live at high altitudes hyperventilate because of hypoxemia, and inhalation of O_2 depresses their breathing more than that of men breathing air at sea level, but their ventilation is still greater than normal (see p. 63).

ROLE IN REGULATION OF RESPIRATION AND CIRCULATION IN THE FETUS AND THE NEWBORN. Cross, Brady and Purves have shown that O_2-sensitive receptors are active at birth in regulating breathing in the newborn human and other species; inhalation of O_2 regularly causes a depression of breathing somewhat similar to that in the adult. Stimulation of the carotid and aortic bodies by low Po_2, high Pco_2 or increased (H^+) may therefore play an important role in initiating the first gasp required to bring air into the lungs of the newborn (see p. 244).

Before birth, the aortic bodies may play a role in maintaining pulmonary vasoconstriction. Aortic bodies receive blood from a branch of the pulmonary artery before birth and from the aorta after birth (p. 37). They would be maximally stimulated in fetal life and much less so after birth and the first breath. Since the fetus cannot inflate its lungs in response to hypoxia, hypoxia is more apt to produce reflex bradycardia in it than in the newborn.

CLINICAL IMPORTANCE OF THE CAROTID AND AORTIC BODIES

1. Since they adapt very slowly to a constant stimulus (low Po_2), the carotid and aortic bodies are responsible for much of the hyperventilation of chronic hypoxemia caused by living at a high altitude or by cardiopulmonary disease.

2. They are responsible for the violent hyperpnea of cyanide poisoning. Hydrocyanic acid blocks O_2 uptake in cells, including those of the carotid and aortic bodies, through paralysis of intracellular oxidation. Although complete hypoxia stimulates these specialized cells, it causes death of all others, despite the higher-than-normal arterial Po_2

caused by hyperventilation. (Even the capillary and venous blood are well oxygenated because of inability of cells to use O_2.)

3. Cyanide, given intravenously in very small doses, has been used to test the arm-to-carotid circulation time. It causes transient hyperpnea, and is then very rapidly detoxified in the blood unless given in overwhelming doses. Other chemicals that stimulate the peripheral chemoreceptors (lobeline, papaverine) have also been used to test arm-to-carotid circulation time.

4. The carotid and aortic bodies are responsible for part of the hyperventilation in patients with hypotension.

5. The *lack* of hyperpnea in certain conditions in which blood O_2 content is low (chronic anemia, methemoglobinemia and HbCO poisoning) can be explained by the normal arterial Po_2, normal blood flow and lack of chemoreceptor stimulation.

6. The chemoreceptor stimulant action of drugs such as lobeline has been used to initiate breathing in newborn infants who are slow to assume normal respiratory activity immediately after birth. Whatever stimulation occurs is brief and acts only as a sudden "kick" to a sluggish respiratory center. However, its ability to produce a few gasps may aid materially in expanding airless lungs. A longer-lasting carotid body stimulant, doxapram, has been used to increase breathing in patients with pulmonary insufficiency.

7. Vascular, neural or fibrous carotid body tumors occur in man, but apparently they neither increase nor eliminate chemoreceptor function. No aortic body tumors have been studied. It is unlikely that *all* chemoreceptor tissue could be destroyed by disease, because of the distance separating the carotid and aortic bodies.

8. Surgeons have removed one or both carotid bodies for the treatment of asthma. Unfortunately, they have done no control or sham operations and few careful measurements to determine whether the asthma was really improved. The operation does involve some risk. It may deprive the patient of some

or most of his protection against hypoxemia; most of the hyperpnea of hypoxemia comes from the carotid bodies and only a minor part of it from the aortic bodies. When man has no chemoreceptors and becomes hypoxic (because of cardiopulmonary disease or life at high altitude), he has a lower arterial Po_2 than normal man and is more apt to develop severe polycythemia and pulmonary vasoconstriction and hypertension. (In the cat, chemosensitive nerve endings regenerate after surgical removal of the carotid body; whether regeneration occurs in man is unknown.)

In addition, surgical removal of carotid bodies may cause "carotid sinus hypertension." The nerve fibers from the carotid sinus pressoreceptors and carotid body chemoreceptors join and enter the glossopharyngeal nerves; any attempt to block, denervate or extirpate carotid bodies may partly or completely denervate the carotid sinuses and, presumably, result in hypertension. The aortic arch has a "buffer" function similar to that of the carotid sinuses, but its receptors seem to have a higher threshold and maintain blood pressure at a higher than normal level in the absence of the carotid sinuses.

9. Nicotine in its lowest effective dose acts only on the carotid and aortic bodies; much larger doses are needed to stimulate sympathetic or parasympathetic ganglion cells directly, even though the ganglionic action is usually thought to be the characteristic action of nicotine. Thus, the cardiovascular and respiratory effects following the pulmonary absorption of small amounts of nicotine during smoking can be explained entirely by reflex effects initiated in the carotid and aortic bodies.

5

The Response to Carbon Dioxide

SINCE THE LUNGS excrete excess CO_2, a metabolic product, it is logical to believe that the level of CO_2 in blood or tissues might be an important controller of respiration—as CO_2 increases, alveolar ventilation might increase; as it decreases, alveolar ventilation might decrease. This is true; inhalation of CO_2-rich gases increases CO_2 concentrations in the body and increases ventilation.[1]

Some characteristics of the respiratory response of man to inhalation of a constant concentration of CO_2 in the inspired gas are shown in Figure 5-1. The tidal volume increases *slowly* to a maximum during the inhalation, even though alveolar and arterial blood P_{CO_2} reach a plateau quickly. Tidal volume also returns *slowly* to previous levels when air replaces the CO_2 mixture, even though alveolar and arterial blood P_{CO_2} decrease quickly. Frequency of breathing also increases as the concentration of CO_2 increases.

The ventilatory response to inhalation of increasing concentrations of CO_2 in air is quite different from that to decreasing concentrations of O_2. With CO_2, respiration increases slightly with slight increases in the concentration of CO_2 inhaled and continues to increase steadily (linearly) as the CO_2 concentration becomes higher over a wide range (Fig. 5-1). With low O_2, the response is not linear—there is a long, "flat" portion of the response curve, over which moderately large decreases in P_{O_2} produce little response, and then there is a steeply rising portion, over which relatively small changes in P_{O_2} can produce large changes in ventilation.

SENSITIVITY TO CARBON DIOXIDE

Sensitivity is determined by measuring the output of a system for a given input. For the respiratory center, the output is the frequency of action potentials in all motor nerve fibers to the muscles of respiration (since this is impossible to measure, physiologists instead determine the minute volume of breathing), and the input is the sum of all stimuli affecting the center. The sensitivity of the respiratory mechanism to changes in CO_2 is determined by measuring the minute volume of ventilation while changing only the alveolar or arterial P_{CO_2}, trying to keep all other known stimuli constant. The unit of sensitivity is the change in minute volume (in L) for a change of 1 torr in alveolar or arterial P_{CO_2}. It is best to measure *arterial* P_{CO_2}, though one can use P_{CO_2} of end-expired gas instead if it really is alveolar gas (it is if the anatomic dead space has been thoroughly flushed and if gas distribution is uniform). It is also necessary to make the measurements only when ventilation is in a

---

[1]The first experiment demonstrating that CO_2 can stimulate breathing was made by Pflüger in 1868 (Arch. ges. Physiol. 1:61, 1868), but it was not until 1905 that Haldane and Priestley demonstrated the specific importance of CO_2 in the regulation of breathing (J. Physiol. 32:225, 1905).

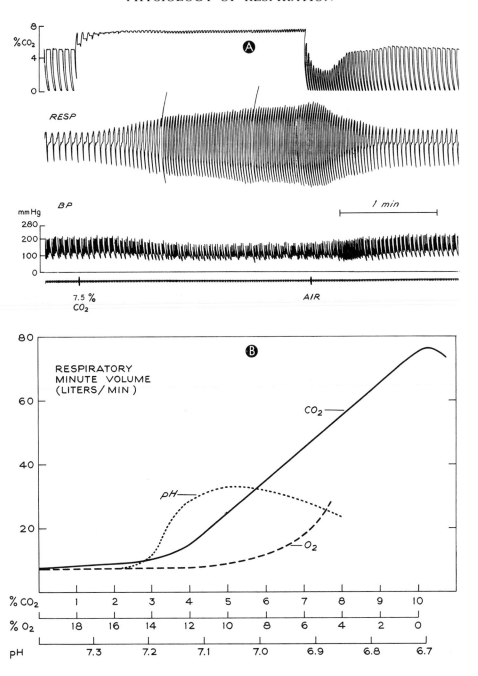

Fig. 5-1.—Respiratory response to inhaled CO_2. **A,** effects of inhalation of 7.5% CO_2 in air by a lightly anesthetized dog. Although alveolar CO_2 (*upper record*) and therefore arterial CO_2 reach maximal values within 1 or 2 breaths, tidal volume and frequency of breathing increase only gradually toward maximal values. Note that abrupt removal of the CO_2 stimulus does *not* lead to abrupt depression of breathing. (Contrast with abrupt removal of the low O_2 stimulus in Figure 4-10 and with the abrupt removal of stimulation of the carotid body by CO_2 in Figure 5-4.) Blood pressure often decreases during inhalation of CO_2 in air by anesthetized dogs but usually increases in awake man. **B,** the response of awake, healthy men to inhalation of increasing concentrations of CO_2 in air. (From Dripps, R. D., and Comroe, J. H., Jr.: Am. J. Physiol. 149: 43, 1947.)

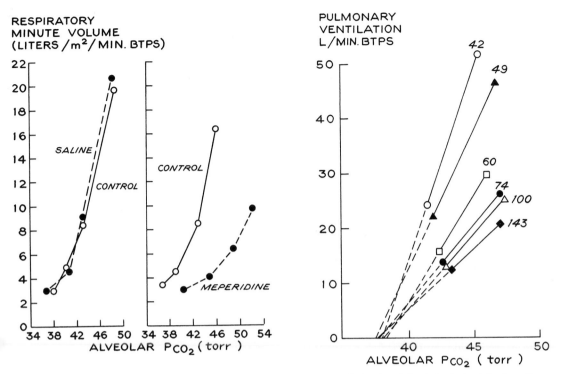

Fig. 5-2 (left).—Effect of meperidine on the CO_2 response curve. *Left*, after injection of physiologic saline solution; *right*, after injection of meperidine. (Redrawn from Loeschke, H. H., *et al.*: J. Pharmacol. Exp. Ther. 108:376, 1953.)

Fig. 5-3 (right).—Effect of varying degrees of hypoxia on the CO_2 response curve. The number at the top of each line is the alveolar Po_2 during the inhalation of high CO_2 mixtures. The *dashed lines* do not represent measured values; they are extrapolated from the two measured points. (Redrawn from Expt. 26 of Lloyd, B. B., Jukes, M. G. M., and Cunningham, D. J. C.: Q. J. Exp. Physiol. 43:214–227, 1958.)

steady state. The average value for healthy men is about 2.5 L/minute for a change of 1 torr Pco_2, though there is wide variation among individuals.

Analysis of CO_2 response curves enables one to determine whether drugs, procedures or altered circumstances change the sensitivity of the respiratory mechanism to CO_2 (assuming that no other excitatory or inhibitory factors affecting respiration are involved). Figure 5-2 shows that in this case sensitivity to CO_2 is reduced by a depressant drug such as meperidine from a control value of 2.3 to 1.0 (L/minute)/torr; morphine produces a similar effect. Figure 5-3 shows how the sensitivity changes from 2.2 to 7.9 (L/minute)/torr Pco_2 as arterial Po_2 changes from 143 to 42 torr. It may also change with change in arterial pH, in arterial blood pres-

sure, in body temperature, in concentration of blood catecholamines or with changes in alertness (wakefulness vs. sleep). Because of differences among healthy men and inability to determine or control other stimuli affecting respiration, it is difficult to know whether the respiratory response of any one patient to inhaled CO_2 is "normal" unless the response is unusually great or unusually slight.

WHERE ARE THE CO_2-SENSITIVE RECEPTORS?

Pumping blood rich in CO_2 through the arteries of the limbs does not stimulate respiration. Nor does total ischemia of one or all four limbs, even though there is a marked local accumulation of CO_2 and of H^+

ions. There seem to be no CO_2-sensitive receptors in the pulmonary circulation that respond by reflexly increasing breathing. In 1927, Heymans and Heymans perfused the isolated pulmonary circulation of dogs with blood unusually rich in CO_2 and observed no change in the respiratory movements of the head even though it was still connected to the trunk by its nerves. Respiration does increase, however, if blood rich in CO_2 is pumped through an isolated left ventricle and aortic arch or through isolated carotid bodies.

So far, the CO_2 story sounds like the O_2 story, but here the similarity ends. Inactivation of the carotid and aortic bodies does not abolish or even significantly reduce the total respiratory response of animals to inhaled CO_2 as it does that to low O_2 mixtures. The chief action of CO_2 seems to be elsewhere, probably on intracranial structures. For this reason, we must consider the *quantitative* effects of the action of CO_2 on peripheral and central chemoreceptors.

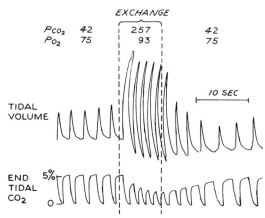

Fig. 5-4.—Stimulation of a dog's carotid body by blood with high Pco_2. Between the *dashed lines*, blood equilibrated with a high Pco_2 was infused into the common carotid artery, while an equal amount of the dog's arterial blood was withdrawn elsewhere. Note the abrupt onset of hyperpnea at the beginning, and cessation at the end, of the infusion. After denervation of the carotid body, the same infusion had no effect on breathing. (From Cropp, G. J. A., and Comroe, J. H., Jr.: J. Appl. Physiol. 16:1029, 1961.)

Carotid and Aortic Bodies

Increase in the Pco_2 of blood flowing through the carotid and aortic bodies stimulates breathing. This is reflex; the ninth and tenth cranial nerves carry the afferent impulses. Figure 5-4 shows how quickly this response can occur when blood with a very high Pco_2 is injected into the common carotid artery toward the carotid body; there is no response after the carotid body nerve is cut, even though the same blood, rich in CO_2, flows through the internal and external carotids to the brain. (In the cat, the dog and man, the medullary respiratory centers normally receive their arterial blood through the vertebral arteries, so that blood flowing through the common carotid usually does not reach the medulla.)

The stimulus shown in Figure 5-4 represents an enormous increase in Pco_2. Do changes in Pco_2 that occur during inhalation of 10% CO_2 in air or during severe CO_2 retention in patients stimulate the carotid and

aortic bodies? Inhalation of 10% CO_2 by man increases respiration in the time required for blood to pass from the lungs to the carotid artery. This is also true in unanesthetized dogs if their chemoreceptors are intact, but not if they have been denervated. In addition, perfusion of isolated carotid bodies with blood rich in CO_2 results in large increases in ventilation if the Pco_2 has been increased considerably (by 20 torr or more). We conclude that the chemoreceptors do respond to large, but still tolerable, changes in arterial Pco_2.

A more important question is whether the carotid and aortic bodies respond to much smaller physiologic changes—are they *the* structures that are exquisitely sensitive to CO_2, that cause the 2-fold increase in ventilation when alveolar and, presumably, arterial blood Pco_2 rise by 2–4 torr? The answer is no. Here is the evidence. Give an animal 1–5% CO_2 in air to breathe and measure the maximal respiratory response of the whole animal. At this point, collect arterial blood, making sure that no CO_2 escapes. Now allow the animal to breathe air. When respiration has returned to normal, perfuse the blood through the isolated carotid bodies of the same animal and measure the maximal *reflex* respiratory response. Studies such as this have shown that (1) chemoreceptor-induced hyperpnea does not occur until Pco_2 is increased by 10 torr, though the whole animal (anesthetized) responds to changes of 3 torr, and (2) when reflex increase in breathing does occur, it is considerably less than that for the whole animal. Or do the reverse experiment. Measure the response of unanesthetized animals to inhalation of CO_2 before and after denervation or block of known peripheral chemoreceptors. After denervation, the ventilatory response to inhaled CO_2 is similar to that of the whole animal.

The conclusion is that the peripheral chemoreceptors are not essential for the characteristic respiratory response of the *whole animal* to CO_2. However, they could be important in 3 conditions:

1. Since the peak response of the chemoreceptors occurs quickly (within 1 second) and that of central chemoreceptors more slowly (a few minutes), any rapid respiratory change in response to a sudden large increase in arterial Pco_2 could be mediated reflexly.

2. Chemoreceptors *could* help maintain ventilation when central CO_2-sensitive receptors are depressed. For example, an overdose of barbiturates or morphine may depress the central receptors so that breathing may depend entirely on a reflex drive from the hypoxic carotid and aortic bodies. But inhalation of CO_2 in air at this time will not usually stimulate breathing, even though the carotid and aortic bodies respond vigorously to the low O_2 stimulus. Further, inhalation of O_2 at this time (physiologic denervation of the O_2 receptors) results in abrupt depression of breathing or apnea, even though CO_2 is still accumulating. Blood with a very high Po_2 does not normally prevent chemoreceptor discharge in response to increased Pco_2. We do not know why CO_2 fails to act reflexly in this case.

3. Figure 5-3 shows that the respiratory response to inhaled CO_2 (increase in minute volume per torr change in Pco_2) becomes greater when alveolar Po_2 is lowered. This potentiation (sometimes called interaction) may occur both within the carotid and aortic bodies and centrally.

Central Chemoreceptors

It is clear that the characteristic ventilatory response to CO_2 is not due to stimulation of peripheral receptors and must therefore be due to stimulation of cells within the central nervous system. Where are these? Are they the same medullary neurons that constitute the medullary respiratory centers (see Fig. 3-1)—those that receive information from all parts of the body, act on it and produce an integrated, appropriate, coordinated respiratory sequence? We formerly thought so because (1) inhalation of CO_2 increases breathing even after the brain stem above the medulla is cut; (2) inhalation of CO_2 increases the volume of the prolonged apneustic inspiration that occurs after section through the lower pons (see Fig. 3-5); (3) injections of minute amounts of bicarbonate solution (which presumably yield CO_2 molecules) cause rhythmic increase in ventilation when injected into this medullary center, and (4) electrical activity synchronous with the respiratory cycle has been detected in this general region of the medulla when an animal inhales a CO_2-rich gas.

However, there is now good evidence that the central chemoreceptors are anatomically quite separate from the reflex center. This new concept has been developed by Winterstein, Leusen, Loeschke, Lambertsen, Robin, Mitchell and Severinghaus. The first direct evidence of the existence of central chemoreceptors in regions other than in the reflex center was Leusen's observation that perfusion of the cerebral ventricles with simulated cerebrospinal fluid (CSF) with a high Pco_2 or (H^+) stimulated breathing and that perfusion with fluid with a decreased Pco_2 or (H^+) depressed it. This led to the belief that there must be sensitive cells, on or near an internal or external surface of the brain, that could be readily influenced by the chemical composition of the CSF as well as by that of blood. In the cat, the chemosensitive cells or their sensory nerve endings seem to be located not in the classic medullary center and not in the cerebral ventricles, but on the lateral surfaces of the upper medulla, near the exit of the ninth and tenth nerves (see Fig. 3-1), or slightly below this. Not everyone agrees that the receptors are on or near the surface, and so far no one has histologically identified these receptors, their cell bodies or nerve fibers running from them to the medullary reflex center or to higher or lower parts of the brain. But application to the surface of solutions with added CO_2, H^+, acetylcholine or nicotine stimulates respiration within a few seconds.

Severinghaus and Mitchell believe that the receptors respond to changes in (H^+) rather than to P_{CO_2}. Gesell postulated in 1925 that central regulation of CO_2 depends on the (H^+) of the *interior* of the cells of the medullary respiratory center, which are beyond the blood-brain barrier. Gesell argued that, since CO_2 is readily diffusible, it penetrates cell membranes quickly. Inside the cell, $CO_2 + H_2O \rightleftharpoons H_2CO_3 \rightleftharpoons H^+ + HCO_3^-$, and so intracellular (H^+) increases. According to Gesell, CO_2 *appears* to be a *specific* respiratory stimulant only because blood H^+ ions do not pass the blood-brain barrier readily and do not penetrate into the cells of the medulla. The same reasoning applies to the action of CO_2 on the carotid body.

A simple, beautiful demonstration of the rapid diffusion of CO_2 and slow diffusion of bicarbonate ions across cell membranes was made by Jacobs, who studied color changes in the interior of cells of flowers that contained an indicator dye. When he immersed these cells in an alkaline solution of $NaHCO_3$, he noted an immediate change of intracellular color, indicating that the interior was now *acid* (due to rapid diffusion of CO_2), and a delayed change to alkaline

color (due to slow diffusion of bicarbonate ions). Presumably, the same mechanism operates across the blood-CSF barrier and sensitive cells of the medulla.

These medullary CO_2- and H^+-sensitive receptors are not *centers* as defined on page 24. They are central *chemoreceptors*, since they are stimulated by changes in their natural chemical environment. To distinguish them from the carotid and aortic bodies discovered 30 years earlier, those bodies are now called *peripheral* chemoreceptors. Central and peripheral chemoreceptors have certain similarities. Both respond to changes in their chemical environment, and both send afferent impulses to the medullary respiratory center, where they are added to all other incoming impulses to determine the total motor response of the respiratory muscles. There are, however, differences between peripheral and central chemoreceptors:

1. Central chemoreceptors are not known to affect the cardiovascular system in any consistent way.

2. They are not stimulated by decreased P_{O_2} or by applications of cyanide.

3. They can be influenced more by the chemical composition of cerebrospinal fluid (CSF) than by that of blood. The CSF differs from blood in lacking a protein buffer, such as hemoglobin, which accepts H^+ ions (see Chapter 16). Carbon dioxide, being freely diffusible, moves rapidly across the blood-brain and blood-CSF barriers, and the P_{CO_2} of CSF and internal jugular venous blood are approximately equal. This means that inhalation of CO_2 leads immediately to an increase in arterial P_{CO_2} and, a few minutes later, to a similar increase in the P_{CO_2} of CSF. However, the (H^+) of CSF will rise more than that of blood because CSF lacks hemoglobin buffer. Lowering arterial blood P_{CO_2} by prolonged hyperventilation will decrease CSF P_{CO_2} an equal amount, but the (H^+) of CSF will decrease more than that of blood.

4. The central chemoreceptors respond

more slowly to abrupt changes in the Pco_2 of arterial blood than do the peripheral receptors (see Figs. 5-1 and 5-4).

5. The location of the central chemoreceptors near the surface of the medulla and their response to changes in the (H^+) of CSF suggest that their function is to guard the pH or (H^+) of CSF, which bathes the central nervous system, while the carotid and aortic bodies regulate the Po_2 and, under extreme conditions, the Pco_2 and pH of the systemic arterial blood.

The central chemoreceptors occupy a strategic position for the performance of their function. If cerebral blood flow stopped, the environment of the H^+ receptors would be influenced largely by the composition of extracellular fluid and CSF — especially by CSF, since the H^+ receptors are fairly close to the surface of the medulla. On the other hand, if cerebral blood flow became unusually rapid, the environment of the receptors would be influenced largely by the composition of plasma.

Medullary Chemoreceptors vs. Medullary Reflex Center

A separation of central chemoreceptors from the medullary respiratory center permits more reasonable explanations of some of the mysteries that have surrounded the control of breathing for many years and brings the medullary respiratory center into line with other centers.

1. For many decades, the medullary respiratory center was in a special category. It not only received, integrated and transmitted nerve impulses (nervous regulation) but was itself profoundly influenced by specific chemical factors, particularly the Pco_2 of the arterial blood (chemical regulation). The discovery of separate intracranial chemoreceptors sensitive to CO_2 or H^+ means that there is no longer any need to assign to the medullary center this exceptional function of having dual excitability, by chemical agents and by incoming nerve impulses. We may

now think of the medullary center as a typical center, which receives numerous afferent impulses from all over the body, decides on some meaningful pattern of action and puts this into effect by sending out impulses over motor nerves.

2. According to the older view, CO_2 directly stimulated the medullary center, and drugs such as morphine or barbiturates depressed or abolished the response of this center to increased CO_2 without significantly depressing its response to incoming reflex signals, even though these had to be routed through these same depressed neurons. We can now postulate that these stimulant and depressant materials act primarily on the chemosensitive cells rather than on the medullary center. The problem now is not why the medullary center loses its sensitivity to CO_2 during deep anesthesia without losing responsiveness to afferent nerve impulses, but rather why sensitivity to CO_2 is frequently lost both centrally and peripherally during deep anesthesia. Possibly the answer is related to the narcotic action of CO_2, which seems to have the ability first to augment and then to diminish excitability of neurons. In man, 5% CO_2 depresses the corneal reflex, and in animals, even lower concentrations diminish excitability of peripheral nerves. Very high concentrations (30%) can produce surgical anesthesia in man.

3. Separation of central chemoreceptors from the medullary reflex center provides an explanation for the slow increase in breathing during the inhalation of 5–10% CO_2 in air and the slow return to normal when the inhalation is stopped. Lambertsen had previously reasoned that central CO_2 receptors could not be attached to the cerebral arteries in the way that the carotid bodies are attached to the carotid arteries, because when he raised arterial Pco_2 very quickly in dogs (by causing them to inhale 7% CO_2 abruptly), pulmonary ventilation still increased slowly to its final plateau. Dutton noted a similar lag even when blood with a Pco_2 was infused as a "square wave" into

the vertebral arteries. The carotid chemoreceptors have a huge blood flow and a small tissue mass, and a "square-wave" stimulus there increases respiration to its maximum with a lag of less than 1 second (Fig. 5-4). Therefore, the more sensitive and more powerful central chemoreceptors must either be in tissues with a poor blood supply, so that a long time is necessary for equalization of gas tensions between arterial blood and brain tissue, or they must be on the surface of the medulla, exposed to a large pool of CSF, which comes into equilibrium with arterial blood slowly. According to the new concept, after any change in arterial P_{CO_2}, there must be time for changes in the P_{CO_2} and (H^+) of the CSF bathing the chemoreceptors for maximal respiratory effects to occur; the chemical change in CSF must lag behind the blood change.

4. It provides an explanation for the presence of hyper- or hypoventilation in patients at times when analysis of arterial blood for P_{O_2}, P_{CO_2} and pH lead one to expect exactly the opposite ventilatory response. In patients whose level of ventilation cannot be explained by arterial P_{O_2}, P_{CO_2} or pH, or by other drives, it is wise to suspect that a

change in CSF (H^+) may be responsible. For example, when intravenous injections of sodium bicarbonate have corrected the arterial *blood* pH in patients with diabetic acidosis, hyperventilation may continue because the *CSF* remains more acid than normal.

Let us take another example. When a man returns to sea level after several weeks at a high altitude, he continues to hyperventilate for many days, even though the arterial blood has no known chemical stimulus to breathing. In the past, these changes have been explained by invoking the concept of "increased sensitivity of the respiratory center to chemical stimuli," which says in essence, "Something has happened that I cannot explain fully."

We can now explain this, assuming that the following sequence occurs (Fig. 5-5, *left*):

a) When man ascends to a high altitude, his *peripheral* chemoreceptors are stimulated. This causes hyperventilation and decrease in the P_{CO_2} of alveolar gas, arterial blood and CSF.

b) The arterial blood and CSF become more alkaline (Fig. 5-5, line *AB*). Because the *central* chemoreceptors are primarily H^+

Fig. 5-5.—Changes in pH of arterial blood and CSF during hypoxia and acidosis. **Left,** hypoxia. Initially (*A*), the pH of arterial blood is 7.42 and of CSF 7.32. *AB* represents acute hypoxia; *BC*, chronic hypoxia; *CD*, immediate effects of relief of hypoxia; *DA*, delayed return to control values. *Dashed arrows* indicate changes in pH that tend to decrease breathing; solid arrows indicate changes in pH that tend to increase breathing. **Right,** acidosis. *AB* represents acute acidosis (ingestion of NH_4Cl); *BC* represents continued ingestion; *CD* represents acute effects after cessation and *DA* the delayed return to normal. (Redrawn from Mitchell, R. A., and Severinghaus, J. W.: Physiol. Physicians 3:1, 1965.)

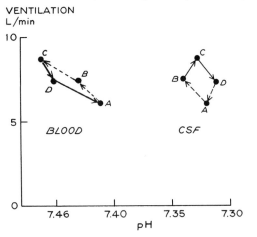

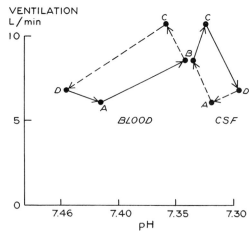

receptors, they now send fewer impulses to the medullary respiratory center. As a result, the total number of excitatory impulses impinging on this center (from peripheral and central chemoreceptors) is less.

c) In a few hours to a day, the (HCO_3^-) of CSF decreases (probably by an active transport mechanism) to match the low P_{CO_2}, and the pH returns to 7.32 (line *BC*). This increases the excitatory impulses from the central chemoreceptors to the medullary respiratory center, and ventilation increases. This explains why *chronic* hypoxemia produces more hyperventilation than acute hypoxemia.

d) When the hypoxemia is terminated (by descent to sea level or by inhalation of O_2), the hypoxemic drive from the *peripheral* chemoreceptors stops, and ventilation decreases. But the decrease in ventilation allows CO_2 to accumulate. Because CSF has no protein buffer and its (HCO_3^-) is now low (because of the homeostatic mechanism described earlier), the increase in CO_2 leads to a more marked increase in (H^+) in CSF than in blood (line *CD*), and the central chemoreceptors are now stimulated. This explains why hyperventilation continues even after termination of the hypoxemic stimulus.

e) The CSF gradually builds its (HCO_3^-) back to normal over a period of days or weeks (line *DA*), and at this time, ventilation returns to normal, there now being no unusual stimulus from either the peripheral or central chemoreceptors.

5. Patients who have required hyperventilation by mechanical respirators for days or weeks continue to hyperventilate when the respirator is no longer needed. This may also be explained by the loss of HCO_3^- ions from the CSF (to match the fall in P_{CO_2} caused by the original hyperventilation) and the subsequent large rise in (H^+) of the CSF when the P_{CO_2} rises at the termination of respirator treatment.

6. Intravenous injection of acids, such as hydrochloric or lactic, produces little change in respiration. For equivalent changes in arterial pH, an increase of arterial P_{CO_2} stimulates respiration far more than does injection of a fixed acid. Presumably this is due to the rapid transfer of CO_2 and the slow transport of H^+ into the CSF.

Peripheral and Central Potentiation and Antagonism

If both groups of receptors are exposed to increased P_{CO_2} or (H^+), their effects should add. If, however, the central receptors are exposed to an increase in (H^+) while the peripheral receptors are exposed to a decrease, the relative time lag, sensitivity and power of the two groups of chemoreceptors will determine the immediate and final effects on ventilation. The pH of CSF is kept fairly constant at 7.32; the pH of blood is kept at about 7.40. It is possible that the receptors exposed to CSF have the primary job of maintaining its pH constant by altering ventilation, and generally do so unless arterial hypoxemia is severe or the pH of systemic arterial blood changes markedly.

Are the Central Chemoreceptors Essential for Breathing?

It has long been known that when arterial P_{CO_2} of anesthetized animals or man becomes low enough, apnea results. In anesthetized animals, even strong peripheral chemoreceptor stimulation by nicotine or cyanide will not initiate breathing if arterial P_{CO_2} is very low. For these reasons, it is believed that a certain level of CO_2 is necessary for rhythmic respiration.

Some experiments indicate that the application of weak procaine solution to medullary H^+ receptors may lead to apnea in anesthetized animals, and that this continues despite strong reflex stimulation of the carotid bodies. This was not true in unanesthetized (decerebrate) cats, in which procaine decreased breathing by only 28%; when the same cats were anesthetized, application of procaine often caused apnea. Unanesthetized men usually do not become apneic when P_{CO_2} is lowered markedly by hyperventilation unless they are trained to relax and be unaware of their surroundings. Presumably, the reticular activating system has an important influence in arousing and altering the reflex medullary centers in awake man. This dramatically illustrates the difficulties one can get into by assuming that what happens in anesthetized cats will happen in awake and alert man.

THRESHOLD FOR CARBON DIOXIDE

The *threshold* for CO_2 is the level of arterial P_{CO_2} at which respiration ceases and apnea begins, or the level at which apnea ceases and breathing begins (assuming that no stimulus has changed except CO_2). Some physiologists "pretend" that the straight lines of the CO_2 response curves, which relate minute volume to arterial P_{CO_2} (shown in Fig. 5-3), can be drawn down to zero minute volume and that the point at which this "pretend" line crosses the abscissa is the threshold for P_{CO_2}. Mathematically, it is correct to describe a line by its slope and its intercept with an x or y-axis, but physiologically, the line has no validity beyond the lowest or highest measured value.

Actually, alert unanesthetized man usually does *not* become apneic even when his arterial P_{CO_2} decreases to 16 torr. In relaxed, unanesthetized patients who have a genuine apnea after hyperventilation and in anesthetized patients (who usually do become apneic after hyperventilation), one can label the arterial P_{CO_2} as threshold when the first spontaneous, involuntary breath ends the apnea. However, if we believe that *CSF* P_{CO_2} is a more important stimulus to the medullary chemoreceptors than is *arterial* P_{CO_2}, and that some time is required for the former to rise, a changing *arterial* P_{CO_2} at any moment cannot represent the stimulus for the central H^+ receptors. But these calculations do make some respiratory physiologists happy and serve as a challenge to others.

IMPORTANCE OF CARBON DIOXIDE REGULATION

1. Although at first thought it would seem more logical to design a respiratory regulatory mechanism that is more sensitive to the P_{O_2} of arterial blood than to blood and CSF P_{CO_2} and (H^+), the CO_2 control system permits the additional control of blood and tissue acidity. As we shall learn in Chapter 14, the shape of the HbO_2 curve insures adequate oxygenation of blood over a wide range of arterial P_{O_2} (from 100 torr down to 60 or 70 torr), and increase in ventilation to raise arterial P_{O_2} above 100 torr does little to increase blood O_2. Thus, free from concern about blood O_2 levels (until blood O_2 is quite low, when arterial chemoreceptors become quite active), the control of ventilation can defend tissues against CO_2 excess or lack and try to maintain acceptable (H^+). If ventilatory control were designed to regulate arterial blood P_{O_2} within narrow limits, there would be no gain for O_2 transport and a loss of fine control of acid-base balance.

2. There is no doubt that increase in tidal volume and frequency of ventilation results from inhalation of CO_2, when the central mechanisms are not depressed. However, many types of hyperpnea occur without any increase in P_{CO_2} of arterial blood. For example, the commonest and largest increase in ventilation — that during muscular exercise (see p. 234) — does not involve a measurable increase in arterial P_{CO_2}. It is undoubtedly important that the level of arterial P_{CO_2} *does not fall* in exercise; maintenance of normal levels may be responsible for maintenance or augmentation of the excitability of the medullary center. Again, increased ventilation in patients is seldom due to increased levels of CO_2. Indeed, the hyperpnea in patients with hypoxemia, fever, hypotension or pulmonary interstitial fibrosis occurs with a decreased arterial P_{CO_2}. Such hyperpnea is undoubtedly influenced by the *level* of CO_2 or, to put it differently, it is limited by a concomitant reduction in arterial P_{CO_2},

because it would be greater if arterial P_{CO_2} were normal.

3. CO_2 inhalation is seldom used therapeutically to increase ventilation. This is because increased P_{CO_2} can depress cells in the brain; most patients who need a respiratory stimulant are hypoventilating and already have an increased arterial P_{CO_2}. The dual effect of CO_2 — stimulating in low concentrations and depressing in high — may explain why lowering the P_{CO_2} by mechanical hyperventilation in patients with respiratory acidosis might actually improve ventilation rather than depress it.

Inhalation of $7 - 10\%$ CO_2 in air for a few minutes may be a useful test to gauge the severity of narcotic depression of the respiratory center and may be used therapeutically in combating the action of gaseous poisons, notably CO (see p. 282).

An increase in arterial P_{CO_2} causes more cerebral vasodilation and increase in cerebral blood flow than any other procedure; inhalation of $5 - 7\%$ CO_2 might be useful in the treatment of cerebral vasospasm if one is sure that there is no concomitant cerebral hemorrhage.

4. The medullary chemoreceptors are more readily depressed than are the synapses in the medullary center. The response to a given level of arterial CO_2 is diminished in sleep and after drugs such as barbiturates, morphine and most general anesthetic agents, particularly cyclopropane and halothane. When other mechanisms that stimulate respiration are inactive, depression of the medullary chemoreceptors may result in complete apnea. This could happen when the reticular activating system is depressed by sleep or anesthesia, when the peripheral chemoreceptors are partly inactivated by inhalation of O_2 or when the Hering-Breuer inflation reflexes are causing tonic inhibition in response to lung distention. However, it is clear that when man is awake and alert, a fall in arterial P_{CO_2} and consequent decreased activity of the H^+ receptors do not lead to apnea.

5. The superficial location of the H^+ receptors and their vulnerability to low concentrations of procaine may explain why high spinal anesthesia may depress breathing even when the concentrations used do not block motor pathways.

6. Depression of respiration due to general or intracranial hypothermia may be due to selective block of these receptors.

7. The depression of breathing that occurs with high intracranial pressures might be caused by pressure on these superficial areas.

8. In inflammatory diseases of the brain, the permeability and selectivity of the brain-CSF barrier may be altered, and materials that are either stimulant or depressant to the medullary chemoreceptors may enter the CSF. This might explain the unusual hyper- or hypoventilation seen in some cases of meningitis or encephalitis (see p. 30). The entry of any material (plasma protein, hemoglobin) into CSF that would increase its buffering capacity would tend to depress respiration because it would minimize the change in H^+ with increasing or decreased P_{CO_2}.

6

The Response to Hydrogen Ions

INCREASED METABOLISM leads to formation of excess H ions, which must be neutralized or excreted. In ordinary circumstances, man's kidneys excrete 40–80 mEq of H^+ per day, and the lungs excrete 13,000 mEq of CO_2 (derived from the chemical reaction of $H_2CO_3 \rightarrow H_2O + CO_2$). It is logical, therefore, to believe that the (H^+) in blood or tissue might be an important factor in regulating ventilation when metabolism is increased (as in lactic acidemia during exercise), when acids are not metabolized completely (as in diabetic acidosis) or when acids formed in normal amounts cannot be excreted completely (as in renal failure). When metabolism increases, both CO_2 and (H^+) increase, and it is hard to separate their effects. Therefore, most studies of the H^+ regulation of respiration have involved measurement of the ventilatory response to addition of acids.

Increasing the (H^+) of peripheral tissues does not increase ventilation; increasing the (H^+) of systemic arterial blood does. A characteristic respiratory response of an anesthetized animal is shown in Figure 6-1. Breathing becomes deep and, with sufficient increase in (H^+), more rapid as well. Deep, labored breathing (Kussmaul) has also been described in patients with severe acidosis.

No good data have been obtained in man because uncomplicated increases in arterial (H^+) are rare. Nielsen changed the pH of arterial blood of normal man by 0.08 units by administering large doses of ammonium chloride; the minute ventilation increased only 0.7 L/minute. Ammonium chloride,

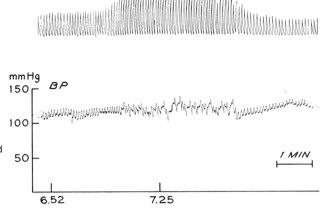

Fig. 6-1.—Effect of acid solutions on isolated carotid bodies. Both carotid bodies of a dog were perfused with phosphate buffers (pH 6.52). The marked increase in tidal volume shown here occurred only when the carotid bodies were innervated. The buffer solutions had no other known stimulus (Pco_2 low; Po_2 high; temperature 37 C). The delay of more than a minute between beginning the acid infusion and the hyperpnea was due to the dead space in the pump and tubing. (From Schmidt, C. F.: Anesth. Analg. 19:261, 1940.)

TABLE 6-1.—EFFECT OF CLINICAL ACIDOSIS ON
PULMONARY VENTILATION*

ARTERIAL BLOOD pH	TIDAL VOL (ML)	FREQUENCY (BREATHS/ MIN)	MIN VENTILA-TION (L/MIN)	ALVEOLAR VENTILA-TION† (L/MIN)	ARTERIAL P_{CO_2} (TORR)	MEAN BLOOD PRESSURE (MM HG)
7.36	500	15	7.5	5.3	30	74
7.21	400	26	10.7	6.5	14	84
7.20‡	770	22	16.9	14.7	14	80
7.17	1,100	19	21	18.0	17	120
7.14			28.4		15	64
7.12			23.9		15	34
7.12‡	920	36	33	29.5	23	79
7.06‡	1,200	25	31	27.5	11	107
7.03‡	880	40	35	31.2	24	58
6.91	1,300	20	26	23.0	17	86
6.86‡	850	24	20	18.0	22	82
6.80‡	780	32	25	21.8	18	72

*Data from Kety et al.: J. Clin. Invest. 27:500, 1948. Each line contains values for 1 patient (12 patients in all).
†Approximate value based on estimated anatomic dead space of 100 ml for females and 150 ml for males.
‡Female patients.

however, is not an ideal agent for this purpose because $NH_4^+ \rightleftharpoons NH_3 + H^+$, and the NH_3 ion passes into the CSF far more readily than the H^+, and makes CSF more alkaline. Acidosis may occur in patients with severe diabetes; Kety found little change in the ventilation of such patients until the pH decreased by 0.2 unit (Table 6-1 and Fig. 5-1). However, their arterial P_{CO_2} was very low because of the hyperventilation (the iso-P_{CO_2} technic was not in use at the time of these studies), blood pressure was often low, body temperature sometimes high, and other stimulant or depressant chemicals may have been present in the blood.

LOCATION AND FUNCTION OF H⁺ RECEPTORS

Carotid and Aortic Bodies

Some believe that there is a single stimulus to chemoreceptors during hypoxemia and increase in P_{CO_2} and that this is an increase in (H^+) within these receptor cells. Certainly, perfusion of acid fluids through isolated carotid bodies does increase respiration, and this is a reflex. However, no stimulation oc-

curs until pH decreases by 0.1 pH unit, and the sensitivity of the cells is low—a change of about 0.4 unit is required to cause a 2- or 3-fold increase in minute volume of breathing. These values may not represent the true capacity of intracellular (H^+) to stimulate the carotid and aortic bodies, or of changes in arterial (H^+) to stimulate chemoreceptors if P_{CO_2} is kept normal (iso-P_{CO_2} technic). However, they are representative of the response of the chemoreceptors to increased (H^+) in blood of patients with renal or diabetic acidosis, because here, too, the arterial P_{CO_2} is low, owing to hyperventilation.

We have no information on the characteristics of cell membranes of the peripheral chemoreceptors and their ability to transfer H^+ ions; changes in (H^+) in arterial blood could be reflected immediately and fully inside these cells or could result in little or no change in their (H^+). A small increase in intracellular (H^+) might be a far more potent stimulus than a large increase of (H^+) in the arterial blood.

No quantitative studies of the respiratory response to intravenous injections of acids before and after chemoreceptor denervation have been done; qualitatively, it is known that hyperventilation still occurs when acids are injected intravenously in animals whose peripheral chemoreceptors are denervated.

H+ Receptors on the Lateral Surface of the Medulla

If these regions are bathed with mock CSF of varied (H^+) and Pco_2, respiration increases when the (H^+) increases, even though Pco_2 is constant or decreased. We do not know the sensitivity of these areas to changing (H^+) in unanesthetized man. In anesthetized animals, the changes in ventilation produced by changes in pH of mock CSF are less than those to inhaled CO_2. On the other hand, Mitchell has shown in a variety of clinical conditions in which arterial (H^+) changes considerably that the (H^+) of CSF is maintained within very narrow limits. If the H^+ receptors are responsible for this remarkable stability, they must be exquisitely sensitive, and it should be possible to demonstrate the sensitivity of the cells by noting hyperpnea following minute changes in (H^+) in their environment; possibly, perfusion experiments damage the sensitive structures under study. Or it may be that the (H^+) of CSF as a whole is not the same as that bathing the chemosensitive area.

PHYSIOLOGIC SIGNIFICANCE OF H+ RECEPTORS

In view of the great interest of both respiratory physiologists and clinicians in acidosis, it is surprising how seldom respiration and circulation have been measured before and during treatment of patients with acidosis. If the respiratory and circulatory responses are attributable wholly or largely to chemoreceptor reflexes, sudden inactivation of these could lead to respiratory and circulatory depression similar to that observed in severely hypoxemic patients when O_2 is administered. Some cases of circulatory collapse have occurred following intravenous administration of alkali to patients with se-

vere diabetic acidosis. In the light of present knowledge, this may be explained by postulating a depressant action of uncompensated acidosis on the vasomotor centers that is counteracted only by reflex stimulation due to the action of decreased pH on peripheral chemoreceptors. However, *respiratory* depression does not occur in such patients; treatment restores arterial pH to normal, but the patient *continues to hyperventilate.*

Mitchell has measured the ventilatory changes that occur during acute and chronic acidosis (produced by ingesting NH_4Cl) and related these to the pH of arterial blood and CSF. Figure 5-5 (*right*) shows the control ventilation (A), the small increase with acute acidosis (line AB), the further increase with chronic acidosis (BC), the immediate decrease with correction of the pH of arterial blood (CD) and the further decrease, over a period of days, to normal (DA). While the arterial blood pH decreased from 7.42 to 7.34 and stimulated the carotid and aortic bodies, the pH of CSF increased from 7.32 to 7.34 because hyperventilation occurred and lowered Pco_2. The increased pH of CSF limited the full response to arterial blood acidosis, but when the (HCO_3^-) of CSF decreased and the pH of CSF returned to normal (7.32), the full hyperpnea occurred (BC). Overcorrection of arterial blood acidosis by administration of $NaHCO_3$ abolished the carotid and aortic body response; ventilation decreased, and Pco_2 rose in blood and CSF. CSF pH became more acid (CD), and the return to normal ventilation was delayed until CSF (HCO_3^-) rose to normal values and CSF pH became 7.32 again. Again, we see that knowledge of CSF pH helps to explain certain types of hyper- and hypoventilation.

We mentioned previously that the pH of CSF is maintained within narrow limits, either by changes in its Pco_2 (effected by changes in alveolar ventilation) or in its (HCO_3^-) (effected by active transport mechanisms). Marked decrease in the pH of CSF is often associated with coma. This may be the cause of stupor and unconsciousness seen in patients with severe pulmonary insufficiency. Since such patients cannot increase their ventilation, and since intravenous bicarbonate changes pH of CSF only slowly, it is important to increase ventilation mechanically in such patients, to decrease blood and CSF P_{CO_2} and CSF pH promptly.

7

Cerebral Blood Flow and Respiratory Regulation

SO FAR we have discussed the effects of changing the *chemical composition* of arterial blood. What happens to respiration when only the *rate* of cerebral blood flow changes? To answer this we must remember that blood flow is essential not only to supply O_2 and substrates to cells but also to remove waste products such as CO_2. The chemical environment of cells, therefore, depends on (1) their own rate and type of metabolism; (2) the rate of blood flow to them; (3) the chemical composition of arterial blood; (4) the chemical composition of their extracellular fluid, and (5) special characteristics of the cell membrane that limit or permit transport of ions or molecules.

If the blood flow to chemoreceptors is very rapid and the mass of the cells exceedingly small — as in the carotid body — then the Po_2 and Pco_2 of arterial blood, tissue cells and end-capillary or venular blood are almost identical. If blood flow is less abundant in relation to the mass of tissue cells, the Pco_2 of the cells will be higher, and their Po_2 lower, than that of arterial blood; in this case, end-capillary or venular blood has a chemical composition much closer to that of the tissues than does arterial blood.

Let us apply this to the central chemoreceptor cells. First let us consider the effect of increasing or decreasing cerebral blood flow, while all other factors such as metabolic rate of the cells and the composition of arterial blood are held constant. The intracellular Pco_2 and (H^+) will increase with decreasing blood flow and decrease with increasing blood flow.

Blood flow decreases as a result of severe systemic arterial hypotension, of increased intracranial pressure (generally or locally) or of thrombosis, embolism or narrowing of one or more cerebral arteries; this results in hyperventilation unless (or until) the cells are depressed by hypoxia, lack of substrates or excessive accumulation of metabolic products.

Blood flow increases during the intravenous injection of pressor drugs (epinephrine, norepinephrine), and this depresses breathing; systemic hypertension can also depress breathing reflexly, via aortic arch and carotid sinus pressoreceptor mechanisms (see p. 86). Blood flow also increases during cerebral vasodilation; severe arterial hypoxemia (arterial blood Po_2 less than 50 torr) or a relatively small increase in the arterial blood Pco_2, or both together, dilates these vessels. Cerebral vasoconstriction occurs when arterial blood Pco_2 decreases, but, according to Lambertsen, does not occur as a direct result of an increase in the Po_2 of arterial blood.

When cerebral vasodilation occurs as a result of inhalation of CO_2, the increased blood flow cannot decrease intracellular

Pco_2 and (H^+), but increases them; the more rapid blood flow hastens the final equilibration of blood and tissue Pco_2.

Inhalation of 100% O_2 at one or more atmospheres of pressure is a special case. Because the amount of *dissolved* O_2 in arterial blood is increased and tissues use this first (see p. 210), less HbO_2 is dissociated and less reduced Hb is available to buffer H^+ ions. Therefore, inhalation of O_2 leads (after a brief period of hypoventilation due to physiologic inactivation of peripheral chemoreceptors) to a slight increase in ventilation.

During hyperventilation, alveolar and arterial Pco_2 decrease and cerebral vasoconstriction occurs. Lambertsen emphasizes that the cerebral vasoconstriction that follows increase in arterial Po_2 is not primary (it does not occur if arterial Pco_2 is kept constant) but secondary to changes in ventilation. Inhalation of O_2 at a pressure of 3 – 4 atmospheres causes so much O_2 to be dissolved in the blood that *no* O_2 is unloaded from HbO_2; as a result, the Pco_2 of jugular venous blood increases from 51 to 54 torr, and presumably the Pco_2 of central chemoreceptors increases a similar amount. The resultant hyperventilation lowers arterial Pco_2 from 41 to 34 torr.

It is well established that an increase in arterial Pco_2 dilates cerebral vessels and increases *overall* cerebral blood flow. However, when *overall* cerebral blood flow changes, blood flow in the highly specialized medullary chemoreceptors need not necessarily change by the same amount or even in the same direction. Similarly, blood from the internal jugular vein draining the brain need not have the same composition as that coming from the very few medullary chemosensitive cells.

8

Reflexes from the Lungs

TWO DRAMATIC DEMONSTRATIONS in the physiology laboratory are (1) severing both vagus nerves in midneck in an anesthetized animal, which leads instantly to very deep and very slow breathing (Fig. 8-1) and (2) electrical stimulation of the peripheral end of a cut vagus nerve, which leads immediately to marked slowing of the heart or even cardiac standstill. These effects, probably because they are so striking, are apt to lead to some misconceptions:

The first is that the *only* efferent fibers in the vagi are cardioinhibitory fibers to the sinoatrial node. This is incorrect because the vagi also carry efferent fibers to the larynx, bronchi, blood vessels, mucous glands and cilia of the respiratory tract, to the atria and ventricles and to muscles and glands in the alimentary tract.

The second is that the *only* afferent fibers in the vagi come from pulmonary receptors that send messages centrally to prevent maximal lung inflation (presumably by cutting off inspiratory activity at a smaller volume and permitting expiration to occur earlier). This is incorrect because these fibers are a very

Fig. 8-1.—Effects of bilateral vagotomy on expired CO_2, tidal volume and systemic arterial blood pressure of the dog.

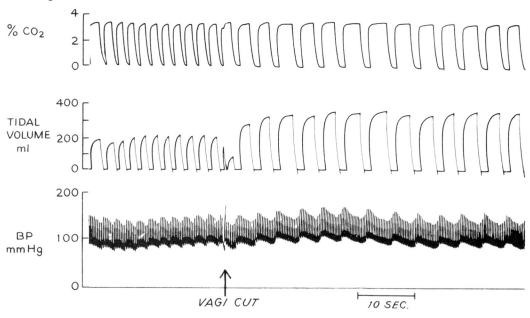

72

small minority of afferent fibers in the vagi; the majority carry impulses from other tracheopulmonary receptors and from receptors in great veins, right atrium and ventricle, pulmonary arteries, arterioles, venules and veins, left atrium and ventricle, aorta, esophagus and gastrointestinal tract.

The third is that vagal reflexes must be the most important single factor controlling breathing. Since vagal reflexes were known long before there was any knowledge of the chemical control of breathing, they were thought to effect "self-regulation of respiration"—inspiration inflated the lungs, stretched the receptors and generated inhibitory impulses, which traveled up the vagus nerves, "turned off" the inspiratory center and permitted (or activated) expiration. (This was one of the earliest forms of negative feedback in physiologic thinking.) It is difficult today to understand how earlier physiologists attributed the *main* regulatory role to these reflexes. If we agree that the important function of the lungs is to supply the body with adequate O_2 and remove excess CO_2, it is obvious that pulmonary stretch reflexes cannot serve this function because they have no way of adjusting respiration to keep pace with metabolic activity of tissues. Inflation or deflation of the lungs simply cannot supply the proper information to the respiratory centers so that they know how well the lungs are doing their primary job of arterializing the mixed venous blood. Phillipson has proved this point conclusively by showing that unanesthetized dogs trained to run on a treadmill have the same increase in respiration during exercise whether their vagi are intact or blocked; however, their response to inhalation of low O_2 or high CO_2 mixtures is less if the vagi are blocked.

The fourth is that if anesthetized cats, dogs and rabbits breathe very slowly and deeply as soon as their vagi are blocked, man must do the same. Guz, Widdicombe and Noble have shown that this is incorrect because neither the rate nor tidal volume of breathing changes in unanesthetized man when both vagi are blocked.

A great deal has been learned in the last decade about the function of lung reflexes in experimental animals, and much of this is now being applied to understanding respiratory control in normal man (including the newborn) and in patients with a wide variety of cardiopulmonary diseases.

IDENTIFICATION AND EVALUATION OF REFLEXES FROM THE LUNGS

Some of the technics used to study lung reflexes are:

1. NERVE SECTION OR BLOCK. Section or block of the vagus, although it gives information only about the dominant activity in that nerve at the time of section, has been performed in man. *Differential* nerve block permits better analysis of the individual components of a mixed nerve. This can be done by cooling the vagus trunks in steps to 0 C. Some fibers carrying impulses from specific sensory receptors may be blocked at 10–15 C and others not until 0–4 C. In these cases, cooling permits clear separation of reflexes.

2. ELECTRICAL STIMULATION. Whitteridge has stated that electrical stimulation of a complex, mixed nerve, such as the vagus, is a "punishable offense." No matter how precise and how varied the frequency, pattern or strength of stimulation may be, it excites more than one type of nerve fiber that carries one specific reflex. Electrical stimulation of afferent fibers below a precise differential cold block is more selective. Anodal block is a technic using direct current that results in block of large fibers in a mixed nerve and permits observation of the effects of stimulation of small fibers; this has not yet been performed on the vagus nerves of man.

3. RECORDING OF ACTION POTENTIALS IN AFFERENT NERVE FIBERS is a better analytic device. However, if one tries to record and analyze electrical activity in a whole nerve trunk, one becomes hopelessly confused. So the neurophysiologist begins to cut across the trunk, teases smaller and smaller

bundles of fibers from the whole nerve and places these in turn on electrodes to record electrical activity until he obtains a record with only a single fiber firing. But it is impossible to know the destination of any individual nerve fiber before it is cut; it is difficult to identify the sensory receptor attached to this nerve fiber even after it is cut, and it is a monumental task to record from hundreds of fibers whose receptors are activated by the same type of stimulus in order to determine the threshold and sensitivity of each. Also, important respiratory reflexes seem to travel in fine, nonmedullated fibers, and these are the hardest of all to study by single-fiber technics. Langrehr has recorded from the vagus nerves of man, and Guz and associates have used the "collision" technic of Douglas and Ritchie to determine vagal activity in man during lung inflation.

Electrical recordings may also be used to map out the central and motor paths excited by the afferent impulses. To accomplish this, microelectrodes may be placed in the medulla, supramedullary regions of the brain and the motor nerves descending to the respiratory muscles.

4. USE OF CHEMICAL AGENTS TO STIMULATE OR BLOCK. The use of specific chemical agents is obviously essential in finding true chemoreceptors. Oddly enough, some chemicals, such as veratridine, even in minute dosage, *stimulate* stretch or mechanoreceptors (initiate an electrical discharge); when used just in threshold dose, they are helpful in identifying pathways for many reflexes. Others, such as halothane, *sensitize* receptors (permit stimulation by the natural stimulus at a lower threshold), or increase their *sensitivity* (produce a greater response to the same natural stimulus), and some, such as procaine, *block* them (indeed, a few chemicals, such as halothane, that stimulate or sensitize in low concentration may, in high concentration, block these same receptors). Some chemicals, such as phenyldiguanide and serotonin, seem to be specific for ferreting out special receptors attached to fine,

nonmedullated vagal C fibers and have little or no effect on stretch receptors attached to large A myelinated fibers.

At present there is clinically useful information on six different types of bronchopulmonary receptors that initiate reflexes affecting respiration and circulation: stretch receptors, irritant receptors, "J" receptors, and the receptors initiating the pulmonary (and coronary) chemoreflex, the deflation reflex and the paradoxical reflex of Head.

STRETCH RECEPTORS AND THE INFLATION REFLEX

Hering and Breuer noted in 1868 that maintained distention of the lungs of anesthetized animals decreased the frequency of inspiratory effort. They showed this effect to be a reflex mediated by afferent vagal fibers. It is often called the Hering-Breuer reflex. However, they also observed that deflation of the lungs causes augmentation of respiration, and so there are really two Hering-Breuer reflexes. To separate these, the distention reflex became known as the Hering-Breuer *inhibito-inspiratory reflex* and the deflation as the *excito-inspiratory* reflex. Now we simply call them the "inflation" and "deflation" reflexes, though some doubt that there is a separate deflation reflex.

The receptors for the inflation reflex probably lie in the smooth muscle of airways from the trachea to bronchioles; they are blocked by procedures (such as inhalation of aerosols of local anesthetics or of steam) whose effects can be confined to these airways. Their impulses travel up large myelinated A fibers (diameter $5-10$ μ; conduction velocity $35-50$ m/second). They do not cross over, i.e., impulses initiated in the left lung travel only in the left vagus. These fibers are blocked by low concentrations of procaine, by cooling to $8-10$ C and by application of direct current (anodal block), all of which permit continued transmission in smaller C fibers.

The receptors are mechano- or stretch receptors. Most of them fire (Fig. 8-2) when

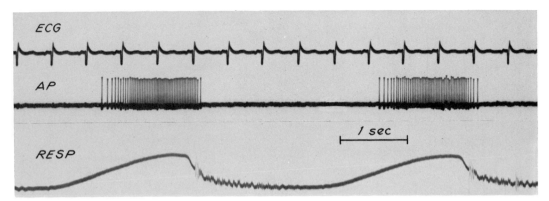

Fig. 8-2.—Inflation reflex in the dog. Record (from above down): ECG, action potentials (*AP*) in a single fiber preparation of the vagus nerve and positive-pressure mechanical ventilation of the lungs (inspiration, up; expiration, down). Note abrupt slowing and then termination of firing at end inspiration. (Courtesy of Dr. John C. G. Coleridge.)

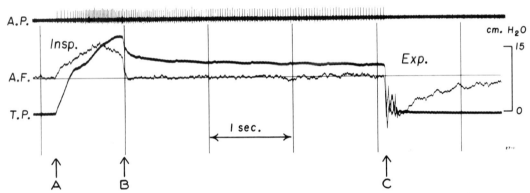

Fig. 8-3.—The inflation reflex. The lungs of a cat were inflated with 100 ml of air at *A*, the point of rise in tracheal pressure (*T.P.*) and beginning of inspiratory air flow (*A.F.*). Note the appearance of action potentials (*A.P.*) in a single vagal nerve fiber. These continued at a lower frequency when air flow stopped and a constant lung volume was maintained at *B* (*A.F.* now zero). The potentials ceased at once when the lungs were suddenly deflated, at *C*. (From Davis, H. L., Fowler, W. S., and Lambert, E. H.: Am. J. Physiol. 187:558, 1956.)

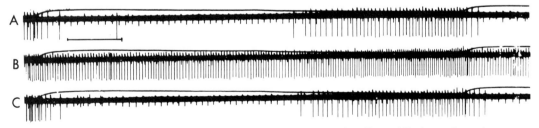

Fig. 8-4.—The inflation reflex during pulmonary vascular congestion. Record **B** shows the action potentials from a single vagal afferent fiber during inflation of the lung while a pulmonary vein was occluded. Note the high frequency compared to **A** (the control period) and **C** (2 minutes after release of venous occlusion). The *continuous line* in **A**, **B**, and **C** is intratracheal pressure; a downward slope indicates lung inflation; time scale = 0.5 second. (From Costantin, L. L.: Am. J. Physiol. 196:49, 1959.)

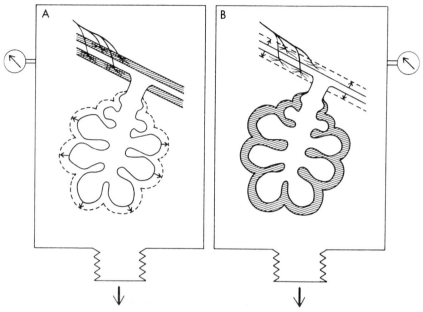

Fig. 8-5.—The inflation reflex in pulmonary disease. If the sensory receptors are in the airway and the airways are stiff (bronchoconstriction, as in **A**), inspiratory effort (bellows moving downward) will distend alveoli more and airways less. If the alveoli are stiff (interstitial fibrosis, as in **B**), it will distend the airways more and the alveoli less.

the lung is stretched during inspiration of normal tidal volume (low-threshold stretch receptors), though some require a greater than normal inflation to activate them (high-threshold receptors). The receptors adapt slowly, i.e., a long-continued stimulus (inflation) leads to long-continued discharge (Fig. 8-3). Since they lie in airways, they are excited by stretch of airways, not by stretch of alveoli. Distention of airways depends on their transmural pressure (difference between air pressure in the lumen and tissue pressure about the airways) and their compliance (change in volume for a unit change in transmural pressure). Factors affecting their distention are illustrated in Figures 8-4 and 8-5.

Physiologic and Clinical Importance of the Inflation Reflex

The two most important discoveries related to the inflation reflex were its initial demonstration in animals by Hering and Breuer and the finding almost 100 years later by Guz and associates that it does not operate in *man* breathing at his normal tidal volume (Fig. 8-6). The reflex is not *absent* in man but requires lung inflation of more than 800 ml above FRC to delay the next breath appreciably (a normal tidal volume is 400 – 500 ml). Curiously, electrical activity is present in the vagus nerves of man when his lungs are at their functional residual capacity and increases in frequency as inspiration increases during a normal tidal volume. This can only mean that the respiratory centers of man have a high threshold to these vagal impulses. In general, it is much more difficult to produce reflex apnea in an unanesthetized, alert animal than in an anesthetized animal. Phillipson found that only one vagus nerve was needed in anesthetized dogs to transmit effective inflation messages but that both were needed (spatial summation?) when the same dogs were unanesthetized. Cross found that the inflation reflex was well developed in unanesthetized newborn babies but decreased in effectiveness during the first 5 days of life, as higher centers became more active.

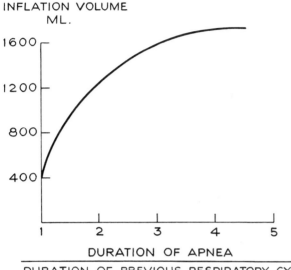

INFLATION VOLUME
ML.

Fig. 8-6.—Inflation reflex in man. The lung must be inflated by large volumes (1,200 ml or more) in man to produce apnea of significant duration. If the cervical vagi are blocked in healthy man during quiet breathing (tidal volume 400–500 ml), no change occurs in tidal volume or frequency of breathing. (After Guz, A., *et al.*: Clin. Sci. 27:293–304, 1964.)

These observations do not mean that the inflation reflex is a mere curiosity in man. It *is* active when tidal volume exceeds 800 ml, when stretch receptors are sensitized and when pathologic conditions lead to less distention of alveoli and more stretch of airways.

What are the likely or possible physiologic roles for the inflation reflex?

1. TERMINATION OF INSPIRATION. We know that impulses traveling up the vagi are required in order to terminate tonic sustained inspiration (apneusis) of animals whose pneumotaxic center in the upper pons has been inactivated. We assume now that the impulses producing this effect are those generated by lung inflation. The inflation reflex thus seems to reinforce the maintenance of respiratory rhythm.

2. TONIC INHIBITION OF THE RESPIRATORY CENTER THROUGHOUT THE ENTIRE CYCLE. The inflation reflex seems also to be able to inhibit central respiratory activity in general. The simplest way to demonstrate this is by breath-holding experiments. A man who has been breathing O_2 can hold his breath longer and to a much higher level of alveolar P_{CO_2} if his lungs are inflated during breath holding rather than deflated. This suggests that impulses travel from the inflated lungs to inhibit the respiratory centers continuously, rather than just to terminate inspiration. A subject at the breaking point of breath holding can continue longer if he is permitted to expire and inspire several times, even if he breathes a gas mixture that neither raises arterial blood P_{O_2} nor lowers P_{CO_2}; presumably, afferent impulses from repeated distention of the lungs inhibit central respiratory activity nonspecifically. Recently, Guz has demonstrated tonic activity from continuously inflated lungs of animals during cardiopulmonary bypass.

3. REGULATION OF THE WORK OF BREATHING. Ideally, regulation not only provides a proper volume of alveolar ventilation, but also accomplishes this with minimal expenditure of energy by the muscles of respiration. More than 90 years ago (1880), Gad stated that the probable function of the Hering-Breuer reflexes was to regulate the work of the respiratory muscles in such a way that the greatest alveolar ventilation occurred for the least muscular effort. It was

TABLE 8-1.—WORK OF BREATHING AT DIFFERENT RATES AND TIDAL VOLUMES*

RATE (f) (BREATHS PER MIN)	TIDAL VOL (V) (ML)	ANATOMIC DEAD SPACE† (D) (ML)	ALVEOLAR VENTILATION PER BREATH (ML)	ALVEOLAR VENTILATION PER MIN (ML)	TOTAL VENTILATION PER MIN (ML)	WORK PER MIN (GM CM/MIN)			
						vs. Elastic Recoil (1)	vs. Airway resistance (laminar flow) (2)	vs. Airway resistance (turbulent flow) (3)	Total
5	1,000	200	800	4,000	5,000	25,000	3,750	375	29,125
10	557	157	400	4,000	5,570	15,510	4,654	518	20,682
15	411	145	266	4,000	6,165	12,667	5,720	706	19,093
20	338	138	200	4,000	6,760	11,420	6,855	927	19,201
30	265	132	133	4,000	7,950	10,530	9,504	1,513	21,547
40	228	128	100	4,000	9,120	10,400	12,476	2,276	25,152
50	206	126	80	4,000	10,300	10,609	15,914	3,278	29,791

*Equations used to calculate work: $(1) = 5,000\, f(V)^2$
$(2) = 150\, [\dot{V}_A + (D \times f)]^2$
$(3) = 3\, [\dot{V}_A + (D \times f)]^3$

V, $\dot{V}_A$ and D are expressed in liters. (Equations from Otis, A. B., Fenn, W. O., and Rahn, H.: J. Appl. Physiol. 2:592, 1950.)

†Note increase in dead space with increasing tidal volume (approximate values).

obvious to him that after both vagi were cut, inspiration became maximal, and the animal seemed to be exerting a tremendous muscular effort with each breath. But this great increase in work does not achieve a comparable increase in alveolar ventilation; in fact, alveolar P_{CO_2} remains about the same (see Fig. 8-1). Therefore, the function of the inflation reflex might well be to regulate tidal volume and rate so that muscle work is minimal.

Since that time, many physiologists have calculated that the intact respiratory systems of different species of animals usually employ a pattern that provides optimal alveolar ventilation with minimal expenditure of energy. Let us give an example: If man requires 4 L of alveolar ventilation/minute, he could achieve this by many combinations of rate and tidal volume of breathing (Table 8-1). The tidal volume determines the work to overcome elastic recoil on each breath (p. 103); the flow rate determines the work to overcome airway resistance on each breath (p. 122). As tidal volume becomes greater, "elastic work" per minute increases, and as rate becomes faster, the "resistive work" increases. Normal man chooses a nice compromise, which performs the least work—a tidal volume of about 400 ml and a rate of about 15/minute.

When airway resistance is increased (as in asthma), more energy is needed to overcome the resistance. Slow, deep breathing keeps flow rates low and avoids excessive resistive work; for some reason, the asthmatic patient breathes in this way. When the lungs become stiffer (as in pulmonary interstitial fibrosis), more work is needed to overcome elastic recoil; shallow breathing keeps elastic work at a minimum. Again, for some reason, the patient with alveolar fibrosis breathes shallowly and more rapidly. The receptors for the inflation reflex could supply some or all of the information needed to achieve the optimal pattern in normal and disease states. When the alveoli are stiffer (see Fig. 8-5, B), transpulmonary pressure stretches the airways more, inspiration is turned off earlier and the rate of breathing increases. When the airways are stiffer (Fig. 8-5, A), transpulmonary pressure stretches them less and the rate of breathing decreases.

A nice question is why the inflation reflex does not prevent the large increase in tidal volume that occurs in exercise, acidosis or hypoxemia in animals that have a well-developed inflation reflex. Perhaps certain reflexes take priority over others (are prepotent). Or perhaps the respiratory center is, among other things, an amazing computer that makes the best possible arrangement under the circumstances.

4. OTHER EFFECTS. Certain inhalation anesthetics, such as halothane, tend to increase the frequency of breathing, probably because of sensitization of inflation receptors and earlier termination of inspiration; this effect, however, is swamped by the direct depressant action of these agents on medullary centers. The sensitization caused by pulmonary vascular congestion (see Fig. 8-4), atelectasis or pulmonary edema seems to be due to physical changes in the lungs. The lungs are stiffer (less compliant), and more of a change in transpulmonary pressure is required to inflate the alveoli a normal amount; this distends the airways to a greater extent, since their compliance is still normal. The sensitization caused by some bronchoconstrictor drugs seems also to be related to physical changes.

Lung inflation also leads to a reflex decrease in bronchiolar tone, which persists for about a minute after a deep breath; if this operates in the normal range of tidal volume, it might be a mechanism that widens bronchioles during inspiration and permits them to narrow during expiration.

A very deep breath leads to closure of the glottis; this may be a reflex action designed to prevent overdistention of the lungs.

The circulatory effects are complex. Modest inflation of the lung leads to tachycardia (Fig. 8-7) and to peripheral vasoconstriction, which are at least partly due to lung reflexes; large lung inflations (40 cm H_2O alveolar pressure) cause bradycardia and peripheral vasodilation.

The contributions of impulses from the lungs to the sensation of dyspnea are discussed on pages 259–261.

IRRITANT RECEPTORS FOR THE COUGH AND IRRITANT REFLEX

These are subepithelial mechanoreceptors located in the trachea, bronchi and bronchioles. Their processes extend between epithelial cells as far as the ciliary layer and seem to be designed to detect delicate deformation of the epithelial surface. They include intrapulmonary epithelial irritant receptors and extrapulmonary tracheal and bronchial "cough" receptors. They are excited by inert particles (dust, smoke), by probing with a fine catheter, by histamine (and by the anaphylactic reaction in airways) and by irritant gases and vapors (such as ammonia, ether and sulfur dioxide), but are not sensitized by anesthetic gases such as halothane. They also fire during unusually large inflations or deflations of the lungs, but whatever the stimulus, the receptors adapt quickly when it is maintained. The receptors send their impulses centrally in the smallest medullated A fibers (diameter about 4 μ, conduction velocity about 13 m/second); in common with other medullated fibers, they are not activated by phenyldiguanide or serotonin.

Fig. 8-7.—Tachycardia during inspiration. Tachycardia occurs simultaneously with the beginning of inspiration in anesthetized dog (*top record*: upstroke = inspiration). The tachycardia is in part central in origin and in part associated with enlargement of the lung and thorax.

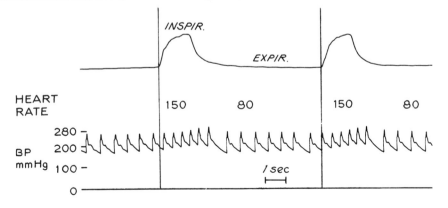

When stimulated, they produce reflex cough or tachypnea and reflex bronchoconstriction. Their cardiovascular effects are not prominent. In pathologic conditions that lead to bronchial secretion or release of chemicals such as histamine or 5-hydroxytryptamine (for example, anaphylactic reactions or multiple embolism), activation of lung irritant receptors may contribute to the reflex respiratory, cardiovascular and bronchomotor changes that develop. It is unlikely that they are activated by distention of the lungs in man, since very large tidal volumes are needed to activate them.

"J" RECEPTORS AND TACHYPNEA

These receptors are believed by Paintal to be present in the interstitial tissue between pulmonary capillaries and alveoli (he calls them "J" receptors as an abbreviation for "juxtapulmonary-capillary receptor"—not because they are J-shaped). He believes that the receptors must be in the pulmonary circulation because he can record impulses in vagal nerve fibers within 2.5 seconds after he has injected phenyldiguanide into the right ventricle, but not after he has injected it into the ascending aorta so that it quickly enters the bronchial circulation. And he believes the receptors lie very close to alveolar capillaries because their nerves fire within 0.3 second after insufflation of halothane into alveoli, even when the circulation of blood has been stopped.

This receptor-afferent-fiber system has not been studied until recently because the fibers are very fine, unmyelinated C fibers and difficult to dissect from the vagus trunk for recording. The system does not respond to inflation of the lung and only feebly and inconsistently to deflation. Paintal believes its unique natural stimulus is pulmonary capillary congestion, capillary hypertension and edema of the alveolar wall and that the "J" receptor is responsible for the increased breathing during exercise and for the tachypnea occurring during pulmonary congestion and edema.

It is certainly of great importance to study vagal reflexes carried in the C fibers because there are so many of these in the vagus nerves. However, much more must be learned before Paintal's interesting ideas are accepted. For example, the "J" receptor cannot be responsible for the hyperpnea of muscular exercise because Phillipson found that dogs, running on a treadmill, had as much hyperpnea during exercise when their vagi were blocked as when they were intact. It is also difficult to believe that these receptors are responsible, even in part, for the dyspnea of pulmonary congestion and edema of man, since Guz injected phenyldiguanide (the stimulus par excellence of "J" receptors, according to Paintal) into the pulmonary artery of man and found no response until the chemical reached the carotid bodies, when it produced typical carotid body hyperpnea but no sensation of dyspnea. Further, the usual respiratory pattern in pulmonary congestion and edema of man is more rapid breathing, whereas chemical activation of "J" receptors causes reflex bradycardia, hypotension and apnea, with either no or delayed tachypnea in cats, and increased tidal volume and bradycardia in dogs.

PULMONARY CHEMOREFLEX

The pulmonary chemoreflex and coronary chemoreflex are excited by minute amounts of certain chemical agents. The characteristic response is reflex hypotension, bradycardia and apnea (Fig. 8-8, 1 and 2). Because similar reflex effects are produced by injections of the same chemicals into the coronary circulation of the same species, the pulmonary chemoreflex is discussed in the next chapter, together with the coronary chemoreflex.

THE DEFLATION REFLEX

There is no doubt that deflation of the lungs leads to an *increased* rate of breathing (Fig. 8-8, 5), but this could be due to lessened activity of receptors serving the infla-

1

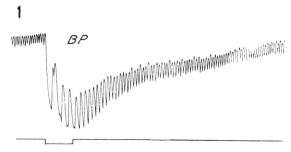

2

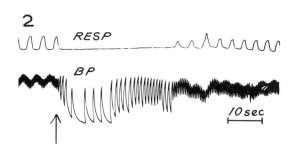

Fig. 8-8. — Other reflexes from the lungs. **1,** pulmonary depressor reflex. At the break in the signal line, the *central* end of the right pulmonary vagus (dog) was stimulated electrically; the record indicates the existence of afferent fibers from the lung capable of causing reflex bradycardia and hypotension. (From Brodie, T. G., and Russell, A. E.: J. Physiol. 26:92, 1900.)

2, pulmonary chemoreflex. Injection of 200 μg of serotonin (at arrow) into the right atrium of a cat caused almost instantaneous apnea, bradycardia and hypotension, reflex in origin, arising from excitation of receptors in the pulmonary circulation.

3

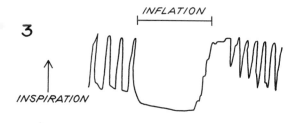

3, inflation reflex; inflation of the lungs leads to apnea in expiration.

4

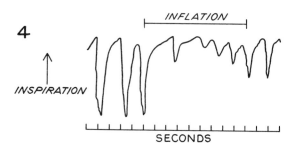

4, paradoxical reflex; inflation of the lungs after vagal cooling (inflation reflex blocked) leads to increase in inspiratory tone (*3* and *4* from Head, H.: J. Physiol. 10:1, 1889, and Cross, K. W.: Brain 84:529, 1961).

5

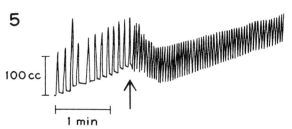

5, the deflation reflex. Injection of air (at arrow) into the thorax of an anesthetized dog decreased lung volume 73 ml and caused immediate tachypnea; pneumothorax did not cause a similar response after bilateral vagotomy. (From Simmons, D. H., and Hemingway, A.: Am. Rev. Tuberc. 76:195, 1957.)

tion reflex rather than to stimulation of specific deflation receptors. (The absence during expiration of electrical activity in the fiber in Fig. 8-2 does not rule out the possibility that other inflation receptors are tonically active when lung volume is at or below functional residual capacity, and that their activity can be lessened or eliminated by further deflation.) Whether the deflation reflex has its own receptors cannot be settled at this time. Irritant receptors and "J" receptors are sometimes activated by pneumothorax; possibly they initiate what has long been called the deflation reflex. If this exists in man as a discrete reflex, it could be responsible for the increased ventilation when the lungs are deflated abnormally (as in pneumo- or hydrothorax [Fig. 8-8, 5]) and for the deep breaths that help to prevent atelectasis. The deflation reflex may also be the mechanism responsible for maintaining inspiratory muscle tone when the lung volume tends to go below the FRC.

THE PARADOXICAL REFLEX OF HEAD

In 1889, Head performed some inflation experiments on rabbits in which he wanted to stop impulses from traveling along the vagus nerves without cutting the nerves, since this excites fibers briefly. He decided to do this by cooling the vagus nerves to 0 C. As he expected, when the vagus nerves were cooled, inflation of the lungs did not inhibit inspiration. However, when the vagus nerves were being warmed, for a time inflation of the lungs produced "a paradoxical effect" — i.e., a further inspiration rather than inhibition of inspiration (Fig. 8-8, 4). This is a nice example of a reflex that is still conducted by certain vagal fibers when those carrying impulses from the inflation receptors are blocked. It is also one of the earliest examples in physiology of "positive feedback."

What is the physiologic role of this reflex? It might provide a mechanism for producing an unusually deep inspiration — possibly to open alveoli wide if they are collapsed as a result of insufficient ventilation. It might be the mechanism involved in sighing. Cross has also suggested that it may play a part in the aeration of the lung of the newborn; he has shown that it is active in the newborn baby. The receptors are known to be in the lung, but their precise location has not been determined.

Reflexes arising in the upper airways are discussed in Chapter 17.

9

Other Reflexes

REFLEXES FROM THE RESPIRATORY MUSCLES

THE MUSCLES moving the thoracic cage are, of course, skeletal muscles. The movement of limb muscles is known to be modified by the stretch reflex. Although little is known about this reflex in the respiratory muscles, evidence is accumulating that their control is similar to that of the limb muscles. The stretch reflex in a limb muscle is elicited by a sudden pull on the muscle (as by tapping its tendon sharply); this is followed almost instantly by contraction of the same muscle. The sensing elements are the muscle spindles that are scattered throughout the muscle parallel with the main muscle fibers.[1] When the main muscle is stretched, the spindle is also stretched, and its stretch receptor fires impulses over afferent nerves that run to the spinal cord, where they end directly on anterior horn motor neurons to form a monosynaptic reflex arc. The motor neurons then send impulses over the motor nerves to the same muscle; these cause the main muscle fibers to contract and shorten, the spindle to shorten, the stretch element to be unloaded and the afferent impulses to stop.

The spindle, however, is not a simple stretch receptor. The sensory element is attached to the spindle muscle fibers, which

have their own motor nerves—the small motor or gamma fibers (Fig. 9-1). The sensory element is functionally in series with the spindle muscle fibers whereas, as indicated above, it is in parallel with the main muscle fibers. (Recently it has become clear that the spindle is even more complicated and contains 2 separate systems—the primary and secondary—each with its own type of gamma fiber, muscle fiber and sensory element. Although the functional significance of these

Fig. 9-1.—Innervation of main muscle fiber and muscle spindle. (See text.)

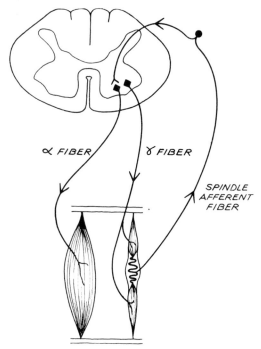

α FIBER   γ FIBER

SPINDLE
AFFERENT
FIBER

---

[1]Neurophysiologists often call the spindle the intrafusal fibers or fusiform fibers and the main muscle the extrafusal fibers. Since "fusiform" simply means "spindle-like," it seems preferable to use the simple terms "spindle" and "main muscle."

is emerging it is not relevant to our present account.) The sensory element generates more impulses when:

1. Stretched by a pull on the main muscle, as by tapping the tendon.

2. Stretched by contraction of the spindle muscles, even though the main muscle remains the same length.

The stretch receptor generates fewer or no impulses when:

1. Relaxed by shortening of the main muscle.

2. Relaxed by lengthening (relaxation) of the spindle muscles.

Descending impulses from the brain excite the large alpha motor neurons that innervate the main muscle fibers; these fibers then contract and shorten to an extent that depends upon the opposing tension. Their shortening is greatest when there is no tension (isotonic contraction) and least when they are opposed by a very great tension (isometric contraction). By contrast, impulses stimulating the spindle muscle fibers through the gamma system cause only stretching of the sensory element. Spindle muscle fiber contraction does not itself directly contribute to change in length or tension of the muscle as a whole. The only action of the impulses in the gamma fibers is to change the length of the sensory element.

Physiologic Importance

In the past 15 years it has become well established that, rather than being just a sensory system, the gamma system is intimately involved in the *control* of movement. Let us consider three ways in which the alpha and gamma systems may cooperate:

1. The gamma system may maintain a constant state of activity so that there is a constant bias on the sensory element. The drive to contract in this case is sent only through the alpha system. Operating in this manner, the sensory elements in the spindles indicate only the change in length obtained as the result of the alpha activity.

2. The drive to contract may be sent through the gamma fibers, which cause the spindle muscle fibers to contract. This contraction stretches the sensory elements and causes an increased afferent discharge of impulses, which in return reflexly excites the alpha fibers. This is now often called the "gamma loop," and this mode of operation is called "the follow-up length servo."

3. The drive to contract may be sent into both the alpha and the gamma systems, in which case the state of the sensory elements will at all times indicate the relative shortenings achieved by the spindle and the main muscle fibers. If the shortening of the main muscle fibers is either too great or too small, it might then be modified through the operation of the gamma loop.

Note that whichever of these modes of operation takes place, the sensory element is all the time signaling the *misalignment* of the spindle and main muscle fibers. This is the key to understanding the mode of operation, and it is common to all three examples.

The Gamma System and the Respiratory Muscles

The diaphragm and intercostal muscles contain spindles. Recently, action potentials arising from muscle spindles in the intercostal muscles have been studied, and a stretch reflex has been demonstrated in the intercostal muscles. Although the diaphragm has not so far received much attention, it too contains spindles and probably has a stretch reflex.

There can, therefore, be little doubt that the gamma system is operative in the control of the respiratory muscles, although the precise way in which it operates can be asserted with no more assurance than for other muscles. But evidence is accumulating to support the view that the functional connection between alpha and gamma systems is like those postulated in 2 or 3 above and that the spindle is not just a mechanism for indicating position. Nathan and Sears studied three patients in whom certain cervical or thoracic sensory roots on one side were cut to relieve pain caused by cancer. In one patient, division of the posterior roots of the cervical segments from which the phrenic nerve arises led to temporary but complete paralysis of half of the diaphragm; it recovered partially in three months. In another patient, a similar operation paralyzed half of the diaphragm, but function returned in 17 days. In the third patient, division of the posterior roots of the fourth to seventh thoracic nerves decreased activity of intercostal muscles, as determined electromyographically. Nathan and Sears concluded that cutting the posterior sensory roots containing afferents from a respiratory muscle stops the firing of the alpha motor neurons to that muscle for some time, but there is gradual recovery. They suggest that sensory input from muscles to the spinal cord may be an important factor in driving anterior horn cells, either directly or by making them responsive to motor impulses descending from the brain or medulla.

Campbell and Howell believe that the functional role of these systems in breathing may be as follows. The respiratory centers decide on the basis of their P_{CO_2} or reflex demands, or both, how much ventilation is needed. On the basis of additional information fed into one or more respiratory centers by the lung afferents, these centers then decide on the optimal combination of frequency and tidal volume to achieve this ventilation with minimal effort. This demand is then fed into those parts of the nervous system responsible for controlling the skeletal muscles. This system decides which respiratory muscles must be activated and perhaps the approximate tension that must be developed. The respiratory muscles then contract, and if there is no unexpected resistance to breathing, they produce the expected change in thoracic and lung volume. If, however, thoracic or pulmonary compliance has decreased or resistance has increased, the gamma loop and small motor fiber system operate as a servo to drive the main muscle fibers to develop additional tension and quickly achieve the proper ventilation.

Campbell and Howell have described how the tidal volume in the breaths following the addition of a mechanical load to the breathing, such as a reduction in compliance, is rapidly restored. The response is too quick to be accounted for by chemical stimulation of the respiratory center and is unaffected by vagotomy in either animals or man. Although these observations cannot be simply interpreted in terms of the operation of the small motor system, they do indicate that there are mechanisms that stabilize the ventilation in the face of changing mechanical conditions much more promptly than the classic servo depending upon the blood gases and that also keep these blood gases and, therefore, the internal environment of the body much more constant.

CHEST WALL REFLEX

A reflex leading to acceleration of breathing can be initiated by light pressure on a small area (1½ in. diameter) of the dog's thorax where the scalenus medius and rectus abdominis muscles insert on the chest cage. The reflex, first described by Whitehead and Draper, cannot be demonstrated in an unanesthetized dog; in fact, it is seen best in a deeply anesthetized dog with a slow rate of respiration. The reflex is strong enough to cause a sustained increase in respiratory rate (Fig. 9-2). It should not be confused with

Fig. 9-2.—Thoracic wall reflex. Very light pressure on the thorax causes increased respiratory frequency in the deeply anesthetized dog. This response does not occur in man or in unanesthetized dogs.

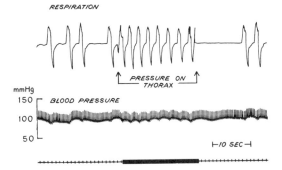

the pulmonary inflation or deflation reflex because it can be reproduced with a pressure so light that it decreases lung volume less than 2 ml; further, dissection of the muscles and their tendons away from the thorax abolishes the reflex. The afferent path has not yet been determined. Accumulation of air outside the lung but within the thorax (pneumothorax) produces the same type of accelerated breathing; here, however, the chest wall expands, the diaphragm moves down and the lung is compressed; in pneumothorax, the inflation or deflation reflex, or both, are probably involved.

REFLEXES FROM THE CAROTID SINUSES AND AORTIC ARCH

The carotid sinuses and aortic arch (Fig. 4-2, p. 35) initiate reflexes that primarily regulate the cardiovascular system. Increase in pressure in these regions stretches the arterial wall and receptors in it. A barrage of impulses travels over the carotid sinus and aortic nerves, and this leads to bradycardia, vasodilation and hypotension. Decrease in pressure leads to less stretch, decreased frequency of impulses and increase in systemic blood pressure. When systemic arterial pressure falls below 40 mm Hg, no impulses can be detected in the nerves.

But these reflexes can affect respiration as well as the cardiovascular system. A convenient way of remembering the effect produced by stimulating these stretch receptors is to regard impulses coming from them as inhibitory. They inhibit (1) the cardio-accelerator center in the medulla and permit greater activity of the vagal or cardioinhibitory center; (2) the medullary vasoconstrictor center and permit vasodilation; (3) the respiratory centers and depress breathing.

Decrease in pressure in the carotid sinuses leads to hyperpnea, and increase to depression of breathing. It is easy to prove this in the dog because the carotid sinuses can be converted into blind pouches completely separated from the carotid body without damaging the innervation of either or altering cerebral blood flow. Increase in pressure in

such pouches decreases respiration as long as the afferent nerve fibers are intact. Increasing the pressure in the carotid sinuses also leads to a decrease in airway resistance and an increase in pulmonary compliance.

The receptors of the carotid sinuses respond to *rate of change* of stretch as well as to the absolute amount of stretch—i.e., they respond to a large pulse pressure and to more frequent pulses, as well as to a change in the level of mean pressure. Increasing the static pressure in the carotid sinuses from 100 to 150 mm Hg will produce a stream of inhibitory impulses in the carotid nerves and a fall in systemic blood pressure, but an alternating pressure with wide pulsations (mean pressure remaining the same) will result in many more impulses per second and considerably more of a reflex fall in blood pressure. An increased number of pulsations per minute also generates more impulses.

We do not know the effects on respiration of varying pulse pressure and pulse frequency in the carotid sinuses, nor do we know the threshold and intensity of the respiratory reflex initiated by these stretch receptors.

Physiologic Role

Some consider that this respiratory reflex has no useful function in man and is merely a vestigial survival of a mechanism that is more important in aquatic animals; fish have stretch receptors in their branchial arches (gill arteries). Others, however, believe that the respiratory component of this reflex does play an important physiologic role in man with low blood pressure: increase in tidal volume lowers intrathoracic pressure more, augments the thoracic pump and increases venous return to the heart. In addition, hyperventilation could improve the P_{O_2} and P_{CO_2} of arterial blood.

THE PULMONARY AND CORONARY CHEMOREFLEXES

In 1867, von Bezold and Hirt showed that an intravenous injection of veratrine in animals caused a large fall in blood pressure and heart rate and apnea; they believed, but did not establish, that this was a reflex from receptors in the heart. In 1900, Brodie stimulated the *central* end of pulmonary branches of the vagi, observed hypotension, bradycardia and apnea and demonstrated that messages from the lungs to the brain cause profound reflex depression of respiration and blood pressure (see Fig. 8-8, *1*). No further studies were done until 1915, when Cramer demonstrated that the von Bezold effect was indeed a vagal reflex. This was, in turn, ignored until 1937, when Jarisch confirmed that the reflex could arise from the heart alone. Finally, in 1947, Dawes showed that there were several components of the total "von Bezold-Jarisch" reflex and that these were initiated by chemical stimulation of receptors in both the pulmonary and coronary circulations. The triad of bradycardia, hypotension and apnea is now called the pulmonary chemoreflex, coronary (or left ventricular) chemoreflex or thoracic chemoreflexes. If the general term "thoracic" chemoreflexes is used, it must be remembered that it does *not* apply to reflexes from aortic body *chemoreceptors* (also within the thorax); the latter are true chemoreceptors and the results of their stimulation are the opposite of stimulation of the pulmonary or coronary chemoreflex.

We call these chemoreflexes rather than chemoreceptor reflexes because they are not excited by chemical change that normally occurs in the body (such as those which stimulate the carotid and aortic bodies). In different animal species, veratridine, nicotine, serotonin, adenosine triphosphate, phenyldiguanide and some antihistaminic agents may activate the pulmonary and coronary chemoreflexes; only serotonin and adenosine triphosphate are body constituents, but they are normally intracellular and are released only when there is damage to cells.

The response is almost certainly due to stimulation of a variety of receptors. For example, at least six types of vagal endings are accessible to drugs injected into the coronary artery: coronary, ventricular, epicardial and atrial receptors, some aortic body chemoreceptors and pulmonary artery endings connected to C fibers. Veratridine also produces reflex apnea by exciting receptors for the lung inflation (Hering-Breuer) reflex; it sends impulses over A fibers that carry impulses initiated by lung inflation. Both stimuli are ineffective when the vagus nerves are cooled to 8 C. Other chemicals continue to produce their effect until the vagi are cooled to 2 C, and their effects are probably carried in vagal C fibers. Still other materials injected into the pulmonary circulation cause only reflex apnea, and some injected into the coronary circulation cause only reflex hypotension and bradycardia.

Physiologic Role

We are, at the moment, left with a reflex that produces a dramatic response, the function of which is uncertain. If the natural stimuli to these receptors are chemicals, the physiologic role of pulmonary chemoreflexes might be to prevent further inhalation of irritant gases into the respiratory tract by causing reflex arrest of breathing on exposure. The simultaneous hypotension and bradycardia are harder to explain. It has been suggested that the effects might be a carryover from our marine ancestors; temporary cardiac arrest would stop circulation through the gills and systemic absorption of toxic materials when a fish comes in contact with chemical poisons. Another possibility is that reflex fall in blood pressure may represent a "protective" collapse mechanism in response to visceral injury. This is typical of stimulation of visceral receptors elsewhere and can be produced by a blow over the solar (celiac) plexus or the testes, irritation of arterial walls or pressure on the eyeballs.

Many physiologists believe that the receptors are stretch receptors, which happen to be stimulated by chemicals that have no relation to the physiologic stimulus. The main problem in identifying them as vascular or left ventricular stretch receptors is that no one has, even by *un*physiologic stretch of the atria, ventricles or pericardium, produced hypotension-bradycardia-apnea approaching the magnitude that can be produced by injection of a few micrograms of chemicals. Possibly, the chemicals stimulate simultaneously, fully and continuously a larger number of receptors than can ever be stimulated by stretch. In this case, the chemicals serve only as a pharmacologic tool to locate sensory nerve endings without providing any clue as to function.

If the receptors are stretch receptors, what purpose does their response serve? What is the function of a depressor reflex caused by increased pressure in the right atrium and ventricle? The typical response in muscular exercise is cardiac acceleration, not slowing. Possibly, reflex systemic peripheral vasodilation serves as a means of transferring blood from the pulmonary to the systemic circulation when pressure rises to a dangerous height in the pulmonary vessels. On the left side of the heart, increased pressure, by acting on pressoreceptors, could supplement the aortic depressor reflex, and there is histologic evidence to support the view that left ventricular and aortic stretch receptors are part of the same system. Excitation of aortic pressoreceptors causes bradycardia, a fall in blood pressure and apnea. What might happen in patients with stenosis of the aortic valve (whose left ventricular pressure is well in excess of aortic pressure) is a mystery.

Clinical Importance

The remarkable species differences in the chemoreflexes make it unwise to transfer observations made in one, or even several, animal species directly to man; for example, in the cat, serotonin causes apnea, hypotension and bradycardia by excitation of the thoracic chemoreflex; in the dog, it causes hyperpnea, hypertension and, usually, tachycardia by excitation of the carotid and aortic bodies. However, it is important for physicians to realize that some or all of these reflexes probably exist in man, and the seriousness of the fully developed triad of reflex bradycardia, hypotension and apnea requires that attention be directed toward establishing the presence or absence of chemoreflex phenomena in various clinical conditions. Some of these are:

HYPOTENSION FOLLOWING RAPID INTRAVENOUS INJECTIONS. The rapid injection of large amounts of fluid, regardless of its chemical composition, may cause an abrupt fall in blood pressure. It now appears possible that this is due to chemoreflexes. Reactions due to rapid intravenous injection of concentrated radiopaque fluids could be due to excitation of chemoreflexes. The reactions that follow infusions of serum in man might be attributed to chemoreflexes because of their drastic effect in cats. Shock after intravenous injection of drugs need not, of course, be reflex in origin, but rapid intravenous injection of any drug should be avoided unless it is known that it does not excite chemoreflexes.

INHALATION OF IRRITANT GASES. There is some evidence that irritant gases, such as chlorine or acid fumes, may cause depression of respiratory movements, bradycardia and hypotension in man, and that certain inhalation anesthetics have a tendency to produce bradycardia and serious cardiac arrhythmias, including cardiac arrest. Nothing, of course, is known about the reflex nature of these reactions in man. It would be of interest to obtain information about the immediate response of man to a variety of gases and vapors used in clinical anesthesia. The effect of procaine in counteracting abnormal rhythms during inhalation anesthesia may be partly due to suppression of chemoreflexes.

CORONARY SHOCK. The effect of intracoronary injection of nicotine is shown in Figure 9-3; apnea, or depressed breathing, is an integral part of this response (though not illustrated). Other chemical substances, acting on receptors in the left ventricular wall, can produce a similar response. It has been suggested, but never proved, that the circulatory collapse so frequently seen after coronary artery occlusion in man is partly reflex in origin. In this condition, chemical sub-

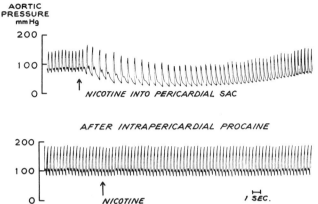

AORTIC
PRESSURE
mm Hg

NICOTINE INTO PERICARDIAL SAC

AFTER INTRAPERICARDIAL PROCAINE

NICOTINE   1 SEC.

Fig. 9-3.—Coronary chemoreflex. A very fine tube is in the pericardial sac of a dog. Nicotine (33 μg) injected into the pericardial sac caused an almost instantaneous slowing of the heart rate and fall in blood pressure. A similar response followed injection of nicotine into the coronary artery supplying the left ventricle. Injection of a local anesthetic (procaine) into the pericardial sac abolished the response to both intracoronary nicotine and intrapericardial nicotine. Nicotine is used here only as a test substance; other chemicals—for example, veratridine—produce the same effect. (From Sleight, P.: J. Physiol. (Lond.) 173:321, 1964.)

stances formed by tissue breakdown or platelet disintegration may accumulate locally in sufficient concentration to stimulate the sensory receptors responsible for chemoreflexes. It has been shown in animals that myocardial infarction reflexly (possibly through the coronary chemoreflex) suppresses sympathetic vasomotor activity and so prevents recovery from hypotension. However, the coronary chemoreflex is not established for man. It is interesting, though, that both adenosine triphosphate and 5-hydroxytryptamine, injected intravenously in man, cause substernal distress or tightness like that frequently experienced by patients with coronary insufficiency.

PULMONARY EMBOLISM. Many investigators believe that embolism of small vessels in the pulmonary arterial circulation causes reflex systemic hypotension, bradycardia, tachypnea or bronchoconstriction (see p. 156). Regardless of the substance injected, blood usually clots around the foreign material (even after injection of heparin), and 5-hydroxytryptamine may be liberated locally, in intimate contact with sensory receptors for the pulmonary chemoreflex. Even if 5-hydroxytryptamine does not excite these chemoreflexes in man, it still is likely to cause bronchoconstriction by direct effects on smooth muscle. The contribution of such chemoreflexes, as modified by species difference and depth of anesthesia, may help to explain the variable results obtained with

experimental pulmonary embolism in animals.

THORACIC SURGICAL PROCEDURES. Thoracic surgeons have observed severe bradycardia and hypotension during manipulation of nerves near the hilum of the lung. The injection of local anesthetics into this area is said to prevent these reactions. However, to date, precise studies on nerve fibers of known origin have not been made in man.

TREATMENT OF HYPERTENSION. Not all the effects of activation of chemoreflexes are potentially harmful. The veratrum alkaloids both slow the heart and lower blood pressure by exciting chemoreflexes in animals, and it is likely that the hypotension they cause in man is also reflex in nature. Probably more attention should be directed to drugs that lower blood pressure in man by this mechanism, for it provides a means of relieving hypertension without paralyzing sympathetic vasoconstrictor pathways and consequent postural hypotension. Unfortunately, veratrum alkaloids produce vomiting in man in doses only slightly greater than those that lower blood pressure; vomiting may possibly be part of the chemoreflex response.

REFLEXES FROM SOMATIC AND VISCERAL TISSUES

Appropriate stimulation of afferent nerves from the limbs can increase rate and depth of breathing. Such hyperpnea may be induced by stimulation of temperature, pain or mechanoreceptors. No one has been able to demonstrate chemoreceptors in the limbs that respond to such physiologic stimuli as low P_{O_2}, high P_{CO_2} or low pH. The chemical agents that stimulate special receptors elsewhere (cyanide, nicotine, serotonin, veratridine, phenyldiguanide) and cause reflex hypo- or hyperventilation, fail to do so when injected into the circulation of the limbs. Materials that stimulate pain endings in unanesthetized man do increase breathing re-

flexly when injected into the limb arteries of anesthetized animals.

Marked hyperventilation follows the sudden application of cold water to large areas of the skin (Fig. 9-4, *B*). When Keatinge gave healthy men showers of cold water (15 C) for 1 minute, their ventilation increased by as much as 20–25 L during the shower, though he did not attempt to keep alveolar or arterial P_{CO_2} constant. The effect is so prompt that it must represent a reflex from cutaneous receptors (for either cold or

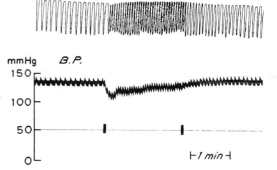

Fig. 9-4. — Effect of afferent stimuli on ventilation. **A,** passive movements of both hind limbs (between marks) cause reflex increase in the rate of breathing in an anesthetized dog. The limbs are connected to the body only by blood vessels and nerves. (From Comroe, J. H., Jr., and Schmidt, C. F.: Am. J. Physiol. 138:536, 1943.)

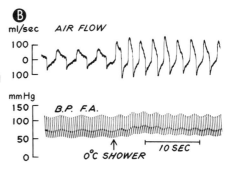

B, cold shower of the trunk (anesthetized cat) instantaneously causes hyperpnea. *B.P. F.A.* = blood pressure in femoral artery. (**B** and **C** from Keatinge, W. R., and Nadel, J. A.: J. Appl. Physiol., 20:65–69, 1965.)

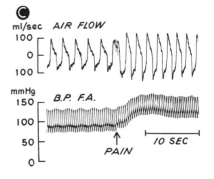

C, painful cutaneous stimuli (anesthetized cat) cause instantaneous hyperpnea. *B.P. F.A.* = blood pressure in femoral artery.

pain). It is not due to surprise, because other startling procedures failed to produce similar responses.

Passive movements of the limbs about a joint increase breathing reflexly in both anesthetized animals and unanesthetized man. The response is largely an increase in the frequency of breathing and not in tidal volume (Fig. 9-4, *A*). It is not due to changes in intrathoracic or intra-abdominal pressure or to vibration caused by back-and-forth movements of the limbs, because it occurs when the limb is severed except for nerves and vessels and the body is firmly fixed. Body vibration also causes hyperventilation.

Visceral pain usually produces effects opposite to those caused by somatic pain. It has been reported that inflation of a balloon in the intestine of a dog causes apnea followed by hyperpnea, that high concentrations of some drugs injected into the mesenteric artery cause apnea, that distention of the gallbladder or biliary ducts inhibits breathing and that traction on some abdominal viscera is associated with apnea. Pressure on the eyeballs produces cardiac inhibition and slower breathing or apnea (unless there is a fall in arterial blood pressure). On the other hand, stretching of the anal sphincter in newborn babies may initiate or increase breathing.

Clinicians have long made use of some of these mechanisms to increase ventilation. An old method for countering the respiratory depression due to an overdose of morphine is to force the patient to walk back and forth. The obstetrician, faced with a nonbreathing baby, often succeeds in starting breathing by slapping the baby vigorously, splashing cold water on its skin or stretching its anal sphincter. All of these procedures increase the input of sensory stimuli to the alerting or reticular activating systems in the medulla and pons.

THE INFLUENCE OF SENSORY STIMULI; WAKEFULNESS AND SLEEP

We have learned most of our respiratory physiology by studying anesthetized animals and have then applied this knowledge to man. Sometimes, however, we get into trouble because different species behave differently. For example, a rabbit exposed to an irritant vapor may hold its breath until it dies, but man does not. Again, a chemical may stimulate the thoracic chemoreflexes and not the carotid and aortic bodies in one species but in another do exactly the opposite — and produce exactly opposite effects on respiration and circulation.

Sometimes anesthesia leads us astray. Every anesthetist is accustomed to judge the depth of anesthesia by noting the continued presence of some reflexes and the absence of others; obviously, some reflexes are depressed by light anesthesia and others are resistant to moderate or even deep anesthesia, but we often forget this in formulating theories of respiratory regulation. We have already noted that hypoxia causes no respiratory stimulation in the anesthetized animal with denervated carotid and aortic bodies, but causes tachypnea in unanesthetized animals similarly denervated.

Here is another classic example. In an anesthetized animal, inhalation of 5 – 10% CO_2 in air increases breathing (if the animal is not too deeply anesthetized); lowering of arterial P_{CO_2}, by hyperventilation, causes apnea. Fink studied a large group of healthy volunteers who did not know that they should become apneic after hyperventilation. To lower their alveolar P_{CO_2} some overbreathed voluntarily and some were hyperventilated with a mechanical device, but at the end of the hyperventilation *none was apneic*, even though the arterial P_{CO_2} was as low as 16 torr. But when subjects were anesthetized, they were always apneic after hyperventilation. Bainton then showed that unanesthetized men did not become apneic at the end of the first or second period of hyperventilation but did after the third or fourth when they had grown accustomed or indifferent to their surroundings.

These observations indicate that the state of alertness, attentiveness and wakefulness acts as an important stimulus to respiration;

when man is awake, alert and attentive, he does not require a high level of arterial P_{CO_2} for continued breathing. The degree of wakefulness or alertness, therefore, must be a factor in the regulation of breathing. It may be determined by the sum of sensory stimuli from the periphery plus impulses from the brain that impinge on the reticular activating system and then on the respiratory center. The variability in CO_2 response curves from day to day in the same man may be an index of the changing activity of his alerting center. Again, the tremendous number of nerve impulses that flow back and forth during maximal exercise may be an important factor in producing the hyperpnea of exercise.

Correlation between activity of the reticular activating system and responsiveness of the respiratory center has been demonstrated. The reticular activating system can be stimulated by CO_2, by electrical currents and by arousal from sleep, and all of these stimulate breathing. It is depressed by anesthetics and by natural sleep.

Respiration has been studied in sleeping man. In deep sleep, alveolar ventilation is decreased, and alveolar P_{CO_2} rises from 40 to 46 torr or more. Sleep, therefore, decreases the responsiveness of the respiratory mechanism to the CO_2 stimulus. On the other hand, hypoxia increases pulmonary ventilation in much the same way in sleeping as in awake man; we would expect this because the carotid and aortic bodies are so resistant to depression by anesthesia.

Other reflexes also operate during sleep. One is the response to obstruction of the nose and mouth. Despite popular belief to the contrary, it is virtually impossible to asphyxiate a child or an adult who is not narcotized or paralyzed, because he wakens instantly and struggles violently for air when his airway is obstructed, even when he is in very deep sleep. (An infant who has not yet learned to breathe through his mouth, however, may die when his nasal passages are completely obstructed.)

Some years ago I wrote, "Sufficient experimental work has accumulated to warrant the revolutionary statement that control of respiration by CO_2 appears to be limited to man at rest or performing mild exercise (and to such laboratory experiments as voluntary hyperventilation and inhalation of CO_2 mixtures). Under all other conditions increased ventilation is caused by other factors than CO_2, and while these may be varied, usually they are of reflex origin." In the light of the work on awake and sleeping persons, Fink believes that the revolution may extend to man at rest, since here also CO_2 appears to play a subsidiary role, and the main respiratory drive appears to be of neural origin.

REGULATION OF THE REGULATORS

Physiology used to be simpler—before physiologists recognized that changes in receptors or in their immediate environment could change the supposedly standard response to supposedly standard stimuli. Let us consider:

1. CAROTID SINUS STRETCH RECEPTORS. The compliance of the vessel wall in which the receptors lie can be decreased by locally applied vasoconstrictor drugs and increased by vasodilator drugs. The receptors can be deformed (stimulated) by a drug-induced increase in vascular tone without any change in arterial pressure within the sinus. Can vasoconstrictor or vasodilator impulses or tolerable doses of drugs given systemically do this?

2. CAROTID AND AORTIC BODY CHEMORECEPTORS. The threshold and sensitivity of O_2 receptors can be changed by a change in the local P_{CO_2} or by an increase in local metabolism. In addition, a decrease in blood flow (metabolism remaining constant) can stimulate them without any change in arterial blood P_{O_2}, P_{CO_2} or pH; conceivably, local decrease in blood flow to chemoreceptors can occur reflexly.

3. INFLATION REFLEX RECEPTORS. These can be sensitized by drugs or by a change in their environment; decreased compliance of

the lungs requires that transpulmonary and transairway pressure be increased to achieve the usual tidal volume, and this produces greater stretch of airway receptors. Contraction of smooth muscle of the bronchioles (as by injected histamine or histamine released during anaphylaxis) leads to a decrease in compliance of bronchi, and they are consequently stretched less per unit of transpulmonary pressure.

4. MUSCLE SPINDLES. Nerve impulses over the gamma fibers can contract the spindle muscles, stretch the spindle receptor and drive the main muscle, even though the latter has not changed its length.

5. THE RESPIRATORY CENTERS. Increase in activity in the reticular activating system can alert the centers and make them more responsive to the incoming stimuli.

10

Mechanical Factors in Breathing

AIR, LIKE WATER, flows from a region of higher pressure to one of lower pressure. When gas pressure in alveoli is equal to atmospheric pressure, no air flows. For inspiration to occur, alveolar pressure must be less than atmospheric pressure; for expiration to occur, alveolar pressure must be greater than atmospheric pressure. There are two ways of producing the pressure difference necessary for inspiratory flow: (1) The alveolar pressure can be lowered below atmospheric pressure; this is called natural or "negative" pressure breathing. (2) The atmospheric pressure can be raised above normal and above resting alveolar pressure; this is called "positive" pressure breathing. Natural breathing in man is accomplished by active contraction of inspiratory muscles, which enlarges the thorax. This further lowers intrathoracic or intrapleural pressure, which is normally less than atmospheric pressure, pulls on the lungs and enlarges the alveoli, alveolar ducts and bronchioles. This in turn expands the alveolar gas and decreases its pressure below atmospheric. Air at atmospheric pressure then flows in the nose, mouth and trachea.

This chapter is concerned with the forces that produce inspiration and expiration as well as the resistances that oppose these forces. Active muscular contraction is needed to provide the force necessary to overcome (1) elastic recoil of the lungs and thorax; (2) frictional resistance caused by deformation of the tissues of the lungs and

thorax, and (3) frictional resistance to air flow through hundreds of thousands of fine air tubes of the conducting airway.

THE FORCES

The Motor Neurons and Respiratory Muscles

The respiratory muscles have no inherent rhythm and do not contract if they do not receive motor nerve impulses. These motor impulses usually originate in the respiratory centers, though some may come directly from higher cortical areas or from the spinal cord in response to sensory impulses from muscle spindles. The fibers carrying excitatory impulses from the respiratory centers apparently cross to the opposite side within the medulla. (Salmoiraghi found that a midline, longitudinal incision separating the right and left halves of the medulla stopped breathing just as surely as complete transection of the lower medulla.) The fibers then run downward in the lateral and anterior columns of the spinal cord. They synapse on the anterior horn cells at appropriate levels, and the motor nerves emerge in the anterior roots. These end on the motor end plates of muscle fibers; discharge of the end plates depolarizes the muscle membrane and initiates contraction of the muscles.

Physiologists have studied respiratory muscle activity by recording electrical impulses in the intercostal and phrenic nerves of animals, by recording the electrical activity of respiratory muscles in man by skin or needle electrodes and by fluoroscopic measurement of the position and motion of the diaphragm in man. Activity of the respiratory muscles, as of other muscles, can be increased by (1) increasing the frequency of discharge in a single motor unit (Fig. 10-1, B); (2) changing the pattern of bursts of activity in a single fiber unit; (3) activating more and more units in a muscle (Fig. 10-1, C), and (4) calling on accessory muscles not ordinarily used.

THE MUSCLES OF INSPIRATION.[1] *The diaphragm.* This large, dome-shaped sheet of muscle that separates the thoracic from the abdominal cavity is the principal muscle of inspiration. In quiet breathing, it may be the only active inspiratory muscle. Its motor nerves leave the spinal cord in the anterior roots of the third to fifth cervical segments and run downward in the phrenic nerves. The diaphragm is anchored all around the circumference of the lower thoracic cage; contraction of the muscle pulls down the central part, much as a piston moves downward in a cylinder. When man breathes qui-

etly, the diaphragm moves downward; during maximal inspiration, its downward stroke may be as much as 10 cm (Fig. 10-2). Its main action is to enlarge the thoracic cavity downward, but contraction of its costal fibers may also elevate the margins of the lower ribs and so increase the circumference of the bony thorax.

The downward motion of the diaphragm tends to increase intra-abdominal pressure; the increase is great if the abdomen is bound tightly or if its walls are already tense because of ascites or pronounced obesity; the increase is small if the abdominal muscles can relax or are flabby.

The diaphragm is the essential muscle of inspiration during deep anesthesia, because the other muscles of inspiration become inactive in the earlier stages of anesthesia. Breathing is then said to be "abdominal," because the descent and ascent of the diaphragm cause outward and inward movement of the abdominal wall. The diaphragm is also essential when the intercostal muscles are paralyzed by disease or when the bony thorax becomes rigid and immobile. However, if the diaphragm is paralyzed, respiration can continue if the thorax and thoracic muscles are normal. Even paralysis of both halves of the diaphragm does not lead to hypoventilation if the thorax is mobile and the thoracic muscles are functioning. Under

---

[1]Much of the work summarized here was done by E. J. M. Campbell and his associates and presented in his monograph *The Respiratory Muscles and the Mechanics of Breathing* (Chicago: Year Book Medical Publishers, 1958).

Fig. 10-1.—Motor impulses in phrenic nerve of a cat. In **A**, a single fiber is active. In **B**, the tidal volume has increased (due to inhalation of CO_2-rich gas), and the frequency of firing has increased. In **C**, both tidal volume and rate of breathing have increased; the neuron of high spike potential (same as in **A**, and **B**) fires still more frequently, and a second neuron of lesser spike potential begins to fire. (From Pitts, R. F.: J. Neurophysiol. 5:403, 1942.)

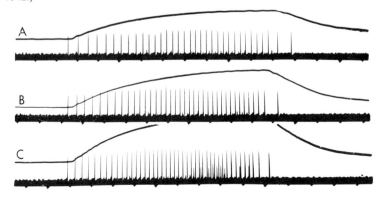

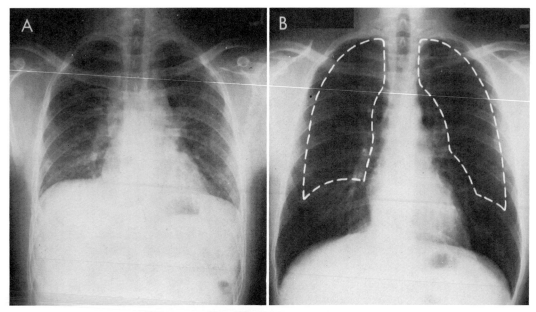

Fig. 10-2.—Roentgenogram of same chest in full expiration (**A**) and full inspiration (**B**). Dashed white line in **B** is outline of lungs in full expiration (as in **A**).

these conditions, however, the paralyzed diaphragm may move up with inspiration instead of down (paradoxical movement); this is because enlargement of the thorax lowers the intrathoracic pressure and pulls the atonic diaphragm upward. Radiologists use the "sniff test" to detect paralysis of one half of the diaphragm because the sniff is a rapid, sharp inspiratory movement that produces a quick upward movement of a paralyzed diaphragm.

In obstructive emphysema, if the thorax is enlarged and if the diaphragm is unable to descend further, its inspiratory contraction shortens the muscle fibers *horizontally*, and this may pull the lower thorax in, producing a motion opposing inspiration.

The diaphragm and other respiratory muscles hypertrophy when they are made to work harder over long periods, just as the heart muscle becomes thicker when made to work harder.

The external intercostal muscles. These are innervated by the intercostal nerves, which leave the spinal cord between the first and eleventh thoracic segments. Contraction of these muscles elevates the anterior end of each rib and pulls it upward and outward, thus increasing the anterior-posterior diameter of the bony thorax. Their contraction also tenses the intercostal spaces and keeps them from being sucked in during inspiration. The intercostal muscles, especially those between the fifth and ninth ribs, contract during inspiration in most normal males, but they are not essential to breathing except when the diaphragm is paralyzed or inactive. If the intercostal muscles alone are paralyzed, there is little decrease in exercise tolerance. Immobilization of the bony thorax by tight binding or by enclosing it in a cast decreases the maximal voluntary ventilation (MVV) by only 20–30%. However, paralysis of these muscles does lead to a loss of rigidity of the intercostal spaces; if descent of the diaphragm pulls in these soft tissues, it expands the lung less.

Other muscles involved in inspiration. The scalene and sternomastoids are the most important accessory muscles of inspiration. According to Campbell's electromyographic studies, they do not contract in quiet breathing—indeed, they are inactive until the minute volume is increased to 50–100 L/minute. (Campbell used skin electrodes. Needle electrodes inserted directly into muscle fibers may detect electrical activity at lower levels of ventilation.) When ventilation exceeds 100 L/minute, as in severe muscular exercise or in maximal voluntary ventilation, all of the accessory muscles are active. These accessory muscles include the posterior neck, trapezius and back muscles.

Other accessory muscles aid inspiration not by enlarging the thorax, but by reducing the resistance to air flow; these include the mylohyoid, digastric, alae nasi, platysma, cheek muscles, levator palati, laryngeal muscles, tongue muscles and the posterior neck muscles.

The maximal contraction of the inspiratory muscles can lower intrapleural pressure to 60–100 torr below atmospheric. Maximal inspiration is terminated abruptly by closure of the glottis, contraction of the abdominal muscles and a rise of intra-abdominal pressure.

THE MUSCLES OF EXPIRATION. Expiration is usually passive. During active contraction of inspiratory muscles, the elastic tissues of the lungs and thorax are stretched, and potential energy is stored in them. Expiration normally occurs by recoil of the stretched tissues and release of stored energy. At very high rates of ventilation or with moderately severe airway obstruction, the expiratory muscles contract actively.

The abdominal muscles. These are the most important of the expiratory muscles. They include the external oblique, rectus abdominis, internal oblique and transversus abdominis. They are innervated by fibers emerging from the lower six thoracic and first lumbar segments of the spinal cord. Contraction of these muscles depresses the lower ribs, flexes the trunk and, above all, increases intra-abdominal pressure and forces the diaphragm upward.

Campbell's studies of normal men show that the abdominal muscles are quiet in normal breathing; they remain quiet even when an expiratory resistance of 10 cm H_2O is added. Man seems to react to a moderate increase in expiratory resistance by inspiring more deeply, stretching the elastic tissues more and generating greater elastic recoil and expiratory force.

The abdominal muscles begin to show activity when ventilation increases to more than 40 L/minute. They contract vigorously (1) when ventilation reaches 70–90 L/minute, (2) during measurement of the expiratory reserve volume or maximal voluntary ventilation and (3) during coughing, straining or vomiting. They are essential for all effort requiring high, expulsive pressures and high linear velocities of air flow. They also contract at the end of a maximal inspiration; along with glottic closure, this cuts off inspiration abruptly.

Abdominal muscle activity may be depressed in patients with emphysema; physical therapists often try to teach patients by breathing exercises to use these muscles more effectively. The abdominal muscles become inactive early in anesthesia, which means that the ability to expire actively is lost. This is unimportant in patients with normal lungs and airways but creates a problem in patients with expiratory narrowing of the airways.

The internal intercostal muscles. This group includes the interchondral and interosseous muscles, the internal intercostals and the innermost intercostals; all are innervated by the intercostal nerves, which originate in the first to eleventh thoracic segments. Contraction of these muscles depresses the ribs, moves them downward and inward and stiffens the intercostal spaces so that they do not bulge during expiratory efforts such as coughing.

The diaphragm. Although primarily an inspiratory muscle, the diaphragm apparently does not relax completely and abruptly at end-inspiration. It is still active during the early part of expiration, presumably to let the thorax decrease in volume less abruptly, so that expiration is smoother. Beyond early expiration, the diaphragm relaxes completely. During quiet expiration, it is pulled upward by the elastic recoil of the lungs; during hyperpnea, it is also pushed up by the increase in intra-abdominal pressure caused by active contraction of the abdominal muscles.

Vigorous contraction of the expiratory muscles can produce a sustained intrapulmonary pressure as high as 120 torr and transient increases up to 300. Maximal contraction of abdominal muscles during straining can produce intra-abdominal pressures of 150–200 torr, enough to stop blood flow through the abdominal aorta. Straining usually involves a sequence of deep inspiration followed by closure of the glottis; contraction of the abdominal muscles then increases intra-abdominal pressure maximally, since it cannot push the diaphragm higher in the thorax.

Maximal Inspiratory and Expiratory Intrapulmonary Pressures

Theoretically, knowledge of the maximal inspiratory and expiratory pressures in the lung should be useful in determining whether patients have respiratory problems because of weakness of the inspiratory or of the expiratory muscles. The pressures are measured by asking the patient to make a maximal inspiratory or expiratory effort with mouth and nostrils closed except for a manometer connected to one nostril (Table 10-1 gives nor-

mal values). They are not often used diagnostically because:

1. The pressure generated varies with the lung volume and previous stretch of muscle fibers. When the thorax is in the expiratory position, the inspiratory muscles are stretched and can contract more; when the thorax is expanded, the expiratory muscles are stretched and contract more vigorously.

2. The test requires the cooperation of the patient. If the pressures recorded are high, the physician can assume that the muscles contract well (if he is sure that the pressures were not generated by contraction of the cheek muscles); however, low pressures may be due to lack of understanding or cooperation.

3. Increased or decreased pressure in the lungs and airways is transmitted through open eustachian tubes to the middle ear and may cause pain from deformation of the eardrums.

4. The great variability among healthy persons or even in the same person at different times makes it difficult to determine whether maximal pressures in any one patient are really low.

Weakness or inadequacy of respiratory muscles may be a cause of hypoventilation or even apnea in (1) prematurely born infants, (2) patients with myasthenia gravis or other generalized diseases of skeletal muscle, (3) patients who have received an overdose of neuromuscular blocking agents, such as succinylcholine, and (4) patients whose

TABLE 10-1. – MAXIMAL EXPIRATORY AND INSPIRATORY PRESSURES AT VARIOUS LUNG VOLUMES*

% OF VITAL CAPACITY DURING TEST	MAXIMUM EXPIRATORY PRESSURE (TORR ABOVE ATMOSPHERIC PRESSURE)		% OF VITAL CAPACITY DURING TEST	MAXIMUM INSPIRATORY PRESSURE (TORR BELOW ATMOSPHERIC PRESSURE)	
	MEAN	S.D.		MEAN	S.D.
9.7	41.5	13.4	3.0	86.0	19.5
25.0	52.5	20.8	21.7	74.6	14.1
43.8	69.9	19.7	34.8	63.3	18.7
60.0	90.0	21.5	55.6	56.8	15.6
75.0	95.3	17.6	75.7	44.8	14.0
83.0	107.0	16.3	91.0	23.6	12.9
100.0	119.0				

*Rahn, H.: Am. J. Physiol. 146:161, 1946.

respiratory muscles receive an inadequate number of motor nerve impulses because of damage or depression of the brain, medulla, spinal cord or motor nerves.

THE RESISTANCES TO BREATHING

Elastic Recoil of the Lungs

How does enlargement of the thoracic cage (by contraction of the inspiratory muscles) enlarge the lungs? The outer surface of the lungs, covered with visceral pleura, is in intimate contact with the inner surface of the thoracic cage, covered with parietal pleura. Both pleural surfaces are covered with a thin film of fluid. Movement of the thorax leads to movement of the lung through the linkage of the thin film of fluid covering the two pleural surfaces. A good analogy is that of two glass slides held together with a film of water. The top slide, when lifted, will carry the lower slide with it; indeed, it is very difficult to separate them by pulling at right angles to the plane of the two slides. However, it is very easy to slide one surface over the other. Because of the ease in sliding the visceral pleura over the parietal pleura,[2] downward movement of the diaphragm enlarges all lobes of the lungs, even when the thorax is fixed.

A healthy lung tends to recoil and pull away from the chest wall. This creates a subatmospheric pressure, just as pulling on the plunger of a closed syringe creates a subatmospheric pressure in it. The more the lung is stretched on inspiration, the more it tries to recoil and the more subatmospheric is the intrapleural pressure. If the lungs were a thin plastic bag with no recoil, intrapleural pressure would be atmospheric at end-expiration and at end-inspiration.

"NEGATIVE" INTRAPLEURAL PRESSURE. The term "negative" is incorrect though firmly entrenched by long use. A negative pressure is less than zero. The correct term is *subatmospheric* because the pressure in the "space" between the lungs and chest wall is normally $4-5$ cm H_2O less than atmospheric pressure (as we shall see later, the pressure is different in different parts of the pleural space). Since there is no air or fluid between the visceral and parietal pleurae of healthy man, how can this pressure be measured? We can create a space by passing a needle between two ribs and injecting a little air or fluid to separate the two pleurae; this is risky in some patients because the needle may puncture the lung. Therefore, when we speak of "intrapleural" pressure, we usually refer to a pressure that would exist in the intrapleural potential space if there were a way of measuring it without actually creating a space. We can push a tube connected to a manometer into the intrathoracic inferior or superior vena cava and measure pressure in it, but the varying pressure of the blood flowing through either of these veins complicates matters. The most convenient way to estimate intrapleural pressure is to ask the patient to swallow a tube until its tip is in the lower intrathoracic esophagus. The tube has a thin-walled balloon, 10 cm long, surrounding its lower end. Pressure measured in the balloon is a good index of intrapleural pressure because (1) the esophagus is in the thorax between the lungs and the chest wall, and (2) the esophagus is a thin tube with little tone and little resistance to the transmission of intrathoracic pressure changes (except during swallowing and peristaltic waves, which are easily identified). Intraesophageal pressure measurements are particularly valuable for estimating *changes* in intrapleural pressure during breathing.

MEASUREMENT OF ELASTIC RECOIL; COMPLIANCE OF THE LUNG. Elasticity is a property of matter that causes it to return to its resting shape after deformation by some external force. A perfectly elastic body, such as the spring in the upper part of Figure 10-3, will obey Hooke's law—when it is acted on

[2]Sometimes the pleural surfaces are fixed to each other by fibrous adhesions. Sometimes they are separated by gas (pneumothorax), and part of the enlargement of the thorax expands the air in the pleural space instead of inflating the lungs. Sometimes the pleural surfaces are separated by large volumes of fluid (hydrothorax).

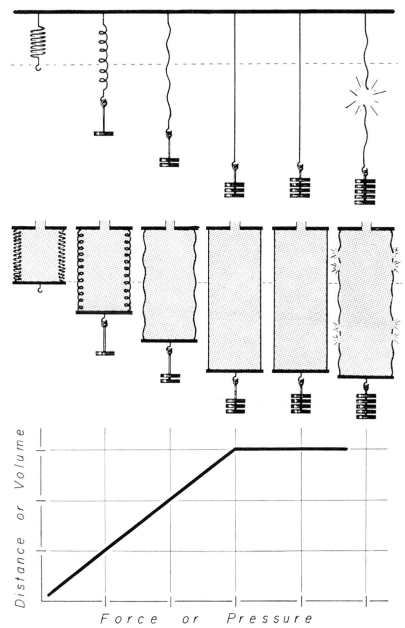

Fig. 10-3. — Hooke's law applied to a spring and to the lungs. For an elastic structure, the increase in length (or volume) varies directly with the increase in force (or pressure) until the elastic limit is reached. This linear relationship applies equally to normal lungs, over the physiologic range. (From Comroe, J. H., Jr., et al.: *The Lung* [2d ed.; Chicago: Year Book Medical Publishers, Inc., 1962].)

by 1 unit of force, it will stretch 1 unit of length, and when acted on by 2 units of force it will stretch 2 units of length, and so on, until the elastic limit is reached or exceeded.

The tissues of the lungs and thorax are not steel springs; they are elastic fibers, collagen, cartilage, epithelial and endothelial cells, smooth muscle, glands, nerves, blood and lymph vessels. But some of these tissues are elastic. Like springs, these tissues must be

TABLE 10-2. — MEASUREMENT OF COMPLIANCE AND RESISTANCE

	DEFINITION	UNITS	MEASUREMENTS REQUIRED	CONDITIONS OF MEASUREMENT
Compliance	Volume change produced by a unit of pressure change	L/cm H_2O	Pressure and volume	Static
Resistance	Pressure difference required for a unit flow change	cm H_2O/(L/sec)	Pressure and flow	Dynamic

stretched during inspiration by an external force (muscular effort); when the external force is removed, the tissues recoil to their resting position. Since elastic tissues obey Hooke's law just as springs do, springs are used in Figure 10-3 to depict the elastic properties of the lungs. (We shall see later that this is a great oversimplification.) The greater the muscular force applied, the more the springs are stretched and the greater the volume change on inspiration. This relation between force and stretch or between pressure and volume is measured under static conditions; the speed with which the new position or volume is attained is not a factor. The slope of the line that results from plot-

ting the external force (pressure) against the increase in volume serves as a measure of the stiffness of the "springs" or the distensibility of the lungs and thorax (as we shall see later, the line for lungs is not straight as pictured in Fig. 10-3). The closer the slope is to a vertical line, the more distensible are the tissues; the closer it is to a horizontal line, the "stiffer" are the tissues.

Physiologists call this the *mechanical compliance* or, more simply, the *compliance* of the tissues; it is defined as the volume change per unit of pressure change, measured under static conditions, and its units are L/cm H_2O. Because resistance involves a relationship between pressure and *flow*

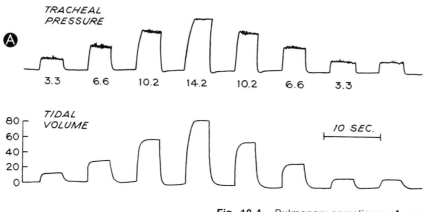

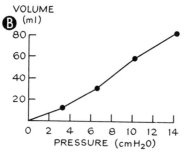

Fig. 10-4. — Pulmonary compliance. **A,** a pump inflates the lungs of an anesthetized animal 6 times/minute with increasing and then decreasing pressures. However, for each inflation, the pressure becomes constant (at 3.3, 6.6, 10.2 or 14.2 cm H_2O) because of an overflow tube set at the desired pressure. Note the increase in tidal volume with increasing pressure. **B,** a static pressure-volume curve has been constructed from the end-inflation values (when there is no air flow).

and is measured during *motion* (not under static conditions), we shall use the term *compliance* in considering *static* pressure-volume relationships and *resistance* in speaking of *dynamic* pressure-flow relationships (Table 10–2).

Pulmonary compliance is easy to measure in an anesthetized animal with a tracheal cannula and an open thorax. Push a known volume of gas into the trachea, then close the trachea and measure the static pressure of lung recoil. Then inject another volume of gas and again measure recoil pressure under static conditions. Repeat at several larger volumes. Or inflate the lungs, using several known pressures, and measure the volume change (Fig. 10-4). The next step in both methods is to plot a line relating pressure change to volume change. The slope of the line expressed as L/cm H_2O is compliance.

Pulmonary compliance can be determined in an unanesthetized man by measuring the pressure in a balloon in his intrathoracic esophagus at the end of a normal expiration and again after he has inspired a known volume of gas and held his breath. Repeat several times with larger inspired volumes. Plot the change in esophageal pressure against the change in lung volume. The slope is again compliance in L/cm H_2O.

Can one estimate the elastic recoil of the lung by determining the intrapleural (intra-esophageal) pressure at just one lung volume, e.g., at end-expiration (FRC)? No, because this requires that the balloon register the *absolute* intrapleural pressure. The intraesophageal balloon records intra-thoracic pressure *changes* more faithfully than it measures *absolute* pressure. The *change* in pressure that produces a change in volume is a reasonably accurate value but requires measurements at two volumes.

It is also possible to measure compliance during breathing. Figure 10-5 shows that there are two points of zero flow during each respiratory cycle, end-expiration and end-inspiration. When there is zero flow, no pressure is required to overcome airway resistance, and all of the transpulmonary pressure

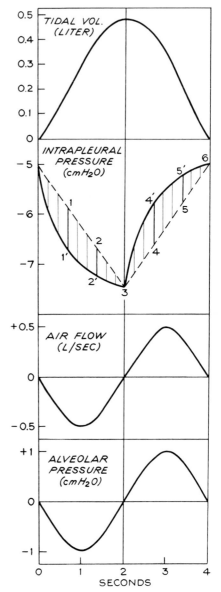

Fig. 10-5.—Volume and pressure changes during a single inspiration-expiration cycle. All measurements are made continuously and simultaneously during 1 cycle. If transpulmonary pressure were needed only to overcome elastic recoil, intrapleural pressure fluctuations during the respiratory cycle would follow the straight *dashed lines*. However, an additional pressure (that between *1* and *1'*, *2* and *2'*, etc., on the intrapleural pressure record) is required to overcome tissue and airway resistance during flow. At end-inspiration (point of no flow), lung volume has increased 0.48 L and intrapleural pressure has decreased 2.4 cm H_2O; compliance = 0.48/2.4 = 0.2 L/cm H_2O. This figure is schematic; inspiration and expiration are not usually equal in time.

at these two points is required to overcome elastic recoil. If pressures are recorded at these two points while the subject makes a series of tidal volumes of increasing depth, a line connecting them is a curve of change in volume vs. change in esophageal pressure, or of compliance. If a subject breathes in and out very slowly while intrapleural pressure and respired volume are measured, flow is so slow that very little pressure is required to overcome airway resistance relative to that needed to overcome elastic recoil, and one line (without a loop) describes the pressure-volume relation during inspiration and expiration. When the subject breathes faster and faster, more and more pressure is required for flow (see p. 122), and the P-V curve now becomes a loop—narrow at lower flows and thicker and thicker as flow gets faster. Still, in a man with normal lungs, the slope of the line joining measurements at end-inspiration and end-expiration remains the same up to rates of 60–90 breaths/minute—i.e., compliance measured during breathing (even fast breathing) equals compliance measured during slow breathing or under static conditions. In many patients with pulmonary disease, pressure-volume curves constructed from

such data obtained during rapid breathing yield values for "compliance" that are much lower than the values obtained under static conditions. When compliance measured during breathing is lower than compliance measured under *known static* conditions, compliance is not really being measured, despite the use of modifying adjectives such as "dynamic." As a rule, tissue or airway resistance is increased in these patients, and these abnormalities prevent complete filling of air units in the short time allowed (Fig. 10-6).

Calculations made from the data in Figure 10-6 show that in *1* (*upper left*) compliance (measured for both lungs) will be the same whether inspiration is complete in 4 seconds (respiratory frequency about 8/minute), in 2 seconds (respiratory frequency about 16/minute) or in 1 second (respiratory frequency about 30/minute). There is essentially no airway resistance and 0.2 L enters *A* and 0.1 L enters *B* without any delay; compliance is $(0.2 + 0.1)/1.0$ or 0.3 L/cm H_2O no matter how high the frequency of breathing. However, in *2* (*upper right*), increased airway resistance slows airflow into *B*; compliance of the two lungs is 0.4 L/cm H_2O if inspiration lasts for 4 seconds,

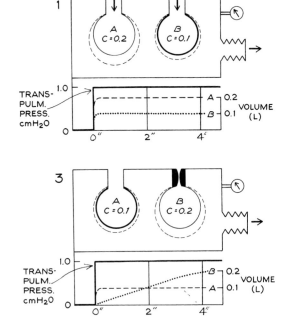

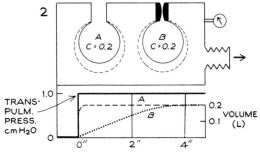

Fig. 10-6. — Effect of changes in lung compliance and airway resistance on lung inflation by constant transpulmonary pressure. C = compliance in L/cm H_2O. In each illustration, transpulmonary pressure (*solid line*) is increased abruptly to 1 cm H_2O and maintained there while air flow into A (*dashed curve*) and B (*dotted curve*) is measured. *Dashed circle* = final volume of each lung at 4 sec. In **1**, only compliance is decreased (in B); in **2**, only resistance is increased (in B). In **3**, compliance is decreased in A and resistance is increased in B; lung inflation is the same in **3** A and B only at 2 seconds (see text).

0.33 if it lasts only 2 seconds and 0.25 if it stops at 1 second. And in *3* (*lower left*), compliance is 0.3 if inspiration lasts 4 seconds, 0.2 if it lasts 2 seconds and 0.15 if it stops at 1 second. It is more precise to measure compliance when there is no flow and to measure pulmonary resistance separately. Little is learned from the finding of decreased "dynamic compliance" except that *something* is abnormal, and better tests must then be used to find out what is abnormal.

Figure 10-6 also illustrates the important ways in which inspired air is distributed unevenly to lungs (or to alveoli) because of uneven airway resistances, non-uniform compliance, or both. Uneven distribution is discussed in Chapter 13.

Compliance is related directly to lung volume. Suppose you inflate the two lungs of a man by 1 L and observe a pressure change of 5 cm H_2O (Fig. 10-7). The compliance is then calculated as 1.0 L/5 cm H_2O, or 0.2 L/cm H_2O. Assume that the right and left lungs originally were equal in volume and elastic properties; then each lung has enlarged only 0.5 L for the same pressure

change of 5 cm H_2O and the compliance of each lung is 0.1 L/cm H_2O. Assume the right lung has three lobes of equal volume and equal elastic properties; then each lobe has enlarged only 0.167 L for a transpulmonary change of 5 cm H_2O, and the compliance of each *lobe* would be 0.033 L/cm H_2O. Now we see clearly the relationship between compliance and lung volume: even though the elastic properties of the tissues are identical throughout the lungs, the compliance calculated for the two lungs together was 0.2, but for one lobe was 0.033 L/cm H_2O. For this reason, compliance is a meaningless figure as a measure of elastic recoil, unless it is related to lung volume. For example, the compliance of the lung of a newborn in absolute values is 0.006 L/cm H_2O, but if it is related to lung volume, it becomes 0.067 L/cm H_2O/L of lung volume, which is almost identical with the compliance of the adult lung when it too is related to lung volume. A decrease in compliance associated with a decrease in lung volume may result from many disorders, ranging from obstructed airways to pulmonary edema or pneumonia.

If you wish to judge whether lung tissue

Fig. 10-7.—Compliance and specific compliance for both lungs, one lung and one lobe. Compliance decreases with decreasing lung volume; specific compliance does not.

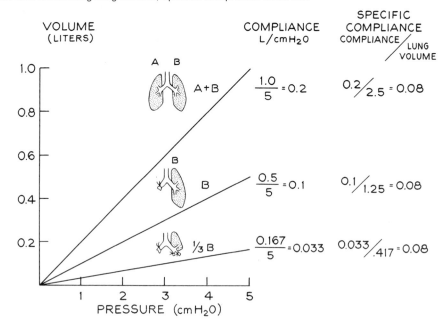

has normal elastic recoil, you must know both the compliance *and* the lung volume at the time compliance is measured. Compliance/lung volume is called *specific compliance.*

If specific compliance is decreased, the tissues of the lung must be more rigid and less distensible. This may occur in some types of interstitial or pleural fibrosis because collagen and fibrous tissue have different length-tension (or pressure-volume) relationships than elastic fibers. Pulmonary compliance may be as low as 0.01 L/cm H_2O, or 5% of predicted normal value, in patients with severe diffuse alveolar fibrosis, partly because of a decrease in lung volume and partly because the tissues are stiffer. In such patients, a transpulmonary pressure of 50 cm H_2O would be required to inflate the lungs with 500 ml of air. Because such pressures are greater than patients can produce over long periods and exceed the capacity of most apparatus designed to produce artificial ventilation, hypoventilation must occur.

An increase in compliance occurs in emphysema when elastic fibers have been lost or damaged without being replaced by collagen or fibrous tissue. The early diagnosis of emphysema, at a time when measures to prevent progression of the disease may still be effective, is an important challenge to pulmonary physiologists. Measurements of elastic recoil of lungs at different lung vol-

umes may point to early stages of emphysema. Normal lungs yield a curve such as *A* in Figure 10-8. Lungs with considerable and widespread loss of elastic recoil (severe emphysema) are more compliant; they yield a curve (*C*) that starts at a higher lung volume (the functional residual capacity of such a lung is well above normal at the usual transpulmonary pressure) and the elastic recoil pressure is less than normal at every lung volume. If the decrease in elastic recoil is patchy in lungs with early emphysema, the curve for such lungs (*B*) should be a composite of curves *A* and *C*: more compliant alveoli fill first; when they are filled, the normal, less compliant alveoli fill. Therefore, at the beginning of inflation (low lung volume) the P-V curve is mainly that of emphysematous alveoli, but later the curve is closer to that of normal lung.

Surface Forces and Lung Recoil

We have assumed that the lung is elastic because of its elastic tissue fibers that can be stained specifically and seen with a microscope. Of equal importance for elastic recoil is a very special surface film that lines the alveoli. The discovery of this surface film and its properties is one of the most fascinating chapters in pulmonary physiology. The story began in 1929, when von Neergaard inflated the lungs of anesthetized cats and

Fig. 10-8. — Pressure-volume curves of normal lungs and lungs with early and advanced emphysema (decrease in elastic recoil). **A**, normal lung. **B**, lung with early (patchy) emphysema (with some normal alveoli). **C**, lung with advanced emphysema. The normal pressure volume curve of **A** is repeated in **B** and **C** as a *dashed line,* for easy comparison with abnormal curves. (See text.) (From Murray, J. F., Greenspan, R. H., Gold, W. M., and Cohen, A. B.: Calif. Med. 116:37–55, 1972.)

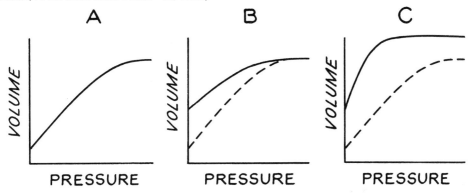

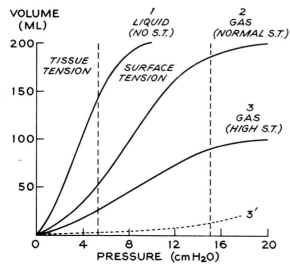

Fig. 10-9.—Air-inflated and fluid-distended lungs. When the lungs (with normal surface tension, *S.T.*) are inflated with gas to a high pressure and then deflated, curve 2 results. If the same lungs are made gas-free, filled with fluid to the same pressure and then allowed to empty. curve *1* results. The *dashed vertical line* at 5 cm H$_2$O shows that the lungs enlarge more than twice as much when fluid-filled (no liquid-gas interface) as when gas-filled (liquid-gas interface present in all alveoli). Curves *3* and *3'* show that the lungs inflate still less when the alveolar lining has a high surface tension; *3'* is a curve obtained during inflation of such a lung and *3*, the curve during deflation.

measured the pressures during deflation. He obtained a relationship between pressure and volume (a pressure-volume curve) similar to that shown in Figure 10-9. He then made the lungs gas-free and distended them with physiologic *fluids*, and repeated the earlier procedure and measurements. The amazing result was that the pressure required to maintain any given lung volume with *fluid*, under static conditions, was *less* than *half* that required to maintain the same volume of an air-filled lung. Filling the lung with a physiologic fluid should not alter its elastic fibers, and there is no reason why these should not recoil with the same force as in an air-filled lung. Why then this remarkable difference? Von Neergaard correctly deduced that each of the hundreds of millions of alveoli has a liquid-air interface, which tends to retract or recoil just as a bubble does. The sum of these recoil forces for the whole lung provides just as much recoil as do the elastic fibers. Filling the alveoli with fluids eliminates the fluid-air interface and replaces it with a fluid-fluid interface that has practically no surface tension. The recoil pressure of the *fluid*-filled lung measures the recoil pressure of only the elastic (or elastic-like) elements. The recoil pressure of *air*-filled lungs measures the recoil of both the elastic elements and the surface film.

WHAT IS SURFACE TENSION? Surface tension is a manifestation of attracting forces between atoms or molecules. In a liquid such as water at rest (Fig. 10-10), the intermolecular forces acting on the molecule in *A* are equal in all directions; molecular forces pull it downward, to the left, to the right and upward. However, the water molecule in *B*, at the water-air surface, does not experience equal attracting forces in all directions. *B* is attracted by water molecules directly beneath it, but there are relatively few molecules in the gas above it to exert an upward force. Therefore, more molecules pull it down than pull it up, and, typical of surface molecules, it tends to dive downward. As a result of this imbalance of intermolecular forces, the surface shrinks to the smallest possible area. The resulting force in the surface is referred to as surface, or interfacial, tension. *Tension* and *pressure* are often used synonymously; for example, we speak of Po$_2$ as the partial pressure of O$_2$ or the tension of O$_2$. However, *surface tension* has the units of force per unit of *length; pressure* has the units of force per unit of *area*. Tension operates in the same plane as the surface; Figure 10-11 shows the tension on a window shade pulling it downward. In the sphere, the tension in the wall tends to make the sphere smaller (Fig. 10-11); to prevent this,

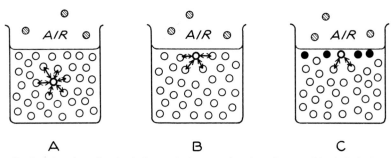

Fig. 10-10.—Surface tension. See text. *Open circles* = molecules of water. *Shaded circles* = molecules of air. *Black circles* = surface-active molecules.

it must be opposed by equal and opposite pressure in the cavity. Laplace's law (pressure = 2 × tension/radius) relates pressure, tension and radius.

The surface tension of a plane film can be measured by a simple Maxwell frame, pictured in Figure 10-12, *A*. A film of liquid is placed on the frame, and stretched by pulling the crosswire to the right; the film tends to pull the wire back to the left. The force on the crosswire necessary to maintain a constant area of film provides a measure of surface tension. The units of surface tension are dynes/cm. At 37 C, pure water has a surface tension of 70 dynes/cm; blood plasma and most tissue fluids at equilibrium have a tension of 50 dynes/cm.

SURFACE TENSION OF THE ALVEOLAR LIQUID-AIR INTERFACE. Some physiologists have used Laplace's law relating tension in the wall to radius of the sphere to calculate the surface tension exerted by the lungs, considering the alveoli as hundreds of millions of tiny bubbles at the ends of capillary tubes. Assuming that the alveolar film exerts a surface tension of 50 dynes/cm (equal to that of plasma), calculations indicate that the surface tension recoil of the lung would be 20,000 dynes/cm² and would exert a pressure of about 20 cm H_2O (1.0 cm H_2O pressure = 980 dynes). This calculated value is reasonably close to von Neergaard's actual measurements for fully inflated lungs but is 5–10 times too large at usual or at low lung

Fig. 10-11.—Tension in a plane surface and a sphere. Tension (*T*) is expressed as force per unit length (*T* = dynes/cm). Pressure (*P*) is force per unit area (*P* = dynes/cm²). The *left half* of the sphere illustrates how wall tension acts; the *right half* illustrates how internal pressure acts. (From Rodbard, S., in Abramson, D. I. [ed.]: *Blood Vessels and Lymphatics* [New York: Academic Press, 1962].)

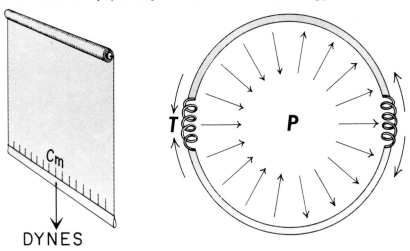

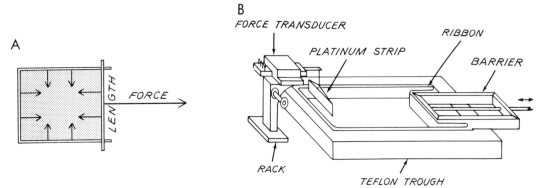

Fig. 10-12. — Measurement of surface tension. **A**, Maxwell frame for measuring surface tension. **B**, Clements' surface balance. Saline is placed in a shallow tray, and the material to be tested is placed on top of it. A platinum strip 0.001 in. thick is then suspended in the fluid from the arm of a sensitive strain gauge (force transducer). The pull of the fluid surface on the strip provides a measure of the surface tension. A barrier driven by a motor then moves from 1 end of the trough toward the other cyclically, first reducing the area of the surface to 20% of its initial size and then expanding it to its original size. The surface tension of the film is measured continuously as the surface area is altered. (From Clements, J. A., and Tierney, D., in Fenn, W. O., and Rahn, H. [eds.]: *Handbook of Physiology* [Washington, D. C.: American Physiological Society, Sec. 3, Vol. II, 1965].)

volumes. The surface tension of the alveolar film at small lung volumes must then be 5 – 10 dynes/cm instead of 50 dynes/cm. This led Clements to suspect that the surface tension in the lung fluid is high when the lungs are inflated and very low when they are deflated. This could occur only if the alveolar lining were something other than saline, plasma or ordinary tissue fluid; it must contain a special type of surface-active material.

Many substances, e.g., detergents, lower surface tension. What is the mechanism involved? Let us say that a liquid contains two kinds of particles: surface-active (black molecules; see Fig. 10-10, *C*) and not surface-active. The former are attracted less strongly to the molecules of the liquid than the latter and therefore accumulate at the surface of the liquid. But surface-active molecules, no matter where they are, exert smaller attracting forces for other molecules; when concentrated at the surface, they dilute the molecules of the liquid and must therefore lower its surface tension. Such substances are called surface-active substances, or surfactants.

We have already said that an ordinary surfactant would not explain the action of the alveolar lining, which requires a high surface

tension when the lung is inflated and a low surface tension when it is deflated. The surface tension of the alveolar lining can be 40 – 50 dynes/cm when the alveoli are large and 2 – 5 dynes/cm when they are small only if the surface tension of the film changes when it is compressed or expanded.

To test this, Clements obtained materials from lungs by repeated rinsing of the airways

Fig. 10-13. — Minimal and maximal surface tensions during a cycle of compression and expansion. The surface tension of pure water is 72 dynes/cm and that of a detergent is 30 dynes/cm. Lung extract is remarkable because its surface tension decreases from about 45 to less than 5 dynes/cm when the film is compressed.

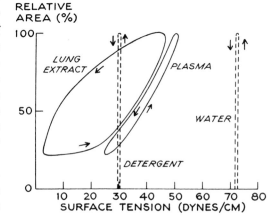

and airspaces, by producing pulmonary edema foam (which presumably contains some of the alveolar film) or by mincing lung tissue. He then placed such material on a trough containing saline (Fig. 10-12, *B*). The surface-active material accumulated on the surface for the reasons given above. He then compressed the surface, to mimic compression of the alveolar lining during expiration, and expanded it, to mimic its expansion during inspiration. The results were remarkable — the surface tension rose to 40–50 dynes/cm when the film was expanded and dropped nearly to zero when the film was compressed (Fig. 10-13).

PHYSIOLOGIC IMPORTANCE OF PULMONARY SURFACTANT. 1. A bubble or alveolus with a low surface tension requires a low air pressure to maintain a given radius or volume; one with a high surface tension requires a large counter-pressure. Low surface tension, therefore, reduces the muscular effort necessary to ventilate the lungs and keep them aerated.

2. A surfactant that changes surface tension as surface area changes helps to stabilize the alveolar gas bubbles and keep them from collapsing. Alveoli vary in size throughout the lungs; some have a radius 3–4 times that of others. If surface tension were the same in all alveoli, regardless of their size, the pressure required to keep air spaces inflated against surface tension would also vary 3–4 times. Since all the conducting tubes to all functioning alveoli communicate with one another, pressures cannot so differ in the alveoli of the lung; pressure must be approximately the same in all. However, Laplace's law shows that if the air pressure were equal in bubbles of different sizes, the smaller bubbles would collapse and the larger ones would overexpand.

Let us consider a bubble blown on the end of a glass tube. For such a system, Laplace showed that the tension (T) in the wall of a spherical bubble tends to contract the bubble and that the air pressure (P) inside the bubble tends to expand it. When there is no

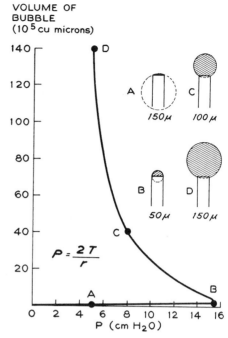

VOLUME OF BUBBLE (10^5 cu microns)

Fig. 10-14. — Pressure-volume curve of a bubble blown at the end of a glass tube. The volume of bubbles *A-D* is the portion of the sphere (*shaded areas*) occupied by the enlarging bubble. The volume continues to increase, but the pressure needed to balance the tension is less as the radius of the sphere increases and more as it decreases. (Modified from Mead, J.: Physiol. Rev. 41:281, 1961.)

movement, there is an equilibrium between the forces tending to enlarge the bubble and those tending to contract it. At this time, $P = \frac{2T}{r}$, where r is the radius of the sphere. If the surface tension in the bubble remains the same, regardless of the radius of the bubble, then the air pressure required to inflate the bubble increases as the radius decreases. The bubble in Figure 10-14 has a large radius as it is being formed (*A*); it is part of the large sphere shown by the dotted line. As the bubble is enlarged, its radius actually decreases and becomes minimal when it equals the radius of the tube (*B*). Therefore, more and more pressure is required to enlarge the bubble from *A* to *B*. Beyond this size, the radius begins to *increase* (*C* and *D*), and less pressure is required to enlarge the bubble. This explains why small bubbles

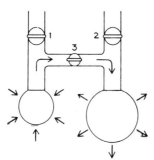

Fig. 10-15.—Dynamics of soap bubbles. Bubbles of different volumes are blown separately (stopcock 3 closed). When connected by turning stopcock 3, the smaller bubble empties into the larger. (From Boys, C. V.: *Soap Bubbles* [New York: Dover Publications, Inc., 1950].)

(small *r*) have a high pressure and large bubbles (large *r*) have a low pressure and why small bubbles can empty into larger ones (Fig. 10-15).

The lung, with hundreds of millions of alveoli of varying size, is inherently unstable. Without some special system to prevent it, the lung would empty its smaller air spaces into larger ones and would then consist only of collapsed alveoli and hyperinflated alveolar ducts. This does *not* occur in healthy lungs because (1) the surface tension of the alveolar lining is considerably less than that of plasma and is lower than predicted, and (2) the surface tension of the alveolar lining decreases markedly as the film is compressed; this probably occurs during expira-

tion, when the alveoli become smaller. Clements has calculated that this factor, acting in conjunction with elastic elements of the tissue, is sufficient to insure the stability and prevent the collapse of small alveoli during expiration and to lead to a stable balance between small and large alveoli. The elastic and other fibers must also contribute to stability, but in actual practice, alveoli collapse when surfactant is absent or inactivated, even though the elastic fibers are normal, unless transpulmonary pressure is high. The combined effect of alveolar size and surface tension on transpulmonary pressure required to maintain lung inflation is shown in Figure 10-16.

When Avery and Mead found that immature fetal lungs and the collapsed lungs of newborn babies dead of respiratory distress syndrome (hyaline membrane disease) contained no surfactant (Fig. 10-17), this material became a substance of great medical as well as physiologic importance. As a result, many investigators have now studied the chemical and biologic characteristics of pulmonary surfactant.

ORIGIN, COMPOSITION, TURNOVER AND REGULATION OF PULMONARY SURFACTANT. Clements and his associates have extracted, purified and determined the chemical composition of pulmonary surfactant. Originally thought to be only a saturated leci-

Fig. 10-16.—Alveolar collapse due to loss of surfactant. **Left**, normal infant. A transpulmonary pressure of only 2 cm H$_2$O is needed to inflate a deflated alveolus with a radius of 50 μ and a minimal surface tension of 5 dynes/cm. **Right**, infant with respiratory distress; 20 cm H$_2$O is required to inflate the smaller alveolus with a high minimal surface tension. The infant must make a maximal effort with each breath to inflate the alveolus.

Note: On converting μ to cm, the pressure on the left = 2,000 dynes/cm^2 and on the right = 20,000 dynes/cm^2; since 1 cm H$_2$O = 980 dynes/cm^2, the pressures are approximately 2 and 20 cm H$_2$O, respectively. (Modified from Avery, M. E., and Clements, J. A.: Physiol. Physicians vol. 1, March, 1963.)

NORMAL INFANT

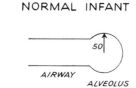

$$PRESSURE = \frac{2 \times TENSION}{RADIUS}$$

$$= \frac{2 \times 5 \ (DYNES/CM)}{50 \ (MICRONS)} = 2 \ cm. \ WATER$$

RESPIRATORY DISTRESS - NEWBORN
(HYALINE MEMBRANE DISEASE)

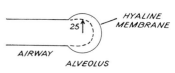

$$PRESSURE = \frac{2 \times TENSION}{RADIUS}$$

$$= \frac{2 \times 25}{25} = 20 \ cm. \ WATER$$

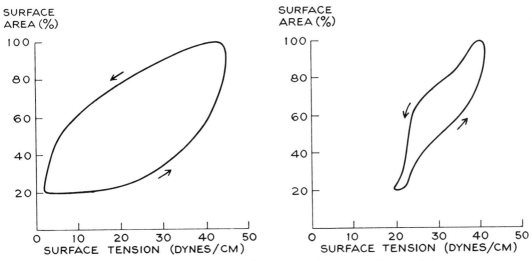

Fig. 10-17.—Surface tension of lung extracts. **Left**, extract from normal lung; minimal surface tension (after compression of film to 20% of original surface) = 2 dynes/cm. **Right**, extract from lung of a newborn baby who died of respiratory distress syndrome (hyaline membrane disease); minimal surface tension is 20 dynes/cm. (Courtesy of Drs. John Clements and William Tooley.)

thin, dipalmitoyl lecithin, it is now known to be a complex lipoprotein, like those in membranes but unique in its high concentration of dipalmitoyl lecithin and in its protein (Table 10-3).

Of the known components, the saturated lecithins give the lowest values of surface tension and the most stable films on compression; they, together with the unsaturated lecithins and cholesterol, account for the property unique to lung extracts of lowering surface tension of compressed films almost to zero. However, surfactant does not cover alveolar surfaces like a coat of paint and stay for years. It is in a state of flux; molecules leave the surface film and newly synthesized molecules enter it. This means that once formed, surfactant must be transported from

the site of formation to the site of action, and ideally the rate of formation and transport should be equal to the rate of loss from the surface. The other components in surfactant, especially the specific apoprotein, may have the important role of speeding the intracellular transport of surfactant and its secretion onto the surface of the alveolar lumen.

Most of the pulmonary surfactant appears to be formed in type II alveolar cells in the lung. (These were originally called "granular pneumocytes" by Macklin, who believed that they discharged granules that somehow regulated the surface tension of alveoli.) These cells have not yet been separated from other pulmonary cells, so the evidence, though strong, is still indirect. Part of the evidence that type II alveolar cells form surfactant comes from studies of maturing fetal lungs. Early in fetal life the lungs have no alveolar cells (when present, these cells can be identified histologically by their characteristic osmiophilic inclusion bodies) and no extractable surfactant; when one appears, the other also is present. Other evidence comes from examination of these cells using the electron microscope; they contain lamellar inclusion bodies (Fig. 10-18) whose ap-

TABLE 10-3.—COMPOSITION OF PULMONARY SURFACTANT

Saturated lecithins (90% is dipalmitoyl lecithin)	41%
Unsaturated lecithins	25%
Cholesterol	8%
Phosphatidylethanolamine	5%
Specific apoprotein	9%
Other components*	12%

*These include glycerides 4%, phosphatidylglycerol + serine 4%, lysolecithin 2%, sphingomyelin 1% and free fatty acids 1%.

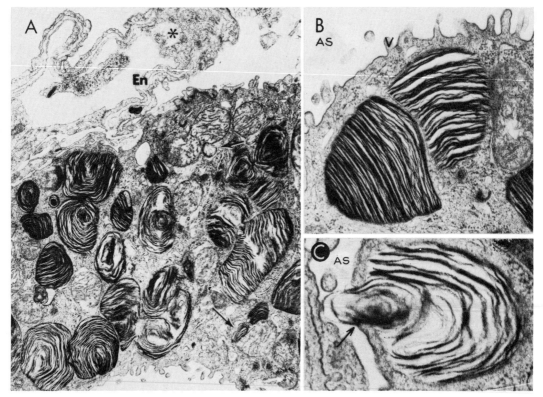

Fig. 10-18.—Electron micrographs of type II alveolar cells. **A**, survey of cell, showing many osmiophilic lamellar inclusion bodies. (Courtesy of Dr. Una Smith.) **B**, × 40,000. **C**, arrow points to material that appears to be extruded from cell into alveolar space. × 60,000. Rat lung. *En* = endothelial cell. *AS* = alveolar space. *V* = microvillus. (From Smith, D. S., Smith, U., and Ryan, J. W.: Tissue & Cell 4:457, 1972.)

pearance is characteristic of phospholipid-rich substances known to be highly surface-active. Presumably material in these bodies passes through the cell membrane and spreads on the surface.

Because this surface film is essential for survival of the newborn, it is crucial that surfactant be formed, stored and available for transport to alveolar surfaces at the earliest moment that a baby born prematurely can survive; this moment is determined in part by the change in alveolar lining cells from thick cuboidal to thin epithelial cells, since only the latter permit easy lung expansion and gas exchange. It appears that lung tissue contains surface-active material as early as the eighteenth to twentieth week of gestation—long before the alveolar cells have matured sufficiently to permit newborn respiratory muscles to expand alveoli.

However, the surfactant does not move onto alveolar surfaces from which it can be extracted without mincing the lungs until about the thirtieth week of gestation (Fig. 10-19); a baby born earlier will probably not survive.

What determines whether there will be enough surfactant on hand at the proper moment in fetal life? Certainly the cells that form it must mature and must receive proper precursors and adequate substrate. The blood supply to alveolar walls, alveolar ducts and respiratory bronchioles comes from the pulmonary circulation (see p. 130). Pulmonary blood flow is low in fetal life (see p. 243); anything that decreases it below minimal requirements for cell growth and surfactant synthesis can interfere with formation, storage or secretion of surfactant. On the other hand, Liggins has demonstrated

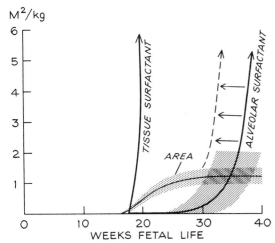

Fig. 10-19.—Appearance time of surfactant in fetal lung. Schema showing early appearance of large amounts of secretable, tissue surfactant and later appearance of surfactant on alveolar surfaces. The area band shows the potential area of the lungs if maximally expanded. When the other band showing the amount of alveolar surfactant exceeds this, there is more than enough to cover all alveolar surfaces. *Dashed vertical line* and *horizontal arrows* show the possibility by therapeutic means of causing earlier release of tissue surfactant (to become alveolar surfactant). Width of bands indicates variability about mean values. (Courtesy of Dr. John Clements.)

that cell maturation and surfactant production can be hastened by hormones, especially adrenal cortical hormones (L-thyroxine appears to act similarly). Sheep with twin lambs provided him with a nice experimental setting, since dexamethasone can be infused into one fetal lamb, leaving its twin as the control. Removal of the pituitary in a fetal lamb delays lung maturation. On the other hand, lungs of a dexamethasone-treated fetus are more mature, easier to inflate and contain more surface-active material than those of the control lamb. Using dexamethasone in fetal lambs, Platzker could force the appearance of surfactant to an earlier time in gestation (Fig. 10-19); nearer term, he could greatly increase its concentration. Presumably this is due to induction of enzymes in the lungs, since both nuclei and cytoplasm of fetal pulmonary cells are rich in glucocorticoid receptors.

The observations just mentioned assume

clinical importance since fluid from the fetal lung drifts from the lung into the trachea and then into the amniotic fluid. The obstetrician can safely remove a sample of amniotic fluid from a pregnant woman near term; using a sensitive test, he can now detect the presence of surfactant in the amniotic fluid. If none is present, it might be possible to delay birth or to try to accelerate formation of surfactant, or both; in any case, the physician can anticipate that the baby will have respiratory difficulties at birth and can prepare for expert intensive respiratory care. When testing amniotic fluid for surfactant, it is necessary to exclude the effect of other materials in amniotic fluid (such as bile, salts of free fatty acids or proteins) that might be surface-active.

BALANCE BETWEEN REMOVAL AND RENEWAL OF SURFACTANT. Little is known of chemical or physical factors that inactivate surfactant or remove it once it is spread on the alveolar surface. Some may re-enter alveolar cells and be recycled; some may enter the "liquid veins" between alveoli and pass into lymphatics; some may be engulfed by alveolar macrophages. Pulmonary disorders that increase the number of these macrophages may increase the amount of surfactant that these cells remove from alveolar surfaces. Some have postulated that cigarette smoking increases the number of alveolar macrophages and so increases the rate of surfactant removal. If so, this would stress surfactant formation to keep pace with removal. It is well to remember that analyses of lung tissue and of tracheo-bronchial-alveolar washings for surfactant do not necessarily give information on the amount of surfactant enacting its physiologic role on alveolar surfaces; surfactant may be within alveolar cells, on its way to the surface, on the surface, in alveolar macrophages or even in pulmonary lymph.

There is also evidence that the lung can be depleted of surfactant when lung volume is decreased or very large. When the lung is deliberately ventilated with low tidal volumes beginning near residual volume, it tends to become atelectatic and needs a new surface film with each inspiration; this is because a film, once collapsed, does not spread out again when stretched unless new molecules enter its surface. When a lung is deliberately overstretched, return to functional residual capacity can also promote film collapse. Large tidal volumes also require additional surfactant. On the other hand, the process of film collapse occurs much more slowly in static lungs than in lungs tidally ventilated. Since lung collapse, lung overdistention and large tidal volumes appear to increase the requirement for formation of new surfactant, it appears that, when slight differences are critical, the best way to maintain balance between loss and gain of surfactant molecules is to maintain a relatively high transpulmonary pressure and permit normal tidal volumes on this base. This is the rationale for treating babies with respiratory distress syndrome with continuous positive airway pressure. This new therapy has strikingly reduced mortality in babies born with this disorder.

PULMONARY SURFACTANT AND CLINICAL DISORDERS. *1. Respiratory distress syndrome of the newborn* has already been discussed. The alveoli tend to collapse and are covered with hyaline membranes. Pulmonary capillaries become congested and leaky.

2. Pulmonary embolism. Alveolar collapse can occur when pulmonary blood flow to alveolar capillaries is completely shut off, thus depriving alveolar cells of precursors and substrate and of a mechanism for eliminating waste products. Alveolar cells may recover their function when the clot is lysed or when bronchial collateral circulation feeds blood into alveolar capillaries.

3. Adult shock lung. It is easy to visualize survival with complete ischemia of *part* of an adult lung (pulmonary embolism) or of *all* of fetal lungs. Because the adult lung has a pulmonary blood flow of more than 5 L/minute

and needs only a very small fraction of this to meet the metabolic needs of alveolar cells, it is difficult to visualize that pulmonary blood flow can be low enough to cause ischemia of these cells in a surviving adult. However, patients in hemorrhagic shock with a very low arterial blood pressure over many hours may suffer from pulmonary ischemia, since their pulmonary artery pressure may be so low that it cannot pump blood to higher regions of the lungs even when the patient is supine (see p. 151). Patients undergoing prolonged cardiopulmonary bypass may develop similar ischemia. Management of such patients requires that their lungs be expanded and ventilated by some form of continuous positive-pressure ventilation and that pulmonary artery pressure be raised high enough to perfuse all of the lung regions.

4. Alveolar proteinosis. In this condition there is an accumulation of protein in the alveolar spaces; this might represent excess production or deficient removal of surfactant by alveolar macrophages or both.

Lung Stability and Interdependence

An organ composed of multiple subunits and continuously changing volume must be stabilized to prevent one portion from moving out of phase with its surroundings. The lung has a number of interrelated physical and chemical properties that tend to prevent asynchronous function. Collateral ventilation (see p. 13) and surfactant are two of these. A recently described property called *interdependence* is another.

During ventilation, if a group of lung units becomes out of phase with its neighbors, it will have a different volume than if it were in phase. To restrain out-of-phase or asynchronous volume changes, stresses are set up within the elastic elements of the segment or of the surrounding parenchyma. Thus it becomes more difficult to inflate a segment asynchronously than synchronously with the rest of the lung. The ratio of the synchronous to asynchronous compliance is a measure of interdependence. In animals, this ratio is probably between 1.5 and 3.0 at normal resting lung volumes and decreases as lung volume increases. It appears that a rigid thoracic cage is necessary for interdependence to be effective in portions of lung subtending the pleural surface.

Interdependence exists not only between adjacent areas of lung parenchyma but also between the parenchyma and intraparenchymal blood vessels and airways. If the lung were perfectly isotropic (i.e., if its physical properties, such as elasticity, were the same regardless of the direction of measurement) and it functioned with perfect synchrony, interdependence would never be manifest.

Since this is not the case, lung stabilization and interdependence may be important in numerous clinical situations. The segment of lung that is expanded despite almost complete occlusion of its bronchus is a good example. In fact, it is possible that the lung bases are not continually collapsing because the lung has inherent properties resisting deformation.

Elastic Recoil of the Thoracic Cage

The tissues of the *thoracic cage* also have elastic recoil. The elastic tissues of the lungs, if not acted on by any external force (such as the pull of the thorax), collapse the lung

Fig. 10-20.—Pressure-volume curves of lung and chest cage. **Left**, pressure-volume curves. P_L = pressure exerted by lung at each volume (expressed as % of vital capacity or % of total lung capacity, *TLC*). P_C = pressure exerted by the chest cage. P_T = pressure exerted by the total system (lungs + chest cage). Line A = minimal air (volume of gas remaining in lungs when the thoracic cage is open to atmospheric pressure); line B = residual volume; line C = FRC; line D = inspiration; line E = deep inspiration. The "lungs-thorax" sketches indicate the direction and magnitude of forces of the two elastic systems at four lung volumes; *dashed arrows* = chest cage tension; *solid arrows* = lung tension. See text for methods of measurement. (Redrawn from Knowles, J. H., Hong, S. K., and Rahn, H.: J. Appl. Physiol. 14:525, 1959.)

Right, schema showing lung "springs" (*L*) and chest wall "springs" (*C*) at each of the five lung volumes, *A-E*. At *A*, neither *L* nor *C* is under tension, (e.g., pneumothorax with no liquid seal between lungs and thorax); at *B*, *C*, *D* and *E*, the lung "springs" are stretched and tend to recoil toward their nonstretched position; at *B* and *C*, the chest wall "springs" are stretched, and at *E* they are compressed beyond the resting position. If, at end-expiration (*C*), all of the muscles of respiration are relaxed (neither pushing nor pulling), there must be a precise balance between the elastic forces of the chest wall and those of the lungs. The forces must be equal or opposite. The intrapleural pressure at *C* (FRC) is 5 cm H_2O; therefore, lung recoil is + 5 cm H_2O and chest recoil is −5 cm H_2O. At *D*, the total and the lung pressures are equal; therefore, the thoracic cage recoil must be zero and all of the recoil pressure is due to lung recoil. At *A*, minimal air volume, lung recoil is zero and the total pressure (which is now less than atmospheric) must all be due to thoracic cage recoil.

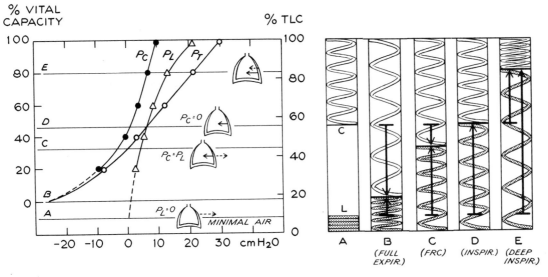

almost to the airless state (beyond residual volume to "minimal volume") (Fig. 10-20, *left, A*). The elastic tissues of the thoracic cage, if not acted on by any external force (such as the pull of the lungs) enlarge the thorax from the resting volume to about 600 ml above it. We know this is so because if we inject air between the parietal and visceral pleura of man (pneumothorax) and break the liquid seal, the lung gets smaller but the thorax gets larger. Therefore, if we think of the lungs and thorax as elastic and springlike, we must think of their springs as having different resting positions. The lung springs are "at rest" when the thorax is open and there are no thoracic springs "pulling on" the lung; the thoracic wall springs are "at rest" when the lungs are removed and no muscular stretching or compressing force is applied (Fig. 10-20, *right, A*).

The thoracic and lung springs are held together by the linkage (cohesion) of the pleural surfaces. At FRC, the thoracic springs have been stretched from their resting position inward, and the lung springs have been stretched from their resting position outward (Fig. 10-20, *left, C*). With increasing inspiration (*D* and *E*), the thoracic springs recoil, but the lung springs must be stretched even more. When the thoracic springs are at their position of rest (*D*), all the relaxation pressure must be due to recoil of the lung springs. At volumes greater than this (*E*), additional force is required, not only to stretch the lung springs more, but to compress the thoracic springs beyond their resting position.

The elastic recoil of the thoracic cage can be measured directly or calculated by subtracting pulmonary compliance from combined pulmonary-thoracic wall compliance (measured simultaneously). Rahn and associates have used both methods (see Fig. 10-20 and Table 10-4). They measured compliance in normal man by two manometers, one connected to an esophageal balloon (to measure changes in intrapleural pressure) and one connected to the mouth or nostril (in a closed, static system, this measures alveolar pressure, or the total pressure exerted by the lung-thorax system). The subject was asked to inspire a known volume of gas and hold his breath with his glottis open; the esophageal pressure change equals the change in recoil pressure of the lung. The subject was then asked to close his nose and mouth and relax all his muscles of respiration. The nose or mouth pressure then equals the total recoil pressure of the lungs and thorax (uninfluenced by active contraction of inspiratory muscles), and the esophageal pressure equals the pressure of the thorax (because the elastic force of the lung is balanced in this closed system by the pressure of the water manometer, which is connected to the nose or mouth).

If data are obtained simultaneously for compliance of the lungs alone and of the lungs and thoracic cage together (total compliance), the compliance of the thoracic cage alone can be calculated by the equation

$$\frac{1}{\text{Total compliance}} = \frac{1}{\text{Pulmonary compliance}}$$

$$+ \frac{1}{\text{Thoracic cage compliance}}$$

TABLE 10-4.—MEAN RECOIL PRESSURE OF LUNGS
AND THORACIC CAGE*

% OF VITAL CAPACITY DURING TEST	RECOIL (RELAXATION) PRESSURE OF LUNGS + THORACIC CAGE (TORR)	RECOIL PRESSURE OF LUNGS ALONE (TORR)	RECOIL PRESSURE OF THORACIC CAGE ALONE (TORR)
20	−8	1.8	−9.8
40	4	5.0	−1.0
60	14	8.9	4.1
80	21	13.3	7.7
100	30	21.0	9.0

*From Knowles, J. H., Hong, S. K., and Rahn, H.: J. Appl. Physiol. 14:525, 1959.

Normal values for a healthy young man are approximately:

Total (lungs and thoracic cage)
  compliance   0.1 L/cm H_2O
Pulmonary compliance   0.2 L/cm H_2O
Thoracic cage compliance 0.2 L/cm H_2O

If the first 2 quantities are known, then

$$\frac{1}{0.1} = \frac{1}{0.2} + \frac{1}{x}$$

$$10 = 5 + \frac{1}{x}$$

$$x = 0.2$$

If a patient appears to be strenuously contracting his respiratory muscles, but his tidal volume is small, the hypoventilation could be due to airway obstruction, to decreased pulmonary compliance or to decreased compliance of his thoracic cage. Thoracic cage compliance may be decreased in all types of kyphoscoliosis (idiopathic, tuberculous and postpoliomyelitic), in scleroderma, in skeletal muscle diseases associated with spasticity or rigidity and in abdominal disorders characterized by marked elevation of the diaphragm (the diaphragm and attached abdominal viscera represent one component of the thoracic cage). It may also be decreased in patients with marked obesity ("Pickwickian" types).

Resistance to Air Flow

Physicists have developed laws that apply to air flow, but for the most part they apply to continuous, one-way flow of gas through rigid cylindrical tubes with a smooth lining and an unobstructed lumen. The real airways are heterogeneous. They start as the upper airways (nose, mouth, pharynx, larynx) that lead into the trachea. They then taper from a trachea of large diameter (18 mm) to terminal bronchioles of small diameter (0.7 mm); they are not rigid, but are distensible, extensible and compressible; they are not a single tube but a remarkable system of branching tubes that starts with a single tube and ends with several hundred thousand tubes (Table 10-5); the branching is not symmetrical and dichotomous but often irregular; the bore is not necessarily circular but in many instances wholly irregular (Fig. 10-21). The diameter of the lumen can change rapidly or slowly; it is subject to narrowing or widening because of changing pressure in or outside the tubes or by contraction or relaxation of bronchial and bronchiolar smooth muscle caused by nerve messages or chemical substances. Furthermore, the terminal airways (respiratory bronchioles and alveolar ducts) are part of the gas exchange system, and constriction of smooth muscle in them affects lung volume and compliance much more than it affects resistance to air flow. The lumen of many of the tubes may also become smaller because of (1) mucosal congestion, edema or inflammation; (2) plugging, partial or complete, of the lumen by mucus, edema, exudate or foreign bodies; (3) cohesion of mucosal surfaces by surface tension forces; (4) infiltration, compression or fibrosis; (5) compression or closure caused by increased intrapleural and decreased transpulmonary pressure, or (6) collapse or kinking of airways due to loss of the normal "widening" pull of pulmonary elastic tissue acting on the airway walls or to loss of structural, supporting tissues of the bronchial or bronchiolar walls ("weak walls").

There has been great interest in the past several years in the quantitative measurement of airway resistance and in the differential diagnosis of obstruction at different levels in the overall airway (alveolar duct versus bronchioles, small airways versus large) and in the mechanisms causing obstruction (compression versus closure versus constriction). This interest has coincided with the realization that some types of airway disease (obstruction of small airways) have gone unnoticed and undiagnosed and that others, such as emphysema, have been diagnosed for the most part only late in the course of disease. As a result, almost as many new tests have been devised as there are pulmonary physiologists (if we include variations in tests and in physiologists).

TABLE 10-5.—CLASSIFICATION AND DIMENSIONAL DATA FOR HUMAN AIRWAYS*†

BRANCHING ORDER NUMBER	COMMON NAME	NUMBER	DIAMETER (CM)	LENGTH (CM)	TOTAL CROSS-SECTIONAL AREA (CM²)	CUMULATIVE VOLUME (CM²)	DESCRIPTION AND COMMENTS
Upper Airways	Nose, mouth, pharynx, glottis						Volume estimate from several sources
Cartilaginous Airways							
0	Trachea	1	1.8	12.0	2.5	30	Main airway; partly in thorax
1	Main bronchi	2	1.22	4.8	2.3	42	First branching of airway; one to each lung
2	Lobar bronchi	4	0.83	1.9	2.1	46	Named for each lobe
3	Segmental bronchi	8	0.56	0.76	2.0	47	Named for radiographic and surgical anatomy
4	Subsegmental bronchi	16	0.45	1.27	2.5	51	Last order of named bronchi; also called medium-sized bronchi
5–10	Small bronchi		0.35–0.13‡	1.1–0.46	3.1–13	77	Decreasing amounts of cartilage; main source of variation in number of branchings. Beyond this level airways enter lobules as defined by elastic lobular limiting membrane
Membranous Airways							
11	Bronchioles	2,048	0.109	0.39	20	85	Unnamed. Major distinction is not size but absence of cartilage. Mucus-secreting elements and cilia decreasing in successive branches. Tightly embedded in connective tissue framework of lung. Are said to have relatively more smooth muscle than bronchi. Most authors designate 2–3 orders as terminal; except for name, they are identical with other membranous bronchioles
12	Bronchioles	4,096	0.095	0.33	29	95	
13	Bronchioles	8,192§	0.082	0.27	44	106	
14	Bronchioles	16,384§	0.074	0.23	69	123	
15	Terminal bronchioles	32,768	0.066	0.20	113	145	

16	Respiratory bronchioles		0.054	Bronchiolar epithelium present but decreasing with successive generations. Scattered small alveoli increasing in size and number peripherally
17	Respiratory bronchioles			
18	Respiratory bronchioles	262,144	0.047	No bronchiolar epithelium; no surface except connective tissue framework
19–23	Alveolar ducts		0.043	Former subgroup names (atria and alveolar sacs) have been dropped. Smooth muscle content of duct rings decreases rapidly after first order
Alveoli				
24	Alveoli	300×10^6	0.02	"... the ultimate respiratory chamber ..." Pulmonary capillaries form an extensive meshwork in the thin alveolar walls

*Modified from Staub, N.C., in Gray, T. C., and Nunn, J.F. (eds.): *General Anaesthesia* (3d ed.; London, Butterworth & Company, Ltd., 1971), vol. 1, chapter 5.

†Data on 5 human lungs fixed at about 75% TLC and treated by statistical sampling methods (Weibel and Gomez, 1962; Weibel, 1963).

‡Dimensions on this line are largest and smallest average values for branches.

§Estimates for dead space calculation purposes.

NOTE: If all branching were dichotomous and symmetrical, it would make no difference if the "order" of airways were numbered from trachea to alveoli or from alveoli to trachea. Since branching is not this orderly, Cumming and associates suggest that airways be numbered from alveolar ducts to respiratory bronchioles to trachea; such numbering permits assignment of the same order number to airways that have the same function.

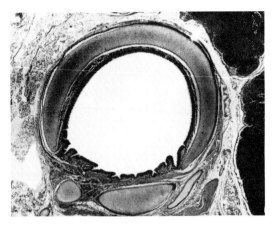

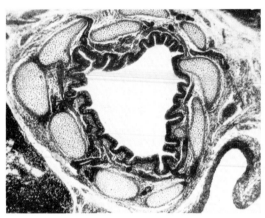

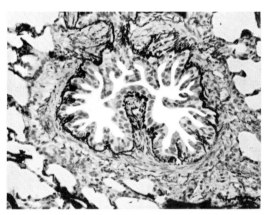

Fig. 10-21.—Histologic sections of large and small bronchi. **Top**, transverse section of extrapulmonary bronchus of adult cat. × 20. Note an almost complete ring of cartilage, as in the trachea. **Center**, transverse section of bronchus to left upper lobe of kitten. × 50. Note numerous discontinuous plaques of cartilage. (Both from Towers, B.: J. Anat. 87:337, 1953.) **Bottom**, transverse section of small, partly constricted bronchiole of rat. × 180. (Courtesy of Dr. S. Sorokin.)

Despite the complexity of the heterogeneous system we call the airways—or maybe because of it—we shall start with a discussion of physical laws that describe frictional resistance to flow in simple tubes.

Most of the work of the respiratory muscles during quiet breathing is used to overcome the elastic recoil of the lungs and thorax. Table 8-1 (p. 78) shows that a man breathing 15 times per minute uses 16,667 gm cm/min to expand the lungs and thorax and only 6,426 to overcome frictional resistance in the air and tissues. However, when respiration becomes rapid or when the air tubes are narrowed, much more work is required proportionately to overcome resistance to air flow.

Figure 10-22 illustrates the force necessary to overcome frictional resistance and to stretch elastic tissues. The upper part of this schema deals with a frictionless system in which work must be done only to stretch a spring (overcome elastic recoil); the graphs at the upper right show that there is a linear relationship between the force exerted and the distance moved. The lower part shows the relationship between force and distance when the force must also overcome frictional resistance; a greater force is necessary at every point *during motion* (*1* or *2*) to move the block equal distances.

If we substitute pressure for force, volume for distance and the lung for the spring, we find that during flow (when there is frictional resistance) the pressure to produce a unit increase in volume is greater than when there is no flow.

Figure 10-5 shows one respiratory cycle (this is schematic; actually expiration is longer than inspiration and flow patterns are not symmetrical sine waves). There are 3 points of zero air flow in this illustration: at the beginning of inspiration (*0*), at the end of inspiration (*3*) (flow is zero before going in the opposite direction), and at the end of expiration (*6*). At these three points, alveolar pressure equals atmospheric. During inspiration, intrapleural pressure would decrease linearly from −5 to −7.5 cm H_2O (along the straight

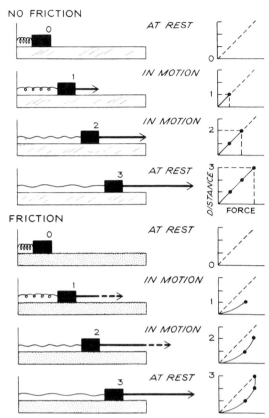

NO FRICTION

FRICTION

Fig. 10-22.—Force required to overcome elastic recoil and frictional resistance. *Solid arrow* shows the force required to move the block a certain distance when there is no friction and only elastic recoil must be overcome. *Dashed arrow* shows the additional force required to overcome frictional resistance, which is present only during motion. The graphs of force vs. distance are straight lines only when there is no frictional resistance. (Redrawn from Comroe, J. H., Jr., *et al.*: *The Lung* [2d ed.; Chicago: Year Book Medical Publishers, Inc., 1962].)

dashed line *1, 2, 3*) if there were no frictional resistance. Instead it is always *more* subatmospheric; it follows line *1', 2', 3* because of the extra pressure required to overcome frictional resistance. During expiration, the pressure is always greater (line *3, 4', 5', 6*) rather than *3, 4, 5, 6*, for the same reason.

PHYSICAL FACTORS DETERMINING RESISTANCE TO AIR FLOW IN RIGID TUBES. Resistance to air flow is determined by the same factors that govern the flow of fluid in tubes (see p. 153), since air at low rates of

flow behaves like a fluid of low viscosity. In 1846 Poiseuille, a French physician, made the first precise measurement of the pressure required to drive fluid through straight, rigid, smooth-bore cylindrical tubes. When flow is laminar or streamline (Fig. 10-23), he found that if the dimensions of the tubes remained the same, the driving pressure (P) to produce a certain flow (V) was directly proportional to the viscosity of the fluid (thus $P = K_1 V$, where K_1 is a constant that includes the influence of viscosity). When he changed the length and radius of the tubes, he found that the pressure to produce a given flow varied directly with the length of the tube and inversely with the *fourth* power of the radius. The radius of the tube is therefore of great importance in determining the resistance to flow: if the length of the tube is increased 4-fold, the pressure must be increased 4-fold to maintain constant flow, but if the radius of the tube is halved, the pressure must be increased 16-fold to maintain constant flow. Poiseuille put this in the form of an equation now known as *Poiseuille's law* for laminar flow (Fig. 10-24).

The physical laws governing resistance to flow in tubes in series and in parallel are similar to Ohm's law for flow of electricity. For resistances in series, add the separate resistances. For resistances in parallel, the reciprocal of the sum equals the sum of the reciprocals of the separate resistances (the reciprocal of R is $\frac{1}{R}$, and this is called *conductance*).

To calculate the total resistance for R_1, R_2 and R_3 in series, add $R_1 + R_2 + R_3$. To calculate the total resistance of R_4, R_5 and R_6 in parallel, add the reciprocals:

$$\frac{1}{R_{\text{total}}} = \frac{1}{R_4} + \frac{1}{R_5} + \frac{1}{R_6}$$

CALCULATION OF AIRWAY RESISTANCE USING OHM'S LAW. In electrical circuits,

$$R = \frac{EMF}{\text{Current}}$$

LAMINAR

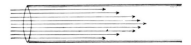

$$P = K_1 \dot{V}$$

TURBULENT

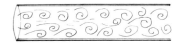

$$P = K_2 \dot{V}^2$$

TRACHEO–BRONCHIAL

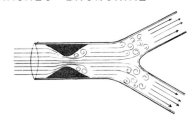

$$P = K_1 \dot{V} + K_2 \dot{V}^2$$

Fig. 10-23.—Types of air flow. Pressure required when flow is laminar or turbulent. The pressure required when air flow is turbulent (or when there are eddies) is considerably greater than when flow is laminar (streamline). For turbulent flow, the density of the gas becomes important and viscosity unimportant, and the pressure to produce a given flow varies with the *square* of the flow rather than directly; hence, $P = K_2 \dot{V}^2$, where K_2 is a constant that includes the influence of density. Flow changes from laminar to turbulent when the Reynolds number exceeds 2,000. (This is a dimensionless number equal to $\left(\dfrac{\text{Density} \times \text{velocity} \times \text{diameter}}{\text{viscosity}} \right)$.)

In smooth, straight tubes, turbulent flow occurs only at high velocities; these usually occur only in large tubes, such as the main bronchi and trachea, and only when there is hyperpnea. The flow rate in the fine tubes is very low because the total air flow is divided among hundreds of thousands of tubes. However, eddy formation may occur at each branching of the tracheobronchial tree, and the pressure required for eddy flow is approximately the same as for turbulent flow. Turbulence (at low flow rates) or eddy formation is particularly apt to occur when there are irregularities in the tubes, such as those caused by mucus, exudate, tumor or foreign bodies or partial closure of the glottis. Sometimes air flow is a combination of laminar and turbulent flow with eddy formation. When there is flow through a narrow orifice, the gas molecules must be accelerated, and this requires a pressure in proportion to the density of the gas and the square of its velocity. Torricelli's theorem applies: rate of discharge through the orifice is proportional to the area times the linear velocity of the fluid. (From Comroe, J. H., Jr., *et al.*: *The Lung* [2d ed.; Chicago: Year Book Medical Publishers, Inc., 1962].)

In fluid flow,

$$R = \frac{\text{Driving pressure}}{\text{Air flow}}$$

To calculate resistance, therefore, one must simultaneously measure the difference in pressure at the two ends of the system of tubes and the flow through the system. Thus,

Resistance across an endotracheal tube =

$$\frac{\text{Pressure at one end} - \text{pressure at the other}}{\text{Flow}}$$

Resistance across the nose =

$$\frac{\text{Atmospheric pressure} - \text{pressure in the nasopharynx}}{\text{Flow}}$$

POISEUILLE'S LAW $\Delta P = \dfrac{\dot{V}\,8\,\eta\,l}{\pi\,r^4}$

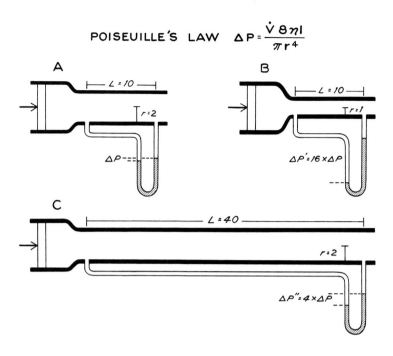

RESISTANCE TO FLOW IN BRONCHI A+B

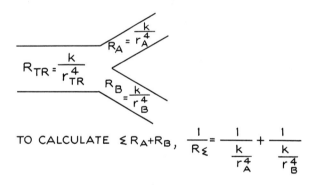

TO CALCULATE $\xi R_A + R_B$, $\dfrac{1}{R_\xi} = \dfrac{1}{\dfrac{k}{r_A^4}} + \dfrac{1}{\dfrac{k}{r_B^4}}$

Fig. 10-24. — Poiseuille's law. **Top,** during constant air flow, with the piston moving forward, ΔP is the pressure difference between the beginning and the end of the tube (dynes/cm²), $\dot{V}$ is the volume of flow (cm³/sec), l is the length of the tube (cm), n is the coefficient of viscosity in poises (dyne-sec/cm², for air the value is 1.9×10^{-4}) and r is the radius of the tube (cm). Since $\dfrac{\Delta P}{\dot{V}}$ = resistance, this equation can also be

written as: $\dfrac{\Delta P}{\dot{V}} = \text{resistance} = \dfrac{8nl}{\pi r^4}$

If $\dfrac{8n}{\pi}$ = a constant, resistance varies as l/r^4. In A, this equals 10/16; in B this is 10/1 (16 times as much); in (C) it is 40/16 (4 times as much). When air flow ($\dot{V}$) is the same, ΔP increases 16 times when the radius of the tube is halved, but only 4 times when the radius is unchanged but length is increased 4 times. (Modified from Fry, D. L., and Hyatt, R. E.: Am. J. Med. 29:672, 1960.)

Bottom, calculations of resistance to flow when a main airway (TR) divides into 2 equal branches, A and B. R = resistance; r = radius.

Resistance across the trachea =

$$\frac{\text{Pressure in the larynx} - \text{pressure at the bifurcation of the trachea}}{\text{Flow}}$$

Resistance across the entire airway =

$$\frac{\text{Mouth pressure} - \text{alveolar pressure}}{\text{Flow}}$$

MEASUREMENT OF AIRWAY RESISTANCE IN MAN. To measure resistance across the entire airway, one needs to measure only two variables—alveolar pressure and air flow (since mouth pressure is approximately atmospheric). Flow can be measured continuously using a pneumotachograph (which, incidentally, operates by measuring the very small pressure difference required for the subject's air to flow through a fixed low resistance screen). Alveolar pressure is the average pressure in the hundreds of millions of alveoli beyond the alveolar ducts. This is not the same as intrapleural (or esophageal) pressure because part of this is used to overcome the frictional resistance in the lung *tissues* themselves, in addition to overcoming the frictional resistance that is involved in the flow of air through tubes.

Pulmonary resistance =

$$\frac{\text{Mouth pressure} - \text{intrapleural pressure}}{\text{Flow}}$$

but this includes airway resistance plus pulmonary tissue resistance. In healthy persons, tissue resistance is about 20% of the total pulmonary resistance, and we could estimate airway resistance as 80% of pulmonary resistance. In patients with increased total resistance, we cannot assume that the tissues are normal and that all of the increase in resistance is in the airways. A more precise way is to use the body plethysmograph, which makes use of Boyle's law relating pressure and volume of gases to measure alveolar pressure directly during inspiration and expiration. The principle of the method is shown in Figure 10-25. The apparatus is widely used in clinical physiology laboratories, not only to measure airway resistance, but also to measure thoracic gas volume (p. 17) and pulmonary capillary blood flow (p. 145). Most of our knowledge of normal values and of changes due to physical, physiologic and

Fig. 10-25.—Schema showing principle of measuring airway resistance by means of a body box (plethysmograph). The patient (only the lung is pictured) is seated within the airtight box; pressure is measured continuously in the box around the patient. One would expect that inspiration of 500 ml of air from the box into the patient's lungs would produce no pressure fluctuations in the box (if precautions are taken to prevent changes due to changes in temperature and humidity of the respired gas); actually the box pressure rises during inspiration. This is simply because gas flows only from a point of higher pressure to a point of lower pressure. At the beginning of inspiration, muscular action has enlarged the thorax and lowered alveolar pressure below atmospheric pressure. Throughout inspiration, alveolar gas (previously at atmospheric pressure) is now at subatmospheric pressure and so occupies more volume; this is the same as adding this increment of gas volume (resulting from the decompression) to the plethysmograph, and so the pressure rises. The pressure change is registered by a very sensitive manometer. The reverse happens during expiration, when alveolar gas is compressed. From this measured pressure and appropriate calibrations, alveolar pressure can be calculated for any moment in the respiratory cycle. From these simultaneous measurements of alveolar pressure and flow (pneumotachograph), airway resistance can be determined.

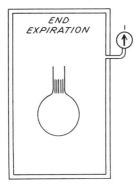
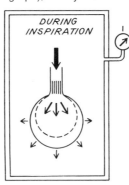
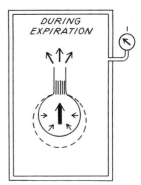

chemical factors has come from the use of this method. When measured by the body plethysmograph, airway resistance is $0.5 - 1.5$ cm $H_2O/(L/second)$ in adults. This measures the resistance when the patient is panting (rapid, shallow breaths) at a slightly greater than normal FRC.

PARTITIONING OF TOTAL AIRWAY RESISTANCE IN MAN. We can determine how much each of the different parts of the airways, from nose to alveolar ducts, contributes to total airway resistance by (1) measuring the dimensions of the airways and using Poiseuille's law, or (2) by measuring the pressure difference required for air flow across each part and then using Ohm's law.

1. Calculations using measured airway dimensions and Poiseuille's law. If we assume that viscosity remains constant, and if we calculate resistance per unit length, the equation in the legend of Figure 10-24 can be simplified to $R = \dfrac{k}{r^4}$ (where k is $\dfrac{8\eta l}{\pi}$). In Figure 10-24, resistance in the trachea is $\dfrac{k}{r_{TR}^4}$. The sum of the resistances in the two branches of the trachea, main bronchi A and B (parallel resistances), is calculated as

$$\frac{1}{R \text{ sum}} = \frac{1}{R_A} + \frac{1}{R_B}$$

$$\frac{1}{R \text{ sum}} = \frac{1}{k/r^4_A} + \frac{1}{k/r^4_B}$$

Using this equation, we learn that a parent tube may branch into two daughter tubes without increase in resistance if the sum of the cross-sectional areas of the two tubes is 1.4 that of the parent tube (this means that the radius of each is 0.85 that of the parent). If the sum of the cross-sectional areas of two branches is less than $1.4 \times$ that of the parent, the resistance to flow through the two daughter tubes increases. For resistance to remain the same, a general formula is that the sum of the cross-sectional areas of all the branches must be $\sqrt{n} \times$ the cross-sectional area of the parent tube, where n is the number of branches. If there are 4 branches, the area must increase 2-fold; if 9 branches, it must increase 3-fold. If a tube divides into branches and the sum of the cross-sectional area of the branches just equals that of the parent, the resistance to flow through a unit length of the two branches is double that through the parent tube. (These calculations take into account the halving of flow in each of the two branches compared to that in the parent branch.) Recently Horsfield and Cumming measured the diameter and length of *every* branch of a human lung from the trachea to tubes 700 μ in diameter and then of samples of the millions of tubes of smaller diameters; from these data, they calculated the contribution of each to total airway resistance.

2. Calculations using Ohm's law. To measure resistance to flow between the trachea and terminal bronchioles, one must measure simultaneously air flow and pressures in the lumen of the trachea and one or more representative terminal bronchioles. Similarly, one can measure resistance between the trachea and bronchi and across the nose, pharynx and larynx.

Methods 1 and 2 have both yielded the same answers: under the conditions of the measurements, only about 10% of the total resistance is in the small airways (< 2 mm in diameter), and most of it is in the nose or mouth (50%), glottis (25%) and trachea and bronchi (15%). Before these measurements were made, we intuitively equated bronchioles and their smooth muscle with arterioles and their smooth muscle and assumed the main resistance to air flow was in bronchioles, just as the main resistance to arterial blood flow is in arterioles; in fact, we must now equate bronchioles with capillaries, in which a large increase in cross-sectional area occurs and leads to a low-resistance segment.

PHYSICAL FACTORS INFLUENCING AIRWAY RESISTANCE IN MAN. In a rigid, smooth-bore, cylindrical straight tube, resistance per unit length of tube is constant because the physical dimensions of the tube do not change, regardless of changes in air pressure within the tube or external forces acting on the tube (Fig. 10-26). The real airways are different: they are distensible and compressible, and pressures within and without can change their physical dimensions and so

Fig. 10-26.—Rigid and collapsible tubes.

The upper 2 schemas show (1) the pressure drop along a rigid, constant bore tube due to frictional resistance and (2) failure of external pressure to influence dimensions of a rigid tube.

The 2 bottom diagrams (redrawn from Campbell, E. J. M., Martin, H. B., and Riley, R. L.: Bull. Johns Hopkins Hosp. 101:329, 1957) represent forced expiration from a normal lung with +2 cm H_2O elastic recoil and an emphysematous lung with +1 cm H_2O elastic recoil. *Circles* = alveoli; *tubes* = airways. *Numbers* refer to intrathoracic (in thorax but outside alveoli and airways), recoil (pressure associated with *arrow*) and airway pressures (cm H_2O). Airways tend to become narrow when lung elastic recoil is diminished; the resulting pressure drop decreases transmural airway pressure and favors collapse of compliant airways. The actual distribution of pressure drop in the airways varies from patient to patient depending on the site of compression, constriction or obstruction. See text.

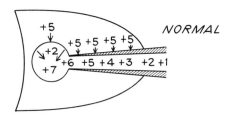

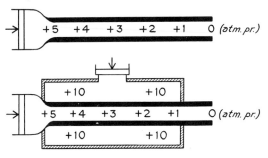

NORMAL

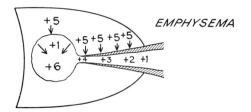

EMPHYSEMA

alter resistance to flow through them; further, pressures that determine transmural airway pressure differ in different parts of the thorax, and compliance (change in dimensions/unit change in transmural pressure) varies from the top to the bottom of the airway.

1. Transmural pressure. Transmural pressure = (pressure within airways) − (pressure surrounding airways). The pressure surrounding the intrathoracic airways is close to intrapleural pressure. Because of gravitational forces, intrapleural pressure in a standing man is about 7.5 cm H_2O higher at the bases than at the apex,[3] and since the effect of gravity on the column of air in airways is very small, gravitational forces result in a higher transmural pressure at the apices than at the bases. This widens airways at the apices relative to those at the bases and in erect man can close airways at the bases while they are still open at the apices. Figure 10-27 shows that if man expires to residual volume, transmural airway pressure at the apices may be +4.5 cm H_2O (airways open) while at the bases, it is −3.0 cm H_2O (airways closed). An inspiration that begins at residual volume and lowers intrapleural pressure 3 cm H_2O everywhere will direct all or most of the inspired gas into the apices (airways open) and none or little into the bases (airways closed); this has been demonstrated experimentally when man has expired to residual volume and then inspired first a bolus of radioactive gas and then room air. This observation is the basis of the "closing volume" test (see p. 136).

Because of gravitational forces, alveoli at the apices contain more air at end-expiration than alveoli at the bases. If the next inspiration begins at FRC (instead of at residual volume), alveoli at the bases receive more

---

[3]Some factors that contribute to this difference are (1) weight of the lung, (2) effects of gravity on the chest wall, (3) support of lung tissue produced by the lung hilum and the abdominal contents and (4) modification of the distribution of these effects by the interdependence of elements of the elastic meshwork of lung tissue.

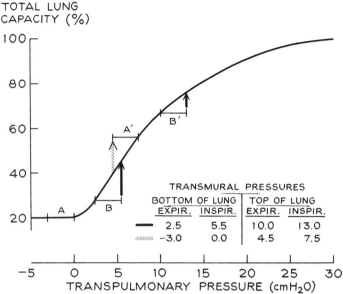

Fig. 10-27.—Transpulmonary pressures at the top and bottom of the lung at several lung volumes. When man, beginning at residual volume (*hatched line and arrow*), lowers pressure by 3 cm H_2O throughout the pleural space and raises transpulmonary pressure by 3 cm H_2O throughout the lung, alveoli at his bases (*A*) receive no inspired gas, but alveoli at his apices (*A'*) do. When man, beginning near FRC (*solid line and arrows*), lowers intrapleural pressure by 3 cm H_2O, more gas enters alveoli at bases (*B*) than at apices (*B'*) because of shape of pressure-volume (compliance) curve. The table shows transmural pressures at the bottom and top of the lung in expiration and inspiration (in each case, the change is 3 cm H_2O) and the differences in transmural pressures between the bottom and top of the lung (in each case the difference is 7.5 cm H_2O).

air than those at the apices (see Fig. 10-27); this is because compliance of the lung is *nonlinear* and alveoli operating in the lower transmural pressure range receive more volume than those at a higher pressure. This is another means of increasing the differences in composition of gases at the apices and bases and is used clinically to demonstrate "closing volume."

2. Compliance, distensibility or compressibility of airways. The compliance of each segment of the airways depends on its structural support. The trachea has almost complete rings of cartilage that prevent complete obstruction (though the lumen can be narrowed if the membranous part is pushed into it [see Fig. 18-1]). The bronchi have incomplete rings or plates of cartilage connected with strong fibrous tissue (see Fig. 10-21). Bronchioles have no supporting cartilage but may become less compliant when their smooth muscle is contracted. Bronchi and

bronchioles altered by disease may be either more or less compliant than healthy airways, and the alteration may be regional or patchy.

3. Dynamic changes during inspiration and expiration. During inspiration, intrapleural pressure becomes more subatmospheric, and this increases transmural airway pressure; airways widen and airway resistance decreases. Further, the walls of the alveoli and airways are part of a 3-dimensional elastic mesh that extends throughout the lung tissue and is anchored at one end to the walls of the airways and at the other to the visceral pleura; during inspiration, the expanding thorax pulls on the lung and on this elastic mesh and elongates and widens the airways. There is little change in airway resistance with quiet inspiration and expiration, probably because the airways become longer as well as wider. A *maximal* inspiration decreases resistance measurably and can, at least temporarily, overcome airway narrowing; part of this is mechanical and part is a reflex widening of bronchioles.

During expiration, particularly forced expiration, some airways are dynamically compressed. The mechanism is illustrated in Figure 10-26. Air flows from alveoli to the nose and mouth because alveolar pressure is greater than atmospheric. Alveolar air pressure comes in part from the positive intrapleural pressure generated by maximal forced expiratory effort. (During inspiration intrapleural pressure is always subatmospheric; during a passive expiration, it is still subatmospheric [see Fig. 10-5], but during a rapid, forced expiration, it becomes positive because maximal effort of expiratory muscles compresses air in alveoli and alveolar ducts faster than air can enter airways and leave the lungs.) In the normal lung pictured in Figure 10-26, alveolar pressure is +7 cm H_2O; 2 of the 7 come from elastic recoil of alveoli, and the other 5 from the positive intrapleural pressure generated by the expiratory effort. The pressure within the airway decreases from +7 to atmospheric. During expiration, transmural pressure becomes negative for portions of intrathoracic airways nearest the trachea, and these are compressed according to their stiffness, rigidity or compliance. (Extrathoracic airways, of course, are not affected by the positive intrapleural pressure and are not compressed.) Intrathoracic airways that have lost their structural support as a result of disease (e.g., emphysema) collapse with less pressure difference. Wright has shown that in patients with emphysema even large bronchi may lose their structural support and act like thin cellophane tubes that open widely during inspiration (when transmural pressure is positive) but collapse readily during rapid expiration (when transmural pressure becomes negative). Narrowing of airways by disease (if the disease does not make them structurally more rigid) favors airway collapse during forced expiration because the pressure drop in narrowed tubes decreases transmural airway pressure downstream to the narrowed portion. In a rigid tube, generating higher pressure always increases flow, but in airways within the thorax, generating higher pressure (by increasing muscular effort) can reduce air flow.

PHYSIOLOGIC FACTORS INFLUENCING AIRWAY RESISTANCE. *Nervous regulation.* This is effected through sympathetic and parasympathetic nerves to smooth muscle. Airways contain smooth muscle all the way from the trachea to the alveoli. In the trachea there are smooth muscle fibers that can narrow it (the rings of cartilage are not complete) and longitudinal bands that can shorten it. The bronchi have plaques of cartilage rather than incomplete rings; constriction of smooth muscle can both decrease the lumen and shorten the bronchi. Bronchioles, terminal bronchioles and alveolar ducts have much more smooth muscle (both circular and longitudinal) relative to the diameter of the lumen; smooth muscle constriction in them can produce almost complete obstruction. The alveolar walls do not contain smooth muscle, but the openings leading from the alveolar ducts to the alveoli are ringed with sphincter-like smooth muscle.

Smooth muscle down to the alveolar ducts is supplied with efferent autonomic nerve fibers and is subject to reflex contraction and dilatation (Fig. 10-28). Sympathetic nerve impulses relax, and parasympathetic impulses contract, airway smooth muscle. It is not known whether the sympathetic postganglionic fibers act mainly on receptors, on smooth muscle or, as in the gut, by inhibiting parasympathetic ganglion cells and so decreasing tonic excitatory impulses to the airway.

These airways are constricted reflexly by inhalation of smoke, dust and chemical irritants (acting on subepithelial receptors responsible for initiating the cough reflex), by arterial hypoxemia (acting through carotid, and possibly aortic, body reflexes), by increase in arterial blood P_{CO_2} (probably through an action on medullary receptors), by cold and by emboli lodging in certain

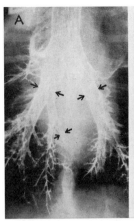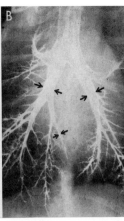

Fig. 10-28.—Effect of vagal stimulation on caliber of airways in dog. **A**, tantalum bronchogram showing diameter of large and small airways. **B**, same airways during electrical stimulation of vagus nerves. The 3 pairs of arrows in each bronchogram indicate the width of the same airways. (Courtesy of Dr. J. A. Nadel.)

parts of the pulmonary circulation. They also constrict reflexly in response to histamine injected into their arterial circulation or that liberated locally by the antigen-antibody reaction or anaphylaxis. The reflex may be initiated by contraction of smooth muscle, by histamine, which in turn excites mechanoreceptors connected to afferent fibers in the vagus nerves, or by a direct action of histamine on sensory receptors in the airway. They are dilated reflexly during deep inspiration and by increase in systemic arterial blood pressure (acting through the carotid sinus). Widdicombe has proposed that there may be continuous regulation of bronchiolar tone to provide the most desirable combination of airway resistance and anatomic dead space; increase in tone lessens dead space, which is desirable, but increases resistance to flow and the work of breathing, which is undesirable.

Chemical regulation. We have already mentioned that chemicals (histamine, increased CO_2 or low O_2) can constrict airways via reflexes. Some drugs and chemicals also affect bronchiolar smooth muscle by stimulating autonomic ganglia, by liberating postganglionic mediators, by stimulating or blocking the receptor sites for postganglionic fibers, or by a direct action unrelated to nerve fibers or their receptors. Isoproterenol, epinephrine and norepinephrine (in order of decreasing potency) stimulate the receptor sites associated with sympathetic postganglionic fibers and cause bronchodilation. Acetylcholine, acting at parasympathetic receptor sites, causes bronchoconstriction, as do anticholinesterase agents, which block the enzyme cholinesterase and permit the accumulation of stimulant concentrations of acetylcholine. Drugs, such as propranolol, that block sympathetic β-adrenoreceptors, cause constriction; atropine, by blocking the effects of postganglionic parasympathetic impulses, reduces or abolishes reflex constriction of airways.

Stimulation of nerves to the airways appears not to affect smooth muscle in the alveolar ducts, nor does local injection of neurohumoral transmitters. However, the alveolar duct sphincters can constrict and do so independently of the bronchiolar smooth muscle. Contraction of these pulls in the alveolar ducts, flattens the alveoli and expels air from the lung, reducing lung volume (Figs. 10-29 and 10-30, *C*), and lung compliance without appreciably increasing airway resistance or decreasing anatomic dead space (the alveolar ducts are part of the gas-exchange system, not of the conducting tubes). Constriction of the terminal bronchioles (Fig. 10-30, *B*), on the other hand, increases airway resistance, decreases anatomic dead space and increases lung volume (because of greater difficulty in expiration).

The action of chemicals on smooth muscle in bronchi and bronchioles can be separated from that in alveolar ducts by intra-arterial injection. Substances injected into the bronchial arteries normally go to bronchioles and bronchi and not to alveolar ducts; substances injected into the pulmonary artery go to alveoli, alveolar ducts and respiratory bronchioles, but not to bronchioles or bronchi. Histamine injected into the pulmonary artery causes marked constriction of the alveolar

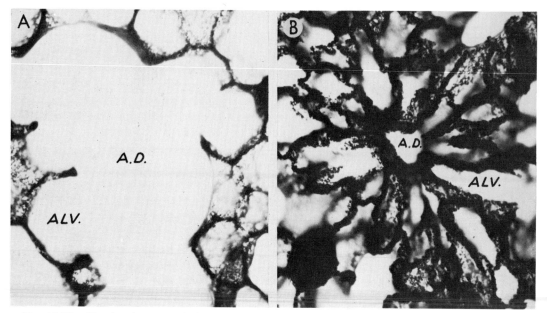

Fig. 10-29.—Alveolar duct constriction. **A**, normal alveoli (*Alv.*) and alveolar duct (*A.D.*). **B**, similar alveoli and ducts after constriction by histamine injected into the pulmonary artery. Similar constriction follows injection of fine emboli of barium sulfate and is presumably due to local liberation of histamine from mast cells. The magnification is the same in both sections of cat lungs. (From Nadel, J. A., Colebatch, H. J. H., and Olsen, C. R.: J. Appl. Physiol. 19:387, 1964.)

Fig. 10-30.—Constriction of bronchiole and of alveolar duct. **A**, the pulmonary artery of the cat supplies the respiratory bronchiole (*RB*), the alveolar duct (*AD*) and the alveoli. The bronchial artery supplies the bronchi, bronchioles and terminal bronchioles. Smooth muscle is present in the bronchioles and in the alveolar ducts (*black ovals*). **B**, stimulation of vagal bronchoconstrictor fibers narrows the bronchioles, increases airway resistance, decreases anatomic dead space, but enlarges the alveoli (*broken lines* show original volume) and the FRC. **C**, contraction of smooth muscle in alveolar ducts decreases alveolar volume and FRC but produces little change in anatomic dead space, bronchiolar size and resistance to air flow. (From Nadel, J. A., Colebatch, H. J. H., and Olsen, C. R.: J. Appl. Physiol. 19:387, 1964.)

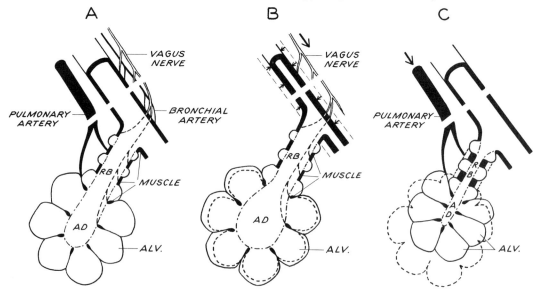

duct sphincters. Microemboli injected into the pulmonary circulation liberate histamine, which in turn causes alveolar duct closure, as pictured in Figure 10-29. When a large artery such as the right or left pulmonary artery is occluded, bronchoconstriction also occurs, but the mechanism is different.

When pulmonary blood flow to one lung stops and alveolar ventilation continues, alveolar gas P_{CO_2} decreases to very low levels (the alveolar CO_2 comes from the mixed venous blood normally flowing through the pulmonary capillaries); this causes constriction of alveolar ducts in the lung whose pulmonary blood flow has stopped. This mechanism shifts ventilation from alveoli with no pulmonary capillary blood flow to those with blood flow and so decreases hyperpnea and prevents a great increase in the work of breathing. The response is initiated by a decrease in alveolar gas P_{CO_2}, since it does not occur if one pulmonary artery is occluded while the gas supplied to that lung is $3-5\%$ CO_2 in air. It is a local response, for it is not abolished by cutting possible nervous pathways. This mechanism may be an important one to insure the proper matching of the supply of air and the supply of mixed venous blood to the alveoli and alveolar capillaries (see Chapter 13).

TYPES OF AIRWAY OBSTRUCTION AND THEIR DIAGNOSIS. Because airway obstruction is a central problem in several of the serious, chronic diseases of the lungs such as emphysema, bronchitis and asthma, it is important to detect early stages of obstructive airway disease, measure the obstruction precisely and determine its response to therapy before disease has become extensive or irreversible.

Vital capacity was the first pulmonary function test available to physicians. However, vital capacity can be normal when a patient with airway obstruction performs the vital capacity test *slowly*. Because repeated, rapid forced breathing accentuates the effect of airway obstruction, the vital capacity test was replaced by a test of maximal voluntary ventilation (maximal breathing capacity); in this test, the patient breathes as deeply and as quickly as he can for $15-20$ seconds, and the expired volume is collected and measured. The test has several disadvantages: it is tiring, even exhausting, for some patients, and it is nonspecific — it measures many factors all at once, including activity of the respiratory centers, motor nerves, respiratory muscles, thoracic and pulmonary compliance, airway and tissue resistance and lung volume. Its main advantage is that, when results are normal, it indicates that all overall mechanical factors are normal.

The maximal breathing capacity test in turn was replaced by tests requiring only one forced maximal breath. Figure 10-31 shows the basic features of one such test. The patient inspires slowly but maximally, then expires as fast and as completely as he can into a spirometer that has minimal resistance and inertia and then inspires as fast and as fully as he can. Movements of the spirometer are recorded on rapidly moving paper. From the record, one can measure the maximal expiratory flow rate in L/second for the early part of the breath (inset A) or the middle part (inset D). Or one can measure the forced expired volume as a percent of actual or predicted vital capacity in 1 second (FEV_1) or 3 seconds (FEV_3) (B and C). One can also determine whether there is obstruction to inspiration. Such a test is simple, inexpensive, does not tire the patient, is easy to repeat and provides a written record of the patient's performance. But, although it is an ideal office procedure to detect moderate to advanced airway obstruction (Fig. 10-32), it is not sensitive enough to uncover early stages of disease.

The use of the body plethysmograph permits specific measurement of airway resistance and does not require forced single or repeated expiration. However, it cannot, as usually employed, detect early obstruction of small airways because these are responsible for only a small fraction of total airway resistance.

For these reasons, physiologists have

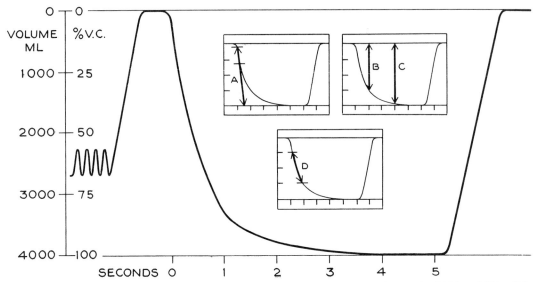

Fig 10-31.—Maximal expiratory and inspiratory flow rates. A subject (vital capacity (*V.C.*) = 4,000 ml) is asked to inspire maximally and then to expire as fully and as rapidly as he can. Then, beginning at full expiration, he is asked to inspire as fully and as rapidly as he can. His expired and inspired volumes are recorded on rapidly moving paper. Note the long tail at the end of the expiratory but not the inspiratory effort. Measurement of maximal flow is used as a clinical test to detect obstructive pulmonary disease. There are many ways of measuring the curve. *A* illustrates "maximal expiratory flow rate" measured as L/min for the first liter of expired gas (after the first 200 ml). *B* and *C* are forced expiratory volumes expired in 1 sec and 3 sec, usually expressed as % of *V.C.* (FEV$_1$ and FEV$_3$). *D* is maximal midexpiratory flow rate (measured as L/min in the middle 50% of the expired volume).

modified present technics and devised new ones (1) to detect obstructive disease in its early stages and (2) to try to determine which airways are obstructed (upper airways, trachea, large bronchi, small airways, alveolar ducts) and by what mechanism (thickening, loss of structural support, constriction, loss of elastic recoil of alveoli). A

brief description of some of these methods follows:

1. Isovolume pressure-flow curves. Airway diameter is a function of the volume of the lung; it is normally greater at large lung volumes and less at small lung volumes. In the conventional tests using forced expira-

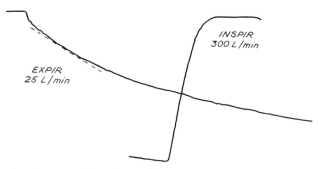

Fig. 10-32.—Maximal expiratory and inspiratory flow rates in a patient with emphysema. This, like Figure 10-31, is a curve of volume (ordinate) vs. time (abscissa); flow rate at any point can be calculated from a tangent to the slope (see *dashed line*). In some patients with emphysema the maximal *expiratory* flow rate may be 25 L/minute or less (normal = 400–600 L/minute), but the maximal *inspiratory* flow rates are near normal. The airways close during forced expiration but open during inspiration.

tion, the patient's lung volume changes at every moment during the expiration, and so does his driving pressure. Neither is measured or recorded. Fry and Hyatt decided to measure maximal flow rates at known lung volumes and known driving pressures. (Driving pressure for expired airflow is alveolar pressure minus mouth pressure; unless the lips are pursed to create an obstruction, mouth pressure = atmospheric pressure, and therefore driving pressure is simply alveolar pressure.) To do this, they measured simultaneously air flow, lung volume and changes in intrathoracic pressure (using an esophageal balloon). A subject, beginning at full inspiration, breathes out slowly to residual volume. He then repeats the maneuver a number of times, breathing out more rapidly and vigorously each time, until finally he breathes out as rapidly and forcefully as he can. Each recorded curve contains values for pressure and flow at each lung volume between full inspiration and full expiration, and the records as a whole contain values for low to high flow and low to high driving pressure at any lung volume. New curves can now be plotted showing the effect of increasing driving pressure on flow when the lung volume is the same, e.g., at near-maximal inspired volume, and at 80%, 60%, 40%, 20% above RV (residual volume) (Fig. 10-33). They are, therefore, *isovolume* curves.

The curves show that when a healthy man increases his effort and driving pressure more and more when his lung is 70–95% inflated, his air flow increases more and more, but when his lung volume is smaller, air flow reaches a maximum despite increasing driving pressure. Since at this time flow remains constant, resistance to air flow must be increasing in direct proportion to the increase in driving pressure (since resistance = *driving pressure*/flow). This change in resistance is due to dynamic compression of the airways. Figure 10-26 shows that when intrathoracic pressure rises during expiration to +5 cm H_2O, at some point along intrathoracic airways, pressure outside the airway exceeds air pressure within the airway

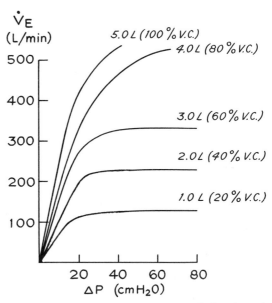

Fig. 10-33.—Pressure-flow curves during forced expiration. Curves are plotted from a series of increasingly vigorous forced expirations (such as those in Figs. 10-31 and 10-32). Pressures and the flows corresponding to them are measured at the same lung volumes (e.g., 20, 40, 60 or 80% of V.C.) for each expiration. Curves show that at lower lung volumes increasing effort and driving pressure do not increase flow progressively—a maximum (plateau) is reached. $\dot{V}_E$ = air flow in L/minute: ΔP = driving pressure during expiration in cm H_2O. (Redrawn from Pride, N. B., *et al.*: J. Appl. Physiol. 23:646–662, 1967.)

(i.e., transmural airway pressure becomes negative); this is because pressure *in* the airway decreases owing to resistance to flow and pressure *outside* the airway does not. However, this small negative transmural pressure does not collapse cartilagenous airways because of their low compliance. Figure 10-34 shows that when the expiratory effort is *greater* and the intrathoracic pressure rises to 25 cm H_2O, the negative transmural airway pressure can now be 15 or 20 cm H_2O, again because air pressure within the tubes decreases along the intrathoracic airways but intrathoracic pressure does not. Dynamic compression can now occur and increase resistance to air flow. The increase in resistance that just matches the increase in driving pressure (as it must if flow reaches a plateau and

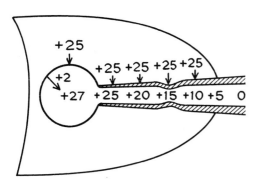

Fig. 10-34.—Dynamic compression of airways during forced expiration. *Circle*=alveoli. *Tube* connected to circle=airways. *Numbers* refer to intrathoracic pressure (in the thorax, but outside the alveoli and airways); recoil pressure (*number associated with arrow*); alveolar pressure (intrathoracic + recoil pressure) and airway pressure, all in cm H_2O. As expiratory effort increases and intrapleural pressure becomes more positive (e.g., 25 cm H_2O), transmural airway pressure becomes more negative because airway pressure must always drop to atmospheric at the nose and mouth. An increase in intrathoracic pressure from +5 cm H_2O (as in Fig 10-26) to 25 cm H_2O (as in this figure) changes the lowest transmural airway pressure from, say, −2 cm H_2O to about −15 cm H_2O. This does not occur in a static, closed system, i.e., if the glottis is closed.

stays there) may be due to more and more narrowing of a small segment of the airway or to increase in length of the narrowed segment.

2. Flow-volume curves. This is a simplification of the previous procedure in that it eliminates the measurement of intrapleural pressure. The subject inspires maximally and then breathes slowly to his residual volume. He then repeats the maneuver several times

(as for the isovolume pressure-flow curves), each time with increasing vigor, until finally he expires with maximal speed and force. During each expiration, air flow and expired volume are measured and plotted against each other. A spirometer is used that provides 2 signals during expiration—one for expired volume and one for instantaneous flow. (The ordinary expired *volume* versus *time* record [see Figs. 10-31 and 10-32] could be used, but this would require calculating instantaneous air flow from slopes of tangents to the curve at many points and replotting the data.)

There are a number of important features of this curve: During the first 20% of the expired volume, the maximal rate of air flow is dependent on the effort generated by the subject. This means that during exhalation of the first 20% of the total expired volume, the harder the subject tries, the greater the flow rate he achieves. Once he has exhaled the first 20% of the vital capacity, however, the flow rate during the remaining portion of the vital capacity is independent of his effort but dependent on lung elastic recoil and airway dimensions. At this point all curves converge onto the heavy outer envelope (Fig. 10-35); this envelope represents the maximal expired air flow at each lung volume, and therefore takes into consideration the change in diameter of airways that normally occurs with changing lung volume.

Two variables determine this flow-volume envelope: (1) elastic recoil pressure generated by the lung at that lung volume; if there

Fig. 10-35.—Maximal expiratory flow-volume curves. The *dotted curves* represent curves produced by progressively increasing effort of a normal subject; note that all four converge onto one down curve ("outer envelope"). In subjects with emphysema, curves of intermediate effort are omitted. See text. (From Murray, J. F., *et al.*, Calif. Med. 116:37–55, 1972.)

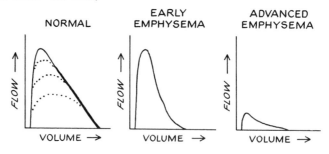

is less elastic recoil, maximal expiratory flow rate is lower; (2) dimensions of the airways; if they are abnormally narrow, maximal respiratory flow rate is lower.

Since this test does not require use of an esophageal balloon to measure intrapleural pressure, it is suitable as a test to screen populations for early obstructive airway disease. It is easy to repeat and can be used to follow the course of disease, treated or untreated. Examination of the curves permits evaluation of abnormalities throughout all of expiration; the information obtained cannot, however, be expressed by a single number.

Figure 10-35 illustrates the changes in flow-volume curve expected in a patient with advanced emphysema and in one with early emphysema. In the advanced stage of the disease, the decided loss in lung elastic recoil at all lung volumes greatly decreases the driving pressure for air flow and also allows intrapleural pressure to be less negative (i.e., closer to atmospheric). For these reasons transmural airway pressure is less and airways are narrower. This results in a decrease in maximal expiratory flow rates at all lung volumes. At an earlier stage of this disease, the changes in flow-volume curves are slightly more complex. At high lung volumes, the recoil characteristics of the lung are virtually normal because the more compliant emphysematous regions fill first, and normal regions, less compliant, fill later. At high lung volumes, driving pressure and airway dimensions are normal so that initial maximal flow rates are likely to be within the normal range. At low lung volumes, on the other hand, the normal regions have already emptied and the areas with high compliance are now emptying. At this point, elastic recoil is less and maximal expiratory flow is decreased, both because of the reduction in driving pressure and the narrowing of the airways.

3. Airway resistance-lung volume curves. Using the body plethysmograph (p. 124), it is easy to measure airway resistance. However, because the small airways contribute so little to overall airway resistance (see p. 125), they must be greatly narrowed to in-

crease overall airway resistance so that it is outside the normal range. Measurement of airway resistance provides more useful data when it is made at several known lung volumes (Fig. 10-36). Normally, airway resistance does not change greatly with large increases in lung volume between functional residual capacity and full lung inflation, but resistance does increase considerably when lung volume is decreased below functional residual capacity toward residual volume. Therefore, the nearer to his residual volume the patient breathes, the more the airways are narrowed and the greater the increase in airway resistance. It is possible to have airway obstruction without primary airway disease if lung elastic recoil is lost. Under these circumstances, the negative pressure in the pleural space at a given lung volume is less (closer to atmospheric) than in the normal chest. As a result, the intrathoracic airways are subjected to a smaller distending pressure and, consequently, the airways of the emphysematous lung are narrower than those of a normal lung at the same volume. Because a lung with little elastic recoil has less support for the intrathoracic airways, airways narrow prematurely at a relatively large lung volume; concurrently, airway resistance increases prematurely as lung volume decreases.

A patient with early emphysema has an

Fig. 10-36.—Airway resistance at different lung volumes in normal man and abnormal (emphysematous) patient whose lungs have diminished elastic recoil. (From Murray, J. F., et al., Calif. Med. 116: 37–55, 1972.)

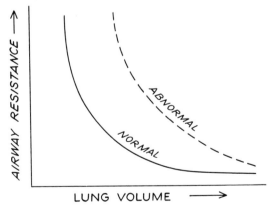

abnormal pressure-volume curve only at low lung volumes, and therefore his resistance-volume curve will be abnormal primarily at low lung volumes; in fact, the airway resistance might be perfectly normal at functional residual capacity or any higher lung volume. Although this measurement is easier to perform than that of lung elastic recoil, it does require cooperation on the part of the patient. Many patients with obstructive airway disease find it particularly difficult to breathe at low lung volumes because of the great increase in resistance to air flow.

4. Functional residual capacity, compliance and specific compliance. When obstruction involves alveolar ducts, it does not appreciably affect airway resistance, because alveolar ducts are essentially parts of the gas exchange system. Contraction of smooth muscle in alveolar ducts reduces alveolar gas volume (FRC) and decreases lung compliance (though specific lung compliance remains normal).

5. Distribution of inspired gas. We learned earlier (p. 125) that the branching of small bronchi into bronchioles is accompanied by a decrease in resistance to air flow, just as branching of arterioles into capillaries is accompanied by a decrease in resistance to blood flow. Since small airways account for only 10% of total airway resistance, tripling resistance in small airways (diameter less than 2 mm) increases resistance of the total airway only 20% (assuming that each category of branching tubes is a resistance in series with the others); therefore, total airway resistance may still be in the normal range and a slight increase be unnoticed. A 10-fold increase in resistance of small airways does not quite double total airway resistance. If small airways with a radius of 1.0 mm constrict to half of that, resistance to flow through these airways increases 16-fold, and the resistance of the total airway increases to 250% of normal. For these reasons, it is useful to try other means of detecting relatively small changes in airway resistance. If small airways narrow more in some regions of the lung than in others, even though overall air resistance does not increase appreciably, distribution of ventilation to alveoli should become uneven, and a sensitive test of uneven distribution of gas may indicate the presence of obstruction of small airways earlier than tests of airway resistance. (See p. 124.)

6. Frequency dependence of value for lung compliance. As stated earlier, in normal lungs, values for compliance remain the same even when the frequency of breathing increases up to 90/minute. When airway obstruction is present, the value measured under static conditions decreases when measured during breathing, especially at high frequency. This measurement requires time, meticulous attention to detail and exactly matched frequency response characteristics of the flow and pressure measuring systems. It also entails considerable patient cooperation and discomfort. It is unsuitable for routine measurements. Further, the compliance of ventilated lung units (as I have defined it on p. 101) is not necessarily decreased, and if not, the test is misleading to those unaware of the careless terminology used; perhaps the word "distensibility" should be used here and "compliance" reserved for its precise meaning.

7. "Closing" volume. When normal man expires fully to residual volume, airways in the dependent lung regions tend to close because of the high intrapleural pressure there, at a time when airways to upper lobes are still open, because intrapleural pressure is about 7.5 cm lower there (see Fig. 10-27). Patients whose lungs have less elastic recoil, whose airways have lost structural supporting tissue or whose airways are narrowed, develop widespread airway collapse and trapping when they breathe between residual volume and functional residual capacity, or even at higher volumes. This trapping can often be detected by procedures deliberately designed to create a different composition of gas in the upper and lower lobes. Because airways to his lower (dependent) lobes are closed when an erect patient has breathed to his residual volume, the first gas entering his lungs on his next inspiration will go preferentially to his upper lobes (Fig. 10-37). (This has been shown for radioactive gases, using external counters.) If the first gas inspired is a foreign gas, such as ^{133}Xe, argon or helium, his upper lobes will have a much higher concentration of it than his lower lobes. On the succeeding expiration, the lung volume at which airways in his lower lobes begin to close will be marked by a sudden rise in concentration of the foreign gas in expired gas, since it is no longer diluted by gas from his lower lobes. The least expensive and simplest way to accomplish this is to use the original "sandwich" technic of Fowler. Ask the patient to breathe out to residual volume and arrange the next inspiration so that the patient first draws into his alveoli his dead-space gas followed by *air* (this goes mainly to his upper lobes and maintains a high N_2 concentration there) and then O_2 (this goes preferentially to his lower lobes and decreases the N_2 concentration there). The concentration of N_2 in the expired gas can then be measured continuously using an N_2 meter (see Figs. 10-37 and 13-1). The vol-

ume of the lungs above residual volume at which this change in expired N_2 concentration occurs is called the "closing" volume; the *total* volume of gas in his lungs at this point is the "closing" capacity. When the volume is high (e.g., "closing" capacity is greater than FRC), presumably airways have closed long before normal airways do, in relation to lung volume. The "closing" volume increases with age between 20 and 80 years, but decreases between 20 and 6 years of age. A high "closing" volume may be an early sign of disease of small airways; it can be high when the conventional test of uneven distribution of gas (see Fig. 13-1) is normal.

8. *Other diagnostic tests.* When obstruction is completely and rapidly reversed by therapy, the obstruction must have been due to smooth muscle constriction, mucosal congestion or edema, or plugging of the lumen. Rapid reversal cannot occur when there is organic narrowing of the lumen (as in peribronchiolar fibrosis) or destruction of tissues resulting in a check valve (as in obstructive emphysema). Relief of obstruction by isoproterenol, which is both bronchodila-

Fig. 10-37.—"Closing" volume measured using nitrogen meter. Before the expiration recorded here, the patient had breathed to residual volume, then inspired some air (which, when inspiration starts at residual volume, goes preferentially to upper lobes) and then O_2 (which at FRC goes preferentially to lower lobes—see Fig. 10-27). With his lungs now maximally inflated (TLC), he expires evenly and fully. A rising N_2 concentration toward the end of expiration indicates that most of the gas is coming from the N_2-rich upper lobes and little or none from the N_2-poor lower lobes. In this case, the change in expired N_2 concentration (once the dead space was washed out—see Fig. 13-1) occurs when there is still 2,000 ml of gas in the lungs (800 ml above a residual volume of 1,200 ml).

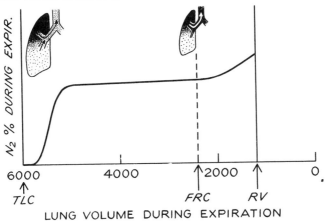

LUNG VOLUME DURING EXPIRATION

tor and vasodilator, suggests that smooth muscle constriction is the mechanism responsible for the obstruction; relief following use of a powerful vasoconstrictor, such as norepinephrine administered as an aerosol, would indicate that vascular congestion is of critical importance.

Airways appear to be obstructed, even though normal, when the respiratory muscles are weak or paralyzed. To learn whether low flow rates are due to weak muscular action, one can determine the maximal force that the respiratory muscles are capable of exerting by measuring the maximal oral or intraesophageal pressures developed during forced expiration.

EFFECTS OF INCREASED AIRWAY RESISTANCE. *1. Effect on FRC and residual volume.* A normal expiration is passive and is complete in less than 3 seconds. If airway resistance increases abruptly during expiration (as at the beginning of an asthmatic attack) and expiration is completely passive, expiration will not be complete in only 3 seconds. This means that the FRC will be greater at the beginning of the next inspiration.

If more time is permitted for expiration, the chest will return to the original resting expiratory level (Fig. 10-38). If the obstruction is very severe, the time for complete expiration would be so long that the respiratory frequency and alveolar ventilation would be reduced. There are two other possibilities: (1) A patient may expire actively rather than passively and so increase the pressure differential available for air flow; this has the disadvantage of tiring the patient and of causing dynamic compression of airways and trapping of gas. (2) As the FRC increases (because the time available is not enough for complete expiration), the elastic force at end-inspiration increases, because this varies directly with the volume of the lung. This increases the pressure available for expiration so that expiration is completed in the time available and inspiratory and expiratory tidal volumes again become equal. Further obstruction will lead to a further increase in FRC and elastic force until a new

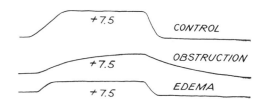

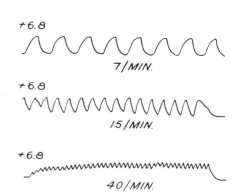

Fig. 10-38.—Airway obstruction and increased FRC. **Top,** change in lung volume during prolonged inflation at constant pressure (7.5 cm H_2O). At the end of the inflation period, the lung is allowed to deflate without any added resistance to expiration. Note the slow inflation (with no plateau during the time allowed) and slow deflation during obstruction (bronchoconstriction induced by a drug). When pulmonary congestion and edema were produced by large intravenous infusions of saline, compliance was greatly reduced (probably owing to reduction in the number of air-filled alveoli), but inflation and deflation were rapid. **Bottom,** effect of changing respiratory frequency from 7 to 15 to 40/minute in an anesthetized cat with bronchoconstriction. (Pressure during inflation is +6.8 cm H_2O in all tracings.) At rapid rates, all of the air entering the lung cannot leave during the time allowed for expiration, and the lungs become hyperinflated (FRC increases).

balance is reached. Figure 10-38 illustrates the increase in a cat's resting expiratory level and in its FRC when the rate of artificial ventilation was increased from 15 to 40 breaths/minute during induced bronchoconstriction.

An increase in FRC is also a disadvantage because the thorax is always larger than normal; because of this abnormal position, some muscular inefficiency and mechanical disadvantage may result. Certainly, a great enlargement of the FRC must lead to a reduction in inspiratory capacity (if the total lung capacity is not enlarged), and this usually limits a patient's ability to increase his ventilation on demand. The anatomic dead space is also larger when the lungs are hyperinflated.

Asthmatic patients usually have a large FRC during periods of airway obstruction, and this returns to normal when vigorous antiasthmatic therapy restores the airway resistance to normal. The lungs of such patients are *hyperinflated* but not necessarily altered structurally. Patients with emphysema have similar or more severe expiratory obstruction and a large FRC, but in them the condition is not reversible because of structural damage to the lungs, which includes loss (or alteration) of elastic tissue, breakdown of alveolar walls, a diminished pulmonary capillary bed and sometimes a loss of supporting tissue in small to medium-sized bronchi.

Patients with severe pulmonary emphysema often present a more serious mechanical problem when anesthetized. They normally achieve expiration in the time available by active contraction of their expiratory muscles; under general anesthesia, expiration becomes passive and can be accomplished only by the recoil of elastic fibers stretched during inspiration.

2. Dyspnea. A normal resting subject in whom bronchial obstruction is induced experimentally by inhalation of histamine or irritant aerosols does not experience any respiratory symptoms until airway resistance is increased 3-fold or more. Severe dyspnea may not result until airway resistance is increased 5–15-fold. It is obvious, then, that patients may have abnormally high airway resistance without any symptoms. Sensitive pulmonary function tests can detect this obstruction and point the way for therapy of disease when it is still mild and may respond better to treatment.

3. Effect on the frequency of breathing. Because resistance increases with the velocity of flow, patients with airway obstruction generally breathe slowly.

Tissue Resistances

In addition to the frictional resistance caused by the flow of gas molecules through the airways, there is frictional resistance in displacement of the tissues of the lungs, rib cage, diaphragm and abdominal contents. Like airway resistance, tissue resistance occurs only during motion, is dependent on the velocity of motion and is a factor during both inspiration and expiration. It is zero also at end-inspiration and end-expiration. The greater the amount of elastic force dissipated in overcoming frictional resistance in the *tissues* during expiration, the less is the elastic force available for overcoming *airway* resistance. When the force available for causing air flow is reduced, expiration is slowed.

Before specific methods for measuring airway resistance were developed, *pulmonary resistance* (which includes two components: *airway* and *pulmonary tissue* resistance) was often used synonymously with *airway* resistance. Tissue resistance cannot be measured independently. However, if *pulmonary* resistance (which is the sum of airway resistance and tissue resistance) and *airway* resistance (body plethysmograph method) are measured simultaneously, pulmonary *tissue* resistance can be calculated.

Pulmonary *tissue* resistance in healthy young men is about 20% of the total *pulmonary* resistance, the remainder being *airway* resistance. Tissue resistance is often increased with pulmonary sarcoidosis, pulmonary fibrosis, diffuse carcinomatosis, asthma and kyphoscoliosis. It is rarely increased to the extent of being an important or limiting resistance.

No measurements of thoracic cage resistance have been made in patients with thoracic disorders, but this may be very great in patients with severe mechanical limitation to movement of the muscles or joints of the thorax, unless breathing is purely diaphragmatic.

Cohesion. In certain abnormal conditions, such as atelectasis or collapse of the lung during thoracic surgery, the surfaces of the smaller air ducts are held together by surface tension forces (cohesion). In such cases, another factor opposes inspiration, because no air movement occurs until an opening pressure has been built up in the airways.

Attempts to overcome atelectasis by high endotracheal pressure are hazardous if some of the airways are open, since the high pressure results in distention of their alveoli and may lead to alveolar rupture. In thoracic surgery, once a lung has been permitted to collapse to "minimal volume," the surfaces of the airways are likely to stick together by cohesion. Probably because of this phenomenon, positive pressure applied to the nose and mouth will inflate only the lung in the closed hemithorax, even though the compliance of a lung and its hemithorax is less than for the lung alone (on the open side). Once this opening pressure is exceeded, the lung on the open side will receive more ventilation than the other.

Inertia. The inertia of the lungs-thorax system is so small that it can be neglected.

The Work of Breathing

In Chapter 8 (p. 78) we discussed regulatory mechanisms that might operate to maintain proper alveolar ventilation with the minimal expenditure of energy by the respiratory muscles.

Work, in the physical sense, is force × distance or pressure × volume. The cumulative product of *pressure* and the *volume* of air moved at each instant is equal to *work* ($W = \int PdV$). If one knew the mechanical work done and the O_2 consumed by the respiratory muscles in doing this work, the efficiency of ventilation could be calculated as follows:

$$\text{Efficiency } (\%) = \frac{\text{Useful work}}{\text{Total energy used}} \times 100.$$

Work of moving only the lungs. This is calculated from records of transpulmonary pressure (Fig. 10-39, *4 − 2*) and volume during breathing. During inflation or deflation of the lungs, the amount of pressure required at any one time depends not only on the pressure to overcome elastic recoil but also on the pressure to maintain movement of air through the airways and movement of the tissues of the lungs. The greater the *rate* of volume change (volume flow/minute), the greater is the pressure used in overcoming friction.

Work of moving the lungs and thoracic cage. This is normally done by the muscles of respiration. It is difficult to estimate by direct means. However, if a patient is no longer breathing spontaneously, as a result of poliomyelitis, deep anesthesia or the injection of drugs that produce neuromuscular block, his ventilation can be maintained by a body respirator.[4] This permits measurements of the work required for normal pulmonary ventilation because, under these conditions, the lungs, thorax and gas are moved by the respirator. It is easy to measure the transthoracic pressure (Fig. 10-39, *4 − 1*) and the volume, and hence easy to measure the work of the body respirator. The respirator must be doing the amount of work that would have been done by the respiratory muscles under these conditions. The normal value is 0.5 kg-m/minute during rest. The work of breathing increases disproportionately as the minute volume increases and reaches a maximum of about 250 kg-m/minute when a subject breathes maximally (about 200 L/minute).

The O_2 consumption of the respiratory muscles. The O_2 consumed by the respiratory muscles in a healthy person is normally such a small fraction of the total body metabolism that it is difficult to measure. It does become measurable as the O_2 cost of addi-

---

[4]Attempts have also been made to measure the work of breathing in subjects who have been instructed to relax voluntarily all the muscles of respiration while they lie in the respirator; it is not certain, however, that such voluntary relaxation is complete.

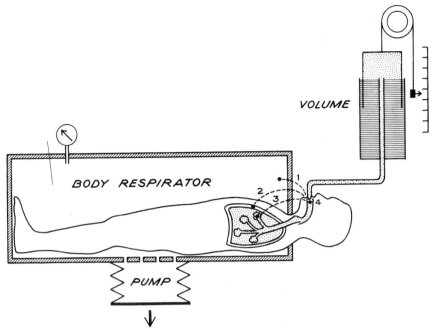

Fig. 10-39.—The work of breathing. A nonbreathing man lies wholly within a body respirator except for his head. On inspiration, the pump (bellows) decreases pressure in the respirator to less than atmospheric, and air at atmospheric pressure enters the man's lungs from the spirometer. On expiration, pressure in the respirator returns to atmospheric, and the unopposed elastic recoil of the lungs-chest cage system produces expiration. Volume of inspired and expired gas and pressure are measured continuously. Pressure 1 = respirator pressure; 2 = intrathoracic (esophageal) pressure; 3 = alveolar pressure, and 4 = mouth pressure. Work = $\int P \, dV$. To calculate work against airway resistance use $4-3$; for work against airway resistance plus tissue resistance plus elastic recoil of lungs, use $4-2$; for total work (including that to move chest cage), use $4-1$.

tional ventilation during maximal voluntary ventilation or when the patient is made to breathe through a known, added resistance. From such measurements and other data, it has been calculated that the mechanical efficiency of the respiratory muscles is low (5 – 10%), so that 10 to 20 times the O_2 is required to perform the mechanical work as would be needed to provide a similar amount of heat energy. It is likely that the respiratory muscles of many patients with cardiopulmonary disease do more work and require more O_2 than those of resting subjects. These muscles hypertrophy, as do other skeletal and cardiac muscles when made to do more work for long periods. To date, a few studies have indicated that the O_2 cost of additional ventilation (above the resting level) is greater than normal in patients with emphysema and in obese patients.

11

The Pulmonary Circulation

THE LUNG has two circulations—a very large pulmonary and a very small bronchial circulation. The pulmonary arteries bring mixed venous blood to the alveolar capillaries; the bronchial arteries supply well-oxygenated blood from the systemic circulation to the tracheobronchial tree.

The main function of the pulmonary circulation is to collect venous blood from all parts of the body and pump it through the alveolar capillaries (where O_2 is added and CO_2 is removed) and on to the left atrium and ventricle for distribution, now as arterial blood, to all organs and tissues. The pulmonary circulation, like the systemic, consists of a reservoir, a pump, a distributing system, an exchange system and a collecting system (Fig. 11-1). The reservoir, the right atrium, accepts venous blood returning to the heart. The pump, the right ventricle, distributes this to the gas exchange vessels through a vast system of low-resistance tubes (Table 11-1).

The exchange system, the capillary bed, is the functional part of the pulmonary circulation. The anatomist defines pulmonary capillaries morphologically; the pulmonary physiologist defines them as vessels that participate in rapid gas exchange. The physiologist, therefore, may include as capillaries vessels that are anatomically pre- and postcapillary; their walls are far thinner than those of similar vessels in the systemic circulation and, although not capillaries, they may permit rapid gas exchange. When Staub almost instantaneously froze the lungs of animals breathing O_2, he found bright red, well-oxygenated blood in pulmonary arterioles with diameters up to 50 μ; these of course contain mixed venous blood that should have a low O_2 content.

The pulmonary capillary bed is a remarkable structure. Normally, at any single moment, it contains only 75 – 100 ml of blood, but this is spread out in a multitude of thin-walled vessels (0.1 μ thick), which have a surface area estimated at 70 m², or 40 times the body surface area. The capillaries in the pulmonary alveoli are so short and so closely knit that some consider that blood in them does not flow in conventional capillary tubes but rather between two sheets of endothelial tissue, held apart by supports of connective tissue (as automobiles might run between pillars in a vast parking garage).

Although the volume of blood in the capillaries is small, the total pulmonary circulation contains 10 times as much. Most of this is in the collecting system, which consists of thin-walled, compliant pulmonary venules and veins that act as a capacitance or a second blood reservoir to back up the left atrium; constriction of smooth muscle in the veins can contract this reservoir and increase the circulating blood volume relative to the internal volume of the vessels.

The pulmonary circulation is sometimes called the "lesser" circulation. Certainly it is not "lesser" in blood flow, since more blood flows through it than through any other organ—indeed, the blood flow though the pul-

142

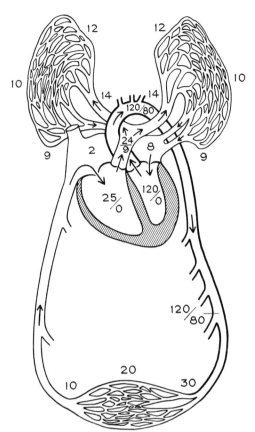

Fig. 11-1.—Blood pressures in the pulmonary and systemic circulations.

normally far less than in the systemic circulation; but even this is not always so, for the pulmonary arterial pressure is quite high in the healthy fetus because of the greater resistance to flow through the fetal pulmonary circulation. Although this pressure decreases to adult levels several weeks after birth, it can return to high levels again in certain circumstances.

The systemic arterial circulation to the lungs is largely through the bronchial arteries, which are branches of the thoracic aorta. They supply blood to the walls of the tracheobronchial tree down to and including the terminal bronchioles, the supporting tissues and nerves in the lung and the outer coats of the pulmonary arteries and veins. Under normal conditions, however, they do not supply arterial blood to the walls of the alveoli, the alveolar ducts and the respiratory bronchioles; these receive pulmonary arterial blood through the alveolar capillaries (see Fig. 1-3 and Fig. 10-30), and the composition of blood flowing to all alveoli is the same.

The pressure in the bronchial arteries is only slightly less than aortic pressure so that, regardless of whether man is erect or supine, it is high enough to supply blood to bronchi, bronchioles and supporting tissue everywhere in the lungs. Although bronchial flow per minute is only 1–2% of pulmonary blood flow, this is appropriate to the mass of the lung that it nourishes (about 475 gm).

When there is a block in the pulmonary circulation to a lung, caused by pulmonary artery ligation, stenosis, thrombosis or embolism, the bronchial arteries enlarge and manage to develop connections with precapillary vessels in the pulmonary circuit. When this occurs, (1) the composition of blood flowing through all alveolar capillaries is no longer the same and (2) blood flowing from bronchial arteries through alveolar capillaries takes up little or no O_2 from alveolar gas (since this blood is arterial and already well oxygenated), but it can still give off CO_2. Much more important is the fact that it brings substrates to the tissues of the alveoli

monary circulation is approximately equal to the combined blood flow through all other organs and tissues. The term "lesser" circulation *is* true most of the time for pressure and resistance, since values for these are

TABLE 11-1.—PULMONARY VESSELS OF A DOG*

PULMONARY VESSEL	No.	DIAMETER (MM)	CROSS-SECTIONAL AREA (MM²)
Pulmonary artery	1	15.5	181
R and L pulmonary artery branches	2	11.5	208
Lobar arteries	8	5.96	223
3d order arteries	1,021	1.0	801
Capillaries	600,000,000	0.007	23,000
3d order veins	1,021	1.22	1,194
Lobar veins	8	6.12	290
Pulmonary veins	4	13.75	756

*From Knisely, W. H., in Abramson, D. I. (ed.): *Blood Vessels and Lymphatics* (New York: Academic Press, 1962), p. 296.

and alveolar ducts, removes waste products of metabolism and so keeps these tissues alive when their pulmonary blood flow is shut off.

Surgeons have occasionally found it necessary in an emergency to tie off one pulmonary artery but still leave the lung in place in the thorax. A year or two later the tissues in these lungs appeared to be healthy and to ventilate normally, though the lungs did not, of course, remove any O_2 from alveolar gas. The surgeons concluded that the pulmonary capillaries were not essential for survival of pulmonary tissues. However, if one experimentally ligates the pulmonary artery to one lung of a dog and examines that lung 24, 48 or 72 hours later, the lung is far from healthy; it is atelectatic, congested and poorly ventilated. This suggests that blood flow through alveolar capillaries is indeed essential for nutrition of the alveoli and alveolar ducts. When such a lung is allowed to remain in the thorax, ventilation improves, and in several weeks the atelectasis and congestion vanish. Since the time required for recovery of the lung is about the same as that needed for the bronchial circulation to establish precapillary connections with the alveolar capillaries, it is a reasonable assumption that the bronchial circulation, by enlargement of existing channels or growth of new vessels, comes to the rescue of tissues normally dependent on the pulmonary circulation for their nutrition. It cannot, however, help the lung oxygenate blood except in patients whose arterial blood, and therefore bronchial arterial blood, is not well oxygenated; the rationale of the classic Blalock-Taussig operation for relief of arterial hypoxemia in babies with tetralogy of Fallot (in which some venous blood bypasses the lungs and goes directly from the right to the left side of the heart) was to send systemic arterial blood directly into the pulmonary artery to improve oxygenation.

Some of the blood flowing though bronchial arteries and capillaries enters systemic veins (such as the azygos) and then goes to the pulmonary circulation for arterialization; some, however, enters pulmonary veins and then flows into the left atrium and ventricle. This is an absolute shunt (see p. 174). Some blood flowing through the coronary arteries also returns directly to the left heart without further oxygenation in the lungs; this also represents an absolute shunt. Because of these shunts, left ventricular output is slightly larger than right ventricular output, and the Po_2 of arterial blood is a little less than its optimal value (see Chapter 13).

VOLUME OF PULMONARY BLOOD FLOW

Four different types of measurements are important.

1. MEASUREMENT OF TOTAL AMOUNT OF BLOOD FLOWING EVERY MINUTE THROUGH THE PULMONARY CIRCULATION. Unless there are pathologic shunts in the circulation, this is approximately equal to left ventricular or cardiac output per minute. Pulmonary blood flow can be calculated by measuring the uptake of a moderately soluble inert gas inhaled into the alveoli at a known concentration, by indicator-dilution methods or by application of the direct Fick principle. The Fick principle states that, in a steady condition, the O_2 removed from the blood by all the tissues of the body each minute is replaced by the same amount of O_2 added to mixed venous blood flowing through the lungs. If one measures O_2 consumption of the body/minute (O_2 removal), this equals O_2 added each minute to mixed venous blood. If one also measures O_2 added to each liter of mixed venous blood (arterial blood O_2 concentration minus mixed venous blood O_2 concentration), one can calculate liters of cardiac output/minute by the equation:

$$\text{Blood flow (L/minute)} = \frac{O_2 \text{ uptake (ml/minute)}}{\text{A-V difference for } O_2 \text{ (ml/L)}}$$

2. MEASUREMENT OF BLOOD FLOW THROUGH THE PULMONARY CAPILLARIES. Figure 11-2 shows schematically how to do

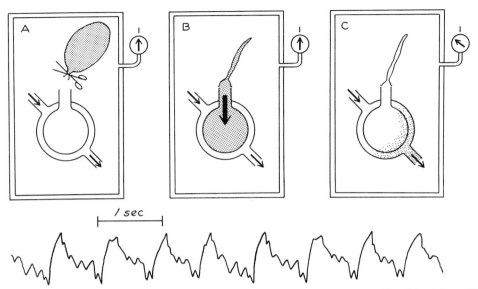

Fig. 11-2.—Body box (plethysmograph) method for measuring pulmonary capillary blood flow. The patient (represented by a schematic lung and pulmonary circulation) sits in an airtight chamber about the size of a telephone booth (**A**). Pressure about the subject is measured continuously by a sensitive electrical manometer (*circled arrow*). On request, the patient inhales 80% N_2O–20% O_2 from a bag into his alveoli (**B**); as N_2O (*black dots*) leaves the gas phase to dissolve in blood flowing through the pulmonary capillaries (**C**), the total gas pressure in the chamber decreases because when *dissolved*, N_2O molecules no longer occupy space, and this decrease is registered continuously by the manometer. Knowing alveolar N_2O pressure, solubility of N_2O in blood and alveolar volume (also measured plethysmographically), one can calculate pulmonary capillary blood flow instant by instant throughout the cardiac cycle, and the pulsatile nature of the capillary volume pulse can be recorded; see tracing. (Redrawn from Comroe, J. H., Jr., *et al.*: *The Lung* [2d ed.; Chicago: Year Book Medical Publishers, Inc., 1962].)

this using a body plethysmograph. Note that the blood flows in pulses into and through the pulmonary capillaries, not as a steady stream. We are accustomed to think that flow through capillaries in all organs is steady and continuous because it is steady in systemic capillaries that are easy to watch under a microscope. But a capillary pulse occurs even there when the pulse pressure (systolic minus diastolic) is very great (as in aortic regurgitation) or the arterioles are widely dilated (as in hyperthyroidism). In the pulmonary circulation, the arteriolar resistance is normally low and the pulmonary artery pulse is transmitted to the capillary blood; indeed, the absence of pulsatile flow may indicate the existence of abnormal pulmonary arteriolar resistance. Pulsatile flow provides more time for gas exchange if the right ventricular stroke volume is less than the volume of the capillary bed. If the stroke volume exceeds the capillary volume, some blood may rush through the capillaries and have less time for gas exchange.

3. MEASUREMENT OF DISTRIBUTION OF PULMONARY BLOOD FLOW TO ALL REGIONS OF BOTH LUNGS. Figure 1-7 shows that the pulmonary vessels ramify to reach all parts of the lung. In a recumbent healthy man, pulmonary blood flow is distributed evenly to all regions. In erect man and in patients with pulmonary disease, distribution is not even. The physician can detect regions of the lung receiving little or no blood by using [133]xenon. This is first dissolved in saline and injected intravenously or into the right atrium. When blood containing [133]xenon passes through alveolar capillaries, it gives off its xenon because this gas is sparingly soluble in blood. By means of external detectors placed on the thorax, or better, by a scin-

tillation camera, one can determine areas of the lung that contain no radioactive gas and therefore have no pulmonary blood flow to ventilated alveoli (see Fig 13-7).

Another way to detect regions of the lung with no pulmonary blood flow is to inject radioactive particles small enough to pass through small arteries but large enough to lodge in pulmonary arterioles. Since the particles go only where blood goes, their presence indicates regions that have pulmonary blood flow, and their absence points to regions that have none. It seems dangerous to block blood vessels deliberately, but only a very few blood vessels need to be occluded in this test and the material used, macroaggregates of albumen, is broken up in a few hours, leaving the arterioles patent again.

4. MEASUREMENT OF THE AMOUNT OF MIXED VENOUS BLOOD SHUNTED AROUND THE ALVEOLAR CAPILLARIES TO ENTER THE SYSTEMIC CIRCULATION WITHOUT FURTHER OXYGENATION. This is discussed in Chapter 13.

Regulation of Pulmonary Blood Flow

The pulmonary blood flow of resting man is about 5.4 L/minute (or 3.2 L/minute/m² of body surface). During exercise, it can increase to as much as 30–40 L/minute. Since pulmonary blood flow or right ventricular output must equal left ventricular output except for very brief periods, it is necessary that the same mechanisms control both right and left ventricular output. Therefore, the pump for the pulmonary circulation behaves very much like the systemic pump. Its beat is slowed by parasympathetic stimulation and accelerated by sympathetic stimulation. It obeys Starling's law of the heart, just as does the left ventricle. This means that, when more blood returns to the right ventricle, it stretches the ventricle more; this increases its energy of contraction, and the ventricle expels more blood. Or if the ventricle cannot empty normally during systole because of increased resistance to flow between the

pulmonic valve and the left ventricle, the normal diastolic filling added to the increased residual blood in the right ventricle stretches it more and allows it to develop a higher pressure during the next systole. The right ventricle also responds to the same chemicals and drugs (acetylcholine, norepinephrine, isoproterenol, digitalis, etc.) that affect the left ventricle. It would be remarkable if this were not so, because different rates and outputs of the two ventricles could not be tolerated for long.

PRESSURES IN THE PULMONARY CIRCULATION

It is well to distinguish three different types of pressures:

1. ABSOLUTE INTRAVASCULAR PRESSURE is the actual blood pressure in the lumen of any vessel at any point, relative to atmospheric pressure.

2. TRANSMURAL PRESSURE is the difference between the pressure in the lumen of a vessel and that of the tissue around it; the transmural pressure is positive when pressure inside the vessel exceeds that outside and negative when pressure inside is less than surrounding pressure. A positive transmural pressure tends to distend the vessel (according to its compliance; see p. 101), just as transmural airway pressure distends the airways (p. 126). A greater pressure in the tissue around a vessel tends to compress or collapse it. The pressure around the pulmonary arteries and veins is the intrathoracic pressure, since these vessels are wholly within the thorax but outside the lung. The pressure around the smaller intrapulmonary vessels (arterioles, capillaries and venules) is difficult to measure because it is neither the air pressure in the alveoli nor the intrapleural pressure, but a pressure in between.

3. DRIVING PRESSURE is the difference between pressures at one point in a vessel and at another point downstream. This is the pressure that overcomes frictional resistance

and is responsible for blood flow between these two points. In a rigid pipe a driving pressure of 10 mm Hg will produce the same fluid flow regardless of whether the pressures at the two points are 25 and 15 or 15 and 5. However, in a distensible vessel the flow will be greater at the higher pressures because the greater transmural pressure widens a distensible vessel and so decreases frictional resistance to flow.

The driving pressure for the total pulmonary circulation is the difference between the pressure at the beginning of the pulmonary circulation (the pulmonary artery) and that at the other end of the pulmonary circulation (the left atrium), except when blood flow is blocked within the lung. It is obvious that when a cuff around an arm is inflated sufficiently to stop blood flow through the brachial artery, tissue pressure around the artery (and not arterial or venous pressure beyond the cuff) limits blood flow. Similarly in the lungs, when alveolar gas pressure regionally or throughout the lungs exceeds alveolar capillary blood pressure enough to close the capillaries, alveolar pressure and not left atrial pressure is the factor that limits blood flow. The same is true for partly blocked vessels, since the reduced flow through them is essentially running into a sink (the veins) that does not limit flow.

What is the normal value for pressure in the pulmonary circulation? There is no *single* value for the pulmonary circulation any more than there is a single value for the systemic circulation. One can, however, measure pressure at several important points. One can place catheters in the main pulmonary artery, the right and left pulmonary artery branches, the pulmonary veins and the left atrium and measure pressure at these specific points. It is not possible to measure intracapillary pressure directly, and there are no precise values for this pressure. But since blood flows from the pulmonary arterioles through the capillaries to the pulmonary venules, the capillary pressure must be less than arteriolar and higher than venular pressure. Since resistance to flow through the

veins into the left atrium is very low, left atrial pressure (which can be measured in man by transbronchial or transseptal puncture) is very close to pulmonary capillary pressure if there is no venous or venular constriction. "Capillary" pressure is sometimes estimated by wedging a cardiac catheter as far as it can go into the finest branch of the pulmonary arterial system and measuring the pressure there; this pressure is approximately equal to pulmonary venous pressure if there is no venular obstruction.

Absolute intravascular pressures in the pulmonary circulation of an adult are pictured in Figure 11-1. Normally, the right ventricle develops a pressure of about 25 mm Hg during its systole, and this is transmitted to the pulmonary arteries. When systole ends, right ventricular pressure falls to atmospheric (zero), but since the pulmonic valves are now closed, pulmonary artery pressure decreases gradually during diastole to a low of about 9 mm Hg as blood flows through the pulmonary arterioles and capillaries; mean pulmonary artery pressure (the average of individual pressures at each instant in systole and diastole) is about 14 mm Hg. Since mean left atrial pressure is about 8 mm Hg, pressure in the arterioles and capillaries must fall from 14 to about 9 mm Hg.

It is important to remember that if there is a high resistance to flow through the arteries or arterioles, pressure can be very high in the pulmonary artery and normal in the pulmonary capillaries. And pressure can be dangerously high in pulmonary capillaries without being dangerously high in the pulmonary arteries. These statements need explanation. There are two main threats from high pressure in the pulmonary circulation. One is that the right ventricle may fail. In a patient with primary pulmonary hypertension, the mean pulmonary artery pressure may be 90 mm Hg (equal to or greater than mean systemic arterial pressure), pulmonary capillary pressure may be normal (13 – 9 mm Hg) because of arteriolar obstruction and left atrial pressure normal (8 mm Hg). The transmural capillary pressure is normal and there is no danger of pulmonary edema, but the high mean pulmonary artery pressure imposes a very heavy work load on the right ventricle and leads to right ventricular strain, hypertrophy and possibly failure. An increased right ventricular pressure does not mean that the right ventricle *must* fail, however, any more than left ventricular failure necessarily follows systemic arterial hypertension. After all, right ventricular pressure and pulmonary arterial pressure are normally high in the fetus and newborn; the muscle of the right ventricle is thick, but it does not fail. However, beyond infancy failure is more likely with a high pressure than if pressure remained normal.

The other threat is pulmonary edema. When transmural capillary pressure exceeds transmural colloidal osmotic pressure (osmotic pressure of plasma proteins minus that of proteins in the interstitial space surrounding the capillaries), the forces favoring filtration or fluid from capillary blood to tissues are greater than those favoring absorption of fluid from tissue to capillary blood. The result is pulmonary edema, which leads to impaired gas exchange, obstruction of airways and uneven ventilation in relation to alveolar blood flow; if it is severe and widespread, death results. For example, in a patient with mitral stenosis and obstruction to flow between the left atrium and left ventricle, the left atrial pressure may rise to 21 mm Hg; as a result, the capillary pressure may now be 26–22 mm Hg and the mean pulmonary artery pressure 30 mm Hg. The increased transmural capillary pressure is high enough to produce pulmonary edema, although the right ventricular pressure is only moderately increased—certainly not to the point of ventricular failure.

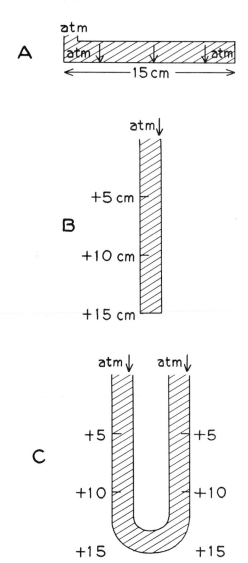

Fig. 11-3.—Effect of gravity on fluid in horizontal and vertical tubes. (See text)

Effect of Gravity on Pulmonary Vascular Pressures

If a horizontal rigid tube, open at one end to atmospheric pressure, is filled with water (Fig. 11-3, *A*), pressure at every point along the tube is atmospheric. The weight of the fluid acting in a vertical direction will increase the pressure at the bottom of the tube, but if the tube has a narrow bore, this effect is small. If a similar tube is now put into a vertical position (Fig. 11-3, *B*), the pressure at the top is still atmospheric, but 1 cm below the top it is 1 cm H_2O greater than atmospheric because of the weight of the column of water; 2 cm below the top the pressure is 2 cm, and 15 cm below (at the bottom of the tube) it is 15 cm H_2O greater than atmospheric. If a fluid-filled, rigid U-tube (each limb 15 cm long) is placed in a horizontal plane and open at one end to atmospheric pressure, the pressure at any point in each limb will again be atmospheric; however, when it is put in a vertical position, the pressure in each limb will be atmospheric only at the top of each limb and 15 cm H_2O at the bottom of each (Fig. 11-3, *C*).

Let us now apply a pressure to one limb of the U-tube by attaching to it a reservoir filled with water to a height of 20 cm (Fig. 11-4, *left*). If we keep the system static by clamping the outlet tube, the pressure at every level in the limbs of the U-tube will now be 20 cm H_2O greater, i.e., the pressure at the top of each will be 20 instead of atmospheric and at the bottom will be 35 instead of 15 cm H_2O. Note that although gravitational forces increase the *absolute* pressure from top to bottom of each vertical tube, they do not create a *difference* in the pressure measured at the same level in the two tubes. Therefore they create no driving pressure in a U-tube.

So far we have discussed only static systems. Let us now consider the same system when fluid is flowing (Fig. 11-4, *left*). To simplify matters, let us keep the pressure head in the reservoir constant by maintaining the fluid level 20 cm above its bottom, and let us assume that the tubes, including the U-tube, offer no frictional resistance to flow except at the fixed resistance *R*. If we now close the tube between *a* and *d* and open the outlet to the atmosphere, fluid will flow from *a→b→c→d→* outlet. If we now close the tops of both U-tubes at *b* and *c* and open the tube between *a* and *d*, fluid will flow from *a→ d→* outlet. *In each case the flow/minute will be the same* because the pressure difference between *a* and the outlet is the same. The same is true if the U-tube is swiveled through 180 degrees so that the connecting limb is now at the top (Fig. 11-4, *center*).

If we have a reservoir, a U-tube and an inverted U-tube, we now have the simplest model of a pulmonary circulation – with a nonpulsatile pump (fluid reservoir), arteries to the top and bottom of the lung, veins from the top and bottom of the lung and vessels connecting arteries and veins (Fig. 11-4, *right*).

However, the U-tubes of the vascular system are not rigid but are distensible arteries, arterioles, capillaries, venules and veins.

Fig. 11-4.—Effect of gravity on pressures and flow. **Left**, flow through a U-tube. **Center**, when the U-tube is rotated 180 degrees upward, flow remains the same as long as the column of fluid in U-tube is unbroken. **Right**, schematic representation of vessels to and from upper (*A*), mid (*B*) and lower (*C*) regions of the lungs. Alveolar gas pressure has its effects first on alveolar capillaries; if it exceeds capillary pressure, it can compress or occlude capillaries.

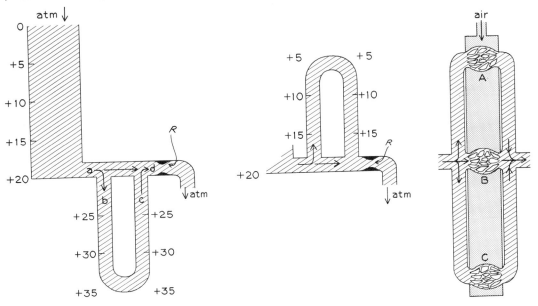

Each will become wider when transmural pressure increases because each is compliant, but each has a different compliance. Although higher pressures toward the bottom of a U-tube and the lower pressures toward the top do not change driving pressure at any level, they do change the transmural pressure. This has two consequences. The first (and now we drop our pretense that our tubes offer no frictional resistance to flow) is that higher transmural pressure toward the bottom of the tubes widens them and, according to Poiseuille's law (p. 123), decreases resistance to fluid flow; flow is therefore greater, not because the driving pressure at any level is greater, but because resistance is less. Since gravitational forces have practically no effect on air in airways (compared to blood in blood vessels), gravity has the effect of increasing blood flow at the bases (relative to ventilation) and of decreasing it at the apices. (Many vessels have the property of autoregulation; i.e., when transmural pressure increases, smooth muscle in the vessels responds by constriction [which opposes passive dilation], and when transmural pressure decreases, smooth muscle responds by relaxing. Within limits, this tends to maintain constant flow. Vessels that are most often subject to the force of gravity and a high transmural pressure tend to develop more smooth muscle and better resist passive distention.)

The second consequence of a higher transmural pressure at the bottom is that transmural capillary pressure must also be higher there. Increase in transmural pressure does not widen fully open, healthy capillaries (see p. 154), but does favor filtration of fluid from them into tissues; this explains why, in ambulatory patients with heart failure and high pulmonary capillary pressure, fluid accumulates at the base of the lungs and why bed rest alone may reduce or eliminate such pulmonary edema.

The real pulmonary circulation differs from the simple model in several ways. In the model, the pressure at the bottom of the reservoir is fixed at 20 cm H_2O; the top of the "lung" is 15 cm above this and the bottom of the "lung" 15 cm below this. In man the pressure in the main pulmonary trunk is not fixed; it varies among individuals and also in the same person during systole and diastole. Further, in man the height of the lung is not 30 cm but varies among individuals, and when the lung is 30 cm high, the distance from the pulmonary trunk (where pulmonary arterial pressure is measured) to the apex is about 11 cm and to the base, about 19 cm.

The systolic blood pressure measured in the main pulmonary arteries of resting man may vary between 15 and 35 cm H_2O.[1] Since some pressure is dissipated overcoming frictional resistance to flow through tubes 15 cm long, the pressure in arteries at the top of the lung may be only 13–33 cm H_2O; 33 cm H_2O is enough to push blood to the top of even the longest lung and through the apical capillaries; 13 cm H_2O is not enough for the longest lungs.[2] And if alveolar pressure rises above atmospheric, higher arterial pressures are required; Figure 11-4 (*right*) shows that high alveolar pressures have their effect first on alveolar capillaries.

Doesn't the "siphon effect" keep blood

---

[1] We can express pulmonary vascular pressures as either mm Hg or cm H_2O. Since we are expressing the heights of columns of blood in pulmonary vessels in cm, it is convenient here to measure pressures in cm H_2O: 1 cm $H_2O = 0.735$ mm Hg.

[2] One cannot simply measure systolic and diastolic pressures in the pulmonary trunk, measure the distance from there to the top of the lung and decide whether blood will or will not perfuse apical vessels, intermittently or continuously. As mentioned earlier, there will be some pressure loss due to frictional resistance to blood flow. In addition, blood does not flow because of the differences in potential energy between two points but because of differences in potential *plus* kinetic energy. The kinetic energy associated with blood flow is about 6% of the total hydraulic power in the pulmonary artery. The pressure that is generated in the pulmonary arterial tree by conversion of kinetic energy (and can then influence pulmonary capillary blood flow) is probably about 1.3 cm H_2O in resting man, but it increases during exercise as blood flow increases. This conversion, rarely considered, may well be important at times in the critically balanced forces that determine patency of capillaries in the apex of the lung. Further, there have been few measurements made of pulmonary artery pressure in normal man in the standing or sitting position.

flowing even when the pressure in the pulmonary trunk is low? No, because a siphon operates only when the tube is completely filled with fluid. Blood vessels are not rigid tubes; thin-walled vessels collapse when the pressure inside them is less than that immediately outside the vessel. When the top of the U-tube is compressed, the vertical column of blood in the vein cannot siphon blood from the artery through the closed segment. In this case, the right ventricle pushes blood through the highest possible artery-capillary-vein system in which the column of blood remains intact. When pulmonary artery pressure, measured in centimeters of H_2O, again exceeds the height of the lungs in centimeters above the pulmonary trunk, it re-establishes flow in apical vessels.

Several factors other than systolic pressure must be considered. First, diastolic pressure in the pulmonary trunk is often not high enough to push blood to the top of the lung in erect man. So somewhere near the top of some lungs, vessels open during each systole and close during each diastole.

Second, the effects of gravity become unimportant when vertical distances are small. When man lies down (supine, prone or lateral position), the distance from the pulmonary trunk to whatever is now the top of the lung is always less than normal pulmonary artery pressure because a lung is not so wide or thick as it is long and blood flow is now continuous through all parts of the lung. And in children or short adults the normal pulmonary artery pressure is enough to perfuse all vessels at the top of the lung (though in very tall people, it may not).

Third, when man exercises and increases the return of venous blood to the right heart, his pulmonary artery pressure increases sufficiently to perfuse the highest vessels, both in systole and diastole, and insure continuous flow and an unbroken column of blood from artery to vein. On the other hand, if he has had a severe hemorrhage and has a low pulmonary artery pressure, the pressure may not be sufficient to raise blood to the top of his lung, even when he lies semirecumbent; this hypoperfusion of regions of the lungs is one cause of "shock" lung, or respiratory distress syndrome in adults. Hypoxemia and acidosis may constrict pulmonary arterioles (see p. 155) and pressure in the alveolar capillaries may fall even lower on this account. (We are speaking here only of pulmonary blood flow to alveolar capillaries; bronchial artery pressure is always sufficient to supply the tracheobronchial tree with blood unless aortic blood pressure is very low.)

Fourth, when man is in outer space, beyond the influence of the gravitational force of earth, intravascular pressures are the same at the top and bottom of the lung. It is also possible to counteract the effect of gravity here on earth. If a U-tube, such as that in Figure 11-3 but with distensible walls, is placed in a jar of water 15 cm deep, the pressure at each level in the water outside the tube will exactly counterbalance pressure in the water column inside the tube because gravitational forces act equally on both; transmural pressure will now be the same from top to bottom. This principle is used to construct antigravity suits for pilots and prevent high transmural pressures in the lower limbs. Obviously, one cannot deliberately surround the lungs or fill the alveoli with fluid to prevent high transmural pressure at the bottom of the lungs. However, in disease, sometimes the visceral and parietal pleura are separated by fluid or blood, and this acts as a water jacket. The fluid-filled lung of the fetus is a physiologic example of precise counterbalancing of the effect of gravity on blood in vessels by fluid outside vessels. And to the extent that lung tissue acts as a fluid, subject to gravitational forces, it will partly counteract the effect of gravity on blood in blood vessels. On the other hand, blood pressures become very high in vessels at the bottom of the lung and very low at the top when astronauts are exposed to strong positive accelerative forces, acting footward $(+G_z)$.

Fifth, we must consider the effect of alveolar pressure. In quiet breathing, mean alveolar pressure is 0 (atmospheric) with a decrease to −1 cm H_2O during inspiration and an increase to +1 cm H_2O during expiration (see Fig. 10-5); these swings increase during forced, deep breathing. Alveolar pressure can be higher throughout the lung during continuous positive-pressure breathing (p. 274) and can be higher regionally during labored expiration in patients with obstructive pulmonary disease or in patients with cysts and bullae. This pressure acts to decrease or stop alveolar capillary blood flow, especially in the upper parts of the lung where pulmonary artery pressure is low owing to gravitational forces. Robin has described patients with shortness of breath who are relieved by lying flat in bed (platypnea), presumably because pulmonary blood can now flow to all parts of the lung and so reduce "alveolar dead space" (see p. 175) and the work of breathing.

Sixth, the level of venous pressure can be important when alveolar pressure exceeds pulmonary capillary pressure and so begins to limit blood flow. For example, stenosis at the mitral valve increases left atrial pressure, and for blood to move forward, capillary, pulmonary arterial and right ventricular pressures must rise. The increased intravascular pressure counteracts the tissue (alveolar) pressure, opens the capillaries and re-establishes continuous capillary flow. It is of interest that ambulatory patients with mitral stenosis are more apt to have uniform blood flow throughout the lungs than healthy people.

West, who has contributed much to our concepts and knowledge of the effect of gravity on pulmonary blood flow, has divided the lung into 3 zones, depending on the relationships among pulmonary arterial pressure, alveolar pressure and venous pressure. Obviously no condition can exist for long in which venous pressure exceeds arterial pressure, but regional alveolar pressure can sometimes be greater than arterial pressure, and it can be less than arterial but greater than venous pressure.

In West's zone 1, the alveolar pressure is greater than arterial or pulmonary capillary pressure and there can be no flow. Here, driving pressure is no longer determined by pulmonary arterial minus left atrial pressure but by pulmonary arterial minus alveolar pressure; since this value is negative, there is no flow. No zone 1 is present in man under normal conditions, but it can be present at the top of the lung (see Fig. 11-4, *right, A*) when alveolar pressure becomes unusually high, when pulmonary artery pressure falls or when accelerative forces have decreased arterial pressure at the top of the lung.

In West's zone 3, arterial pressure is greater than alveolar pressure, and flow is determined by pulmonary artery pressure minus pulmonary venous or left atrial pressure. Since transmural pressure increases toward the bottom of the lung, vessels there are fully open, offer less resistance to flow, and flow increases (Fig. 11-5).

In the intermediate zone 2, arterial pressure exceeds alveolar pressure, but alveolar pressure is greater than venous pressure. Here each vessel acts as a collapsible tube surrounded by a pressure chamber, and the end of the pulmonary capillary, where intracapillary pressure is lowest, is compressed. In this zone, blood flow depends on the transmural pressure; any increase in alveolar pressure or decrease in arterial pressure tends to decrease flow. For this reason, flow increases toward the bottom of zone 2 where arterial pressure is greater.[3]

---

[3]Since venous pressure is low and the veins are far from filled, they accept whatever amount of blood alveolar pressure allows to flow into them, just as a sink accepts whatever amount of water passes through the restriction at the faucet. Some have likened zone 2 conditions to a waterfall on the basis that the amount of water going over the fall is the same regardless of how far the water falls. However, the analogy is not appropriate because there is no restriction to flow at the top of a real waterfall. Others have likened zone 2 to a Starling resistor, which the famous cardiovascular physiologist used to vary resistance to flow in his heart-lung experiments. Since this resistor is jargon to most physicians, who first require a description of a Starling resistor before they can understand the analogy, it may be best just to look at Figure 11-4 (*right*), which contains 3 capillary beds (*A, B* and *C*) surrounded by the same air pressure chamber, and visualize how vessels may be compressed or widened by raising or lowering arterial pressure and simultaneously raising or lowering alveolar gas pressure.

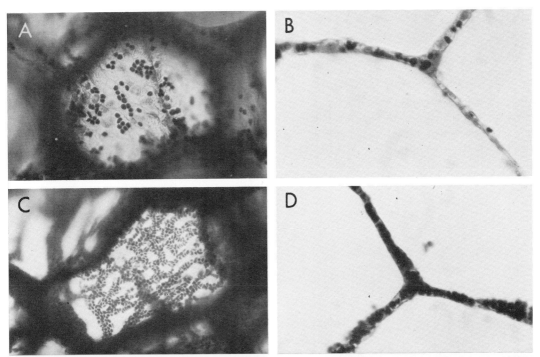

Fig. 11-5.—Range of capillary blood volume in cat lung (approximately fourfold). **A** and **B**, capillaries contain minimal number of red cells. Blood flow is zero because alveolar pressure is higher than pressure in pulmonary artery (Zone 1). **C** and **D**, congested capillaries with 2 or 3 red cells abreast. Both pulmonary artery and vein pressures exceed alveolar pressure (Zone 3). Lungs frozen rapidly at 10 cm H_2O alveolar pressure. **B** and **D** are thin sections (10 μ); **A** and **C** are thick sections (200 μ). Magnification of final pictures varies slightly; approx. ×300. (Courtesy of Dr. Norman Staub.)

Capillary blood flow can also be limited by extravascular pressure caused by tissue edema; because transmural pressure is highest at the bottom of the lung, edema is most apt to occur there.

For a discussion of increased and decreased ventilation in relation to blood flow that occur at the top and bottom of the lung as the result of gravity, see Chapter 13.

RESISTANCE TO FLOW

Just as with airway resistance, vascular resistance is calculated from an equation similar to Ohm's law for electrical circuits relating resistance and current flow to electromotive force. In any vascular system,

$$\text{Resistance} = \frac{\text{Driving pressure}}{\text{Blood flow}}$$

In classic physical terms, pressure is measured in dynes/cm² (force per unit area).

Blood flow is measured as cm³/second.

$$\frac{\text{Pressure}}{\text{Flow}} \text{ becomes } \frac{\text{dynes/cm}^2}{\text{cm}^3/\text{sec}} = \frac{\text{dynes} \times \text{sec}}{\text{cm}^5}$$

$$= \text{dynes} \times \text{sec} \times \text{cm}^{-5}.$$

We avoided this cumbersome term when discussing resistance to air flow, and used units of cm H_2O/(L/second), because this unit is more meaningful to physicians. The unit for blood pressure is usually mm Hg and for flow, L/minute; the resistance unit is then mm Hg/(L/minute). In the systemic circulation with a mean driving pressure of 90 mm Hg and a flow of 5.4 L/minute, the resistance is 90/5.4, or 16.6 mm Hg/(L/minute); this means that a pressure of 16.6 mm Hg is needed to drive 1 L of blood through the resistance in the system in 1 minute. In the pulmonary circulation with a mean driving pressure of less than 9 mm Hg and the same flow, the resistance is 9/5.4, or 1.66 mm

Hg/(L/minute) or 1/10 that in the systemic circulation. (Some use units of ml/sec for flow; in this case systemic resistance would be 90/90, or 1, and pulmonary vascular resistance would be 9/90, or 0.1.)

In the normal pulmonary circulation, most of the resistance to flow is through arterioles and capillaries. The venous system offers little resistance to flow; the pressure difference between the end of the capillaries and the left atrium is believed to be less than 1 mm Hg.

Passive Changes in Pulmonary Vascular Resistance

Passive changes (i.e., not involving primary contraction or relaxation of vascular smooth muscle) occur in pulmonary vascular resistance in several circumstances:

1. WHEN CHANGES OCCUR IN PULMONARY BLOOD FLOW AND PULMONARY ARTERIAL PRESSURE. When man exercises maximally, his right ventricle can pump as much as 30 – 40 L of blood through the pulmonary circulation each minute without raising the pressure high enough to exceed colloidal osmotic pressure and cause pulmonary edema. When pulmonary blood flow doubles during mild to moderate exercise, the driving pressure increases by only 25 – 50%. Similarly, there is no large rise in driving pressure when pulmonary blood flow increases in hyperthyroidism, fever, anemia and artery-to-vein shunts (including left-to-right shunts associated with septal defects and patent ductus arteriosus). Again, removal of one lung in a young patient with strictly unilateral disease usually leads to only a small increase in pulmonary vascular pressures, even though the remaining vascular bed has twice its former flow. Inflation of a balloon in the right or left pulmonary artery forces the whole right ventricular output to flow through the other lung, but the main pulmonary artery pressure rises but little.[4] Since resistance = driving pressure/flow, calculations show in each of these instances that vascular resistance must have decreased, which means that pulmonary vessels have widened. Since no mechanism for *active* dilation has been demonstrated, we assume it is passive. Which vessels are affected? We assume that large vessels and arterioles become wider. Do capillaries widen when their transmural pressure increases? Most physiologists believe that healthy capillaries, once fully open, strongly resist further distention, even by very high internal pressures. However, resistance to flow through capillary beds can be decreased if previously closed capillaries open or if partly compressed capillaries go from a flattened to a round shape and so have a greater cross-sectional area. If erect man has partly or completely closed capillaries in his upper lobes, these may well act as reserve beds that open during exercise.

Normal pulmonary capillaries, fully open, are about 10 – 15 μ in diameter, wide enough for two red blood cells to pass through abreast. Under certain abnormal conditions (disease, severe hypoxia, ischemia or change in their chemical environment), capillaries may become wider. Some have reported seeing pulmonary capillaries with 3 or 4 red cells abreast in patients with mitral stenosis and long-standing increase in left atrial and pulmonary capillary pressure.

2. DURING INSPIRATION AND EXPIRATION, BECAUSE OF CHANGES IN DIMENSIONS OF THE LUNG. The extrapulmonary and large intrapulmonary vessels become

---

[4]The thoracic surgeon who plans to remove one lung from a patient with pulmonary cancer or tuberculosis can make use of this knowledge to determine preoperatively whether the circulation to the other lung is normal. Before operation he can catheterize the pulmonary artery going to the lung to be removed and occlude it by inflation of a cuff around the catheter. This forces the whole right ventricular output to flow through the lung to be spared. If pressure in the main pulmonary artery rises only transiently, the vascular bed in that lung is expansible; if it rises sharply and remains elevated, the surgeon may anticipate that the patient will have high pulmonary arterial and right ventricular pressures after pneumonectomy. The pressure rise in older patients is greater than normal because the aging process alone appears to reduce the size and distensibility of the pulmonary vascular bed. A large rise often occurs in patients in whom bilateral disease has destroyed, compressed or restricted part of the vascular bed.

longer and wider during inspiration (if there is no limit on blood flow to fill them) and shorter and narrower during expiration. Because resistance varies with length/radius[4], widening of vessels more than compensates for the increase in length during inspiration. The small intrapulmonary vessels *in* alveolar walls are probably flattened as the alveoli become larger and those *between* alveoli are enlarged by the stretch of the elastic fibers attached to them. Total pulmonary vascular resistance increases during both maximal inflation and forced deflation of the lungs.

3. DURING CHANGES IN ALVEOLAR PRESSURE. We have already mentioned that increased alveolar pressure can compress alveolar capillaries and stop or reduce blood flow through them. However, not all of the alveolar pressure is transmitted to the vessels. Some is needed to overcome the surface tension of the alveolar lining (see p. 105); since this lining is between the air and the vessels, it "absorbs" some of the alveolar pressure, and this part does not compress vessels. Butler and associates have shown that blood flow through *fluid*-filled lungs (no fluid-air interface) stops when alveolar pressure equals vascular pressure; it continues in *air*-filled lungs when alveolar pressure is well in excess of vascular pressure. The complete transmission of alveolar pressure to the capillaries of fluid-filled alveoli may explain why blood flow is often shifted from alveoli filled with edema fluid to air-filled alveoli.

Active Changes in Pulmonary Vascular Resistance

Even after introduction of the technic of catheterization of the pulmonary artery, there were few who believed that pulmonary vessels could constrict actively in response to nervous impulses, chemical agents or physical changes such as alteration in temperature. Histologists saw very little smooth muscle in pulmonary arterioles of adult animals or man; physiologists found no striking changes in resistance after stimulation of nerves to the lungs; pharmacologists found only small changes after injection of drugs that act as vasoconstrictors or vasodilators elsewhere. Further, teleologists reasoned that there was no need for regulation because in the adult all the cardiac output must flow through the lungs and one resistance (a low one) would permit the right ventricle to pump it through with minimal work; even in the fetus, one resistance (a high one) would prevent most of the combined output of the right and left ventricles from going through fetal lungs, which have very little need for blood flow. The pulmonary circulation seemed to be quite different from the systemic circulation; in the latter, variable resistances and vasomotor regulation *are* essential to shift cardiac output from resting to active tissues, or, in emergencies, from nonessential to vital organs.

It is known now that there *is* enough smooth muscle in pulmonary arterioles to alter resistance (not much is needed in a low-pressure system) and that it can hypertrophy remarkably in pathologic conditions such as mitral stenosis (particularly in the lower lobes, where vascular pressures are high because of the force of gravity). It is also known that drugs can cause vasoconstriction and vasodilation. Further, electrical or reflex stimulation of the sympathetic nerves to the lung causes vasoconstriction. And it is recognized that teleologically, it would be beneficial at times to shunt blood from alveolar capillaries in one region to those in another.

Of the physiologic stimuli that cause active pulmonary vasoconstriction, hypoxia (systemic or local) is one of the most important. Systemic hypoxemia, acting on chemoreceptors in the aortic body (at least in the dog), causes overall pulmonary arteriolar constriction and leads to an increase in right ventricular and pulmonary arterial pressure, with no increase in capillary pressure. This is a regular feature of residence at high altitude (see Table 11-2), of hypoxemia resulting from cardiopulmonary disease at sea level and of normal fetal life.

TABLE 11-2.—PULMONARY ARTERY PRESSURE OF SUBJECTS
LIVING AT DIFFERENT ALTITUDES

LOCATION	ALTITUDE (FT)	BAR PR TORR	$P_{I_{O_2}}$* TORR	$P_{A_{O_2}}$ TORR	$\bar{P}_{PA}$ MM HG
Boston	Sea level	760	148	103	13
Lima, Peru	500	752	147	102	14
Denver	5,250	625	121	80	16
Mexico City	7,400	580	111	81	15
La Paz, Bolivia	12,150	485	92	59	23
Morococha, Peru	14,900	445	83	50	28
Chacaltoya, Bolivia	17,100	398	73	39	36

*Moist (tracheal) $P_{O_2} = (BP - 47) \times .2093$. (From Cudkowicz: Respiration 27:417, 1970.)

Decreased local alveolar P_{O_2} also causes precapillary constriction and increased resistance to blood flow through the hypoxic region (even when the P_{O_2} of systemic arterial blood is normal) and so shifts flood flow to alveolar capillaries exposed to higher alveolar P_{O_2}; this mechanism serves to prevent arterial hypoxemia. It operates even in isolated lungs without nerves and without reflexes. The way in which local hypoxia causes local pulmonary arteriolar constriction is uncertain. Lloyd has shown that pulmonary arteries, freed from surrounding tissue, do not constrict when made hypoxic; this suggests that hypoxia releases a substance from the lung parenchyma and this chemical is responsible for causing vasoconstriction. Some believe that the chemical change is an increase in local $[H^+]$ (which in itself causes pulmonary vasoconstriction), others believe that hypoxia releases K^+ and still others believe that local hypoxia releases histamine from perivascular pulmonary mast cells and histamine is then responsible for vasoconstriction (in support of the last hypothesis is some evidence that alveolar hypoxia degranulates mast cells and that hypoxic vasoconstriction is prevented by antihistaminic agents). Recently, Berkov found that an adequate plasma concentration of angiotensin II is required for hypoxic pulmonary constriction.

Another condition leading to active pulmonary arteriolar constriction is increased left atrial and pulmonary capillary pressure, as in mitral stenosis. Dexter believes that this increase in arteriolar resistance is a reflex designed to protect the capillary bed against sudden increase in pressure and possible pulmonary edema. It is at least partly reversible within two weeks after an operation that corrects the valvular stenosis and decreases left atrial pressure; however, the arteriolar resistance does not decrease immediately after the operation, as one might expect if it were induced reflexly. Possibly the increased resistance is due partly to smooth muscle hypertrophy and partly to atherosclerosis.

Pulmonary vascular occlusion may also cause active changes in pulmonary vascular resistance, even of nonoccluded areas. There is no agreement on this point, and the difference in results may be due to different technics and sites of occlusion (ligation vs. embolization; large vs. small vs. microemboli; inert vs. chemically active emboli). Hypothermia causes increased vascular resistance; the mechanism is not known. Increased alveolar P_{CO_2} increases resistance to pulmonary blood flow.

Norepinephrine, epinephrine, serotonin, histamine, angiotensin and fibrinopeptide B constrict arterioles; serotonin, Escherichia coli endotoxin, histamine and alloxan constrict venules and veins. Isoproterenol and acetylcholine dilate constricted arterioles.

Acetylcholine is often injected into the pulmonary circulation to determine whether it will decrease vascular resistance; if it does, the increased resistance was due at least partly to vasoconstriction rather than to atherosclerosis or other organic obstruction.

This use of acetylcholine is a nice application of basic physiologic knowledge to clinical diagnostic problems. Acetylcholine in the systemic circulation causes marked vasodilation, bradycardia and hypotension. However, it is destroyed very rapidly in blood by a specific enzyme, cholinesterase. A dose of acetylcholine is selected for injection into the right ventricle or pulmonary artery that will act during the time it is in the pulmonary vessels but will be largely inactivated before it reaches the aorta and systemic circulation.

Oxygen inhalation causes dilation when hypoxic constriction is present. Aminophylline, nitrites and papaverine dilate vessels of perfused, isolated lungs but are not useful vasodilators in man. Little is known about the effect of anesthetic gases or vapors or irritant gases.

Pathologic Changes in Pulmonary Vascular Resistance

Pulmonary vascular resistance may increase in many pathologic conditions, and in these the increased resistance may be in the artery, arterioles, capillaries, venules or veins. Among the causes of increased resistance are: (1) intraluminal obstructions, such as thrombi or emboli (blood clots, parasites, fat cells, air, tumor cells, white blood cells or platelets); (2) disease of the vascular wall, such as sclerosis, endarteritis, polyarteritis or scleroderma; (3) obliterative or destructive diseases, such as emphysema and interstitial pulmonary fibrosis; (4) critical closure of small vessels during a period of severe hypotension and (5) compression of vessels by masses of infiltrative lesions.

12

Pulmonary Gas Diffusion

WE HAVE DISCUSSED some general aspects of alveolar ventilation and of pulmonary capillary blood flow. The function of ventilation is to maintain a high alveolar P_{O_2} and a low P_{CO_2}; the function of blood flow is to transport O_2 from the lungs to tissue capillaries and CO_2 from tissues to the pulmonary capillaries. How do O_2 and CO_2 pass between alveolar gas and capillary blood? The process is entirely a passive one brought about by diffusion. No secretory or active transport mechanisms are involved. Although the alveolocapillary membrane does no work to speed the process of diffusion, the respiratory muscles do, because ventilation brings fresh air into alveoli and raises the O_2 concentration in them above that in mixed venous blood. And active body tissues, by aerobic metabolism, lower tissue and mixed venous blood O_2 concentrations and establish a concentration difference between alveolar gas and blood in pulmonary capillaries.

WHAT IS DIFFUSION?

Molecules of gases are constantly in random motion. If the concentration of molecules of a particular gas is greater in one region than in another, there are more collisions and more motion. Although the molecules in both regions are in motion, the net effect is that gas diffuses from the region of higher concentration to the region of lower concentration and the concentrations of the gas in the two regions tend to become equal.

A light gas diffuses faster in a gaseous medium than a heavier gas. Different gases with equal numbers of molecules in equal volumes have the same molecular energy at the same temperature. Therefore, light molecules will travel faster, collide more frequently and diffuse faster. The relative rates of their diffusion are inversely proportional to the square root of their densities (Graham's law). For O_2 (molecular weight 32) and CO_2 (molecular weight 44), the relative rates of diffusion in a gas phase would be

$$\frac{\text{Rate for } CO_2}{\text{Rate for } O_2} = \frac{\sqrt{\text{mol wt } O_2}}{\sqrt{\text{mol wt } CO_2}} = \frac{\sqrt{32}}{\sqrt{44}} = \frac{5.6}{6.6}$$

Thus, in alveolar gas, O_2 would diffuse more rapidly than CO_2. During normal inspiration, ventilation moves fresh air into the alveolar ducts and alveoli. Diffusion occurs between this air and the alveolar gas that was there before inspiration. The alveoli are so small and the maximal distance for diffusion so short (the diameters of human alveoli are about 100 μ) that any difference between the concentration or partial pressure of a gas at the center and periphery of an alveolus would be eliminated in a fraction of a second; calculations show that diffusion of gas in a normal alveolus is 80% complete in 0.002 second if the diffusion distance is 0.5 mm. However, in emphysema, alveolar walls may be destroyed and a group of alveoli may become one air sac; sometimes large sacs (blebs and bullae) form. The distances for

158

diffusion are now much greater, and the P_{O_2} (or P_{CO_2}) may not be the same throughout these abnormal regions. If the diffusion distance in an air sac is 7 mm, 0.38 second would be required instead of 0.002 second. When a gas must diffuse over very long distances, e.g., from an alveolus to the mouth, the rate of diffusion is much too slow to permit any useful gas exchange. This is well illustrated by the accumulation of CO_2 in the alveoli, blood and tissues during a period of respiratory arrest.

The diffusion of O_2 and CO_2 that is essential to pulmonary gas exchange takes place between gas and tissue – between a gaseous phase and a liquid phase. The solubility of the gas in the liquid is an important factor in diffusion in liquids, and Henry's law now applies. This states that the volume (at standard temperature and pressure) of a slightly soluble gas that dissolves in a liquid at a given temperature is almost directly proportional to the partial pressure of that gas. This holds for gases that do not unite chemically with the solvent. At the surface of the liquid or tissue, the gas tension will be equal to that in the gas phase, but immediately below the surface, it will be less because diffusion in the liquid phase sets up gradients of gas concentration. The solubility of CO_2 in water is high, and therefore its concentration in the surface layer will be high. Thus, for CO_2, there will be a large concentration gradient between the surface and deeper layers of the fluid or tissues. Since the diffusion rate within a liquid depends on its *concentration* gradient, the greater the solubility of a gas in a liquid, the more rapid will be its rate of diffusion in the liquid. The relative solubilities of CO_2 and O_2 in water (milliliters of gas that dissolves in 1 ml water at 37 C when the gas pressure is 1 atmosphere) are

$$\frac{\text{Solubility } CO_2}{\text{Solubility } O_2} = \frac{0.592}{0.0244} = \frac{24.3}{1.0}$$

This explains why CO_2 diffuses far more rapidly between alveolar gas and capillary blood than O_2, even though CO_2 diffuses less rapidly *within* alveoli.

If we combine Graham's and Henry's laws to include diffusion both into the liquid surface and through the tissue fluid, we see that the relative rates of diffusion for CO_2 and O_2 are

$$\frac{\text{Rate for } CO_2}{\text{Rate for } O_2} = \frac{5.6}{6.6} \times \frac{0.592}{0.0244} = \frac{20.7}{1}$$

For this reason, from now on we shall discuss diffusion of O_2 rather than CO_2; outward diffusion of CO_2 should never be a clinical problem unless a patient is found whose diffusion is so severely impaired that his life can be maintained only by inhalation of 100% O_2. And from now on, we will talk of differences in partial pressure between gas and blood (instead of differences in concentration), assuming that the solubility of gas in liquid and tissue remains constant.

FACTORS DETERMINING DIFFUSION OF OXYGEN

Difference in Partial Pressure of Oxygen in Alveoli and in Capillary Blood

Figure 12-1 shows these pressures for normal man breathing air and breathing O_2. Increased alveolar ventilation or inhalation of O_2 raises alveolar P_{O_2} and pulmonary capillary P_{O_2}. The pressure difference responsible for the diffusion of O_2 across the alveolocapillary membranes (during air breathing) is not the initial difference $(100-40=60)$, the end-capillary difference $(100-99.99=0.01)$ or the average of these two. It is an integrated mean value that depends on complex factors, including the shape of the Hb-O_2 association curve (p. 184).

Length of Diffusion Path

This is pictured in Figure 12-2. An O_2 molecule in alveolar gas must first pass through the surfactant lining (not shown in Fig. 12-2), then through the alveolar epithelial membrane, the capillary endothelial membrane, a layer of plasma in the capillary

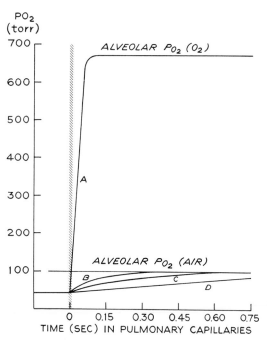

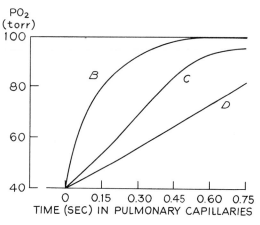

Fig. 12-1.—**Top**, exchange of O_2 in pulmonary capillaries. Curves *A-D* show the rate at which mixed venous blood ($Po_2 = 40$ torr) entering the pulmonary capillaries (at *vertical hatching*) comes into equilibrium with the Po_2 in alveolar gas. When O_2 is inhaled (*A*) and alveolar Po_2 rises to near 670 torr, equilibration is almost instantaneous because of the very large initial difference in Po_2 (670 – 40 torr). When air is breathed and alveolar Po_2 is 100 torr, equilibrium is reached more slowly (*B*) but still well within the time that the blood remains in the pulmonary capillaries. With moderate impairment of diffusion (alveolocapillary block, curve *C*), O_2 uptake is slower, but capillary blood comes into near equilibrium with alveolar gas within 0.75 sec. With more severe impairment of diffusion (curve *D*), blood leaves the capillaries at less than a Po_2 of 100 torr, and systemic arterial hypoxemia results. The impairment pictured in *C* can be detected by CO uptake tests but not by measurement of arterial O_2 saturation (except during exercise, which shortens the time that blood remains in the pulmonary capillaries). **Bottom**, enlargement of the 40 to 100 torr portion of the top figure.

blood, the erythrocyte membrane and, finally, through intracellular fluid in the erythrocyte until it encounters a hemoglobin molecule with which it combines chemically. The minimal distance across normal alveolocapillary membranes is very small ($0.2\ \mu$) – so small that it requires electron microscopy to prove conclusively that the alveolocapillary membrane is really two closely applied, continuous membranes. This is a negligible barrier to the diffusion of O_2; Figure 12-1 shows that the Po_2 in pulmonary capillary blood comes into almost complete equilibrium with

the Po_2 in its corresponding alveolus (99.99 vs. 100 torr).

Note that the distance for diffusion is not this short everywhere. The membranes are living tissues and contain alveolar cells and the nuclei of epithelial and endothelial cells, which occupy 20 – 30% of the alveolar wall; the distances are greater across them.

The path for diffusion may become longer in disease. (1) The alveolar wall may be thickened by the growth of fibrous tissue or of additional alveolar cells (Fig 12-3, *G, I*). (2) The capillary membrane may be thick-

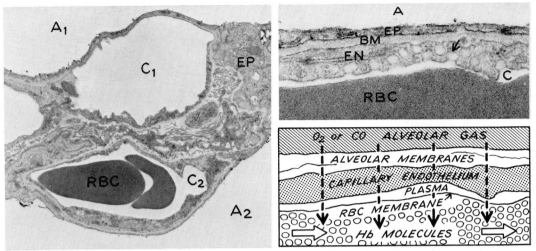

Fig. 12-2.—Blood-air barriers. **Left,** electron micrograph of an adult rat lung. Two capillaries, C_1 and C_2, lie in the wall that separates 2 alveoli (A_1 and A_2). C_2 contains 2 erythrocytes (*RBC*), while C_1 (sectioned tangentially) appears empty. *EP* is a type II alveolar epithelial cell. Note the difference in thickness of tissue separating A_1 from C_1 and A_2 from C_2 or C_1. **Right,** the layers that separate an alveolus (*A*) from the capillary lumen (*C*) are the thin cytoplasm of an alveolar epithelial cell (*EP*), the basement membrane (*BM*) and the capillary endothelial cell cytoplasm (*EN*). An erythrocyte (*RBC*) lies within the lumen of the capillary. Note the many vesicles (*arrow*) within the endothelial cell. (Courtesy of Dr. Judy Strum.) The sketch below shows the diffusion path for O_2 or CO molecules from alveolar gas to chemical combination with hemoglobin within the red blood cell.

ened. (3) The two membranes may be separated by interstitial edema fluid and exudate, which may be replaced by fibrous tissue (*G, 2*). (4) There may be intra-alveolar edema fluid or exudate (*G, 3* and *4*). (5) The intracapillary path may be increased if capillaries are dilated (*F*). (6) The membrane or shape of the erythrocyte may be altered in a way that increases the path for diffusion (no such disturbance has yet been described). In all of these conditions, there is a physical "block" to diffusion, which is called alveolocapillary block. In its proper sense, this term should be used only when there is indeed a block between the alveolus and its capillary bed, namely, a longer pathway across the alveolocapillary membranes. It should not be used in referring to other conditions described later in which pulmonary diffusing capacity is decreased.

Sometimes we become involved in semantics; we do when discussing pulmonary edema. Electron microscopists have demonstrated that—at least in some cases—transudate from pulmonary capillaries first separates capillary and alveolar membranes; this increases the distance for diffusion and causes alveolocapillary block. If edema fluid enters and fills alveoli, this again lengthens the distance for diffusion. When fluid wells up into alveolar ducts, respiratory and terminal bronchioles or even higher into large bronchi, the path for diffusion of O_2 becomes so long that useful diffusion can no longer occur; however, these regions of the lung are now filled with fluid and can no longer be ventilated. Is the defect "impairment of diffusion" or "hypoventilation"? We usually classify this as a problem in ventilation—the alveoli are nonventilated or poorly ventilated.

Area for Diffusion

This is not the total alveolar area or the total capillary area, but the area of functioning alveoli in contact with capillaries with flowing blood. It is estimated to be approximately 70 m² in man. The vast size of this alveolar surface is due to the subdivision of

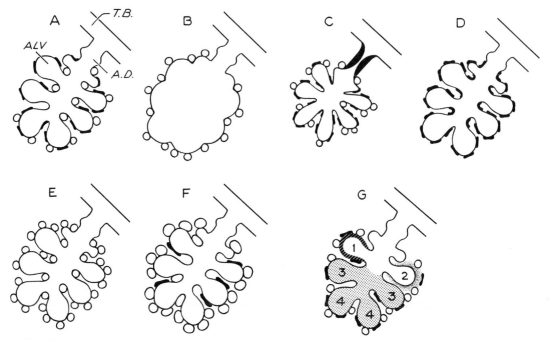

Fig. 12-3. — Area for gas exchange. **A,** normal arrangement of alveoli (*ALV*) clustered about an alveolar duct (*A.D.*); about half of the alveolar capillaries are open and half are closed. *T.B.* = terminal bronchiole. **B,** destruction of alveolar walls and of about half of the total available number of capillaries. **C,** obstruction of alveolar duct and decreased area for gas exchange with no decrease in potential alveolocapillary contact surface. **D,** obstruction of the pulmonary circulation; no alveolocapillary blood flow. **E,** increase in the number of open capillaries, as might occur in exercise. **F,** capillary enlargement, as might occur in chronic mitral stenosis. **G,** longer paths for diffusion due to (*1*) thickening of alveolar epithelium, (*2*) tissue separating alveolar capillary from alveolar epithelium, (*3*) and (*4*) nonventilated alveoli filled with edema fluid or exudate.

air spaces by the alveolar walls; destruction of these walls by disease, such as emphysema, decreases both alveolar and capillary surface, since the walls contained many capillaries (see Fig. 12-3, *B*). In emphysema, the alveolocapillary membranes are not thickened and there is no *physical* alveolocapillary block, but diffusion of O_2 may be limited by a decrease in area for gas exchange. Again, the alveolocapillary membranes may be normal, but the area for diffusion decreased by nonventilation of alveoli, lobules or lobes (see Fig. 12-3, *C*).

An increase (*E*) or decrease (*D*) in the number of open alveolar capillaries also alters the area for diffusion. Occlusion of the pulmonary artery to the left lung immediately decreases the area for diffusion by almost half, but within seconds it may return to normal if an equal number of previously closed alveolar capillaries open in the right lung, and blood flow through it is doubled.

Characteristics of the Alveolocapillary and Erythrocyte Membranes

As stated earlier, gases move from alveoli to capillaries by going from a gaseous state to a state of solution on the surface of tissues and then moving through the tissue because of concentration gradients. Therefore, the solubility of a gas in tissue influences its rate of diffusion across it; it is because CO_2 is 24 times as soluble as O_2 in tissue that the CO_2 in blood and gas always come into equilibrium. We do not know whether the solubility in tissue of any single gas (O_2, CO_2, CO, etc.) changes if the composition of tissues in the diffusion path should change as a result of disease.

PULMONARY DIFFUSING CAPACITY

The physician wants to know whether his patient has impaired diffusion because of a longer tissue path (alveolocapillary block) or a decreased area for gas exchange, or both. To put it differently, he wants to know the ability of the alveolocapillary membranes to transfer or conduct gases.

Conductance is the reciprocal of resistance.

$$\text{Resistance} = \frac{\text{Driving pressure}}{\text{Flow}}$$

$$\therefore \text{Conductance} = \frac{\text{Flow} \quad Q\,(\dot{v})}{\text{Driving pressure} \; \triangle P}$$

In measuring the diffusing characteristics of the lung, we are measuring a kind of conductance:

$$\text{Diffusing capacity} = \frac{\text{Flow}}{\text{Mean driving pressure}}$$

The equation for the diffusing capacity (D) for O_2 is:

$$D_{O_2} = \frac{\text{ml } O_2 \text{ transferred/minute from alveolar gas to blood}}{\text{Mean alveolar } P_{O_2} - \text{mean pulmonary capillary } P_{O_2}}$$

and the units are (ml O_2/minute)/torr P_{O_2}. By expressing the transfer capacity on a basis of transfer *per torr* P_{O_2}, we eliminate the variable of the driving pressure for O_2 and so obtain information about the area and thickness of the tissues. These two factors cannot be separated; a decrease in measured D_{O_2} may be due to decreased area or increased thickness, or both. It is even possible that D_{O_2} may be "normal" if thickness is increased (interstitial edema) but area is simultaneously increased (increase in the number of functioning capillaries). It is possible to calculate the "conductance" of the alveolocapillary tissues separately from the "conductance" for the uptake of O_2 within the erythrocyte (see p. 166). Some of the factors influencing D_{O_2} are shown schematically in Figure 12-3.

Tests of Diffusing Capacity

These require measuring the transfer of gases from alveolar to capillary blood. But not any gas can be used. For most gases, the amount transferred per minute depends not only on the transfer properties of the membranes but also on the quantity of pulmonary capillary blood flow per minute. Some gases (such as N_2O) are used in the measurement of pulmonary *blood flow;* others (O_2 and CO) are used to measure *diffusing capacity.* Why? Gases such as N_2O are soluble to an equal extent in the alveolocapillary membranes and in blood; they almost instantly saturate the pulmonary tissues and blood (Fig. 12-4). Once the P_{N_2O} in pulmonary capillary blood rises to equal alveolar P_{N_2O}, further gas transfer can occur only if capillary blood is flowing and blood entering the capillaries contains little or no N_2O. Since the uptake of a gas such as N_2O is not limited by diffusion but by the volume of blood flow per minute, it can be used to measure pulmonary blood flow (see p. 145).

Two gases, O_2 and CO, have the unique property of being far more "soluble" in blood than in alveolocapillary membranes, because of chemical association between them and hemoglobin (see p. 192). One L of blood with a normal hemoglobin content can combine with 200 ml of O_2 or CO if it contains neither O_2 nor CO initially. Because hemoglobin can combine with larger amounts of O_2 or CO than normally cross alveolocapillary membranes, this chemical combination could keep end-capillary P_{O_2} or P_{CO} low enough that their uptake is not *flow-limited,* and then O_2 or CO could be used to measure diffusing capacity.

OXYGEN DIFFUSING CAPACITY (D_{O_2}). This is difficult to measure because venous blood flowing into the pulmonary capillaries is not O_2-free; it is already about 75% saturated with O_2. As it combines with additional O_2, the P_{O_2} of gas and blood come into equilibrium; as mentioned above for N_2O,

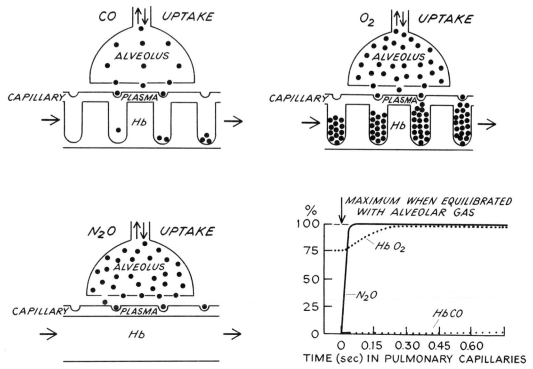

Fig. 12-4.—In each *schema*, the black dots signify gas molecules. The bottom of each alveolus represents the alveolocapillary membrane with numerous pores to permit diffusion of gas molecules. Blood moves from left to right through the pulmonary capillary beneath the pulmonary membrane. The bloodstream, solely for purposes of illustration, is divided into 2 portions: upper portion represents plasma (and all other watery parts of the blood), with a certain number of pockets to indicate its capacity for dissolving each gas; lower portion represents hemoglobin; there are no compartments in the hemoglobin layer for N_2O because it does not combine chemically with hemoglobin, but large pockets are available for CO and O_2. Mixed venous blood enters the capillary with no CO or N_2O in the plasma and hemoglobin compartments (since these are foreign gases) but with the O_2 compartments partly full.

The *graph* presents blood gas content (ordinate) plotted against the time that the blood spends in the pulmonary capillary. The horizontal line at the top indicates maximal gas content of the blood when it is *saturated* at the gas pressure maintained in the alveoli. In the case of CO, there is only a very slight increase in HbCO concentration along the capillary; it never approaches the maximal value because of the low partial pressure of CO in the alveoli. In the case of N_2O, the blood attains maximal concentration before it has gone 1/20 the distance along the capillary. In the case of O_2, saturation increases from 75 to 97% along the capillary. (Redrawn from Comroe, J. H., Jr., *et al.: The Lung* [2d ed.; Chicago: Year Book Medical Publishers, Inc., 1962].)

when this occurs, gas uptake is at least in part *flow*-limited (see Fig. 12-4).

To measure Do_2, one must know the Po_2 of mixed venous blood. Further, the rate of diffusion of O_2 into the blood depends on the difference between the Po_2 of the alveolar gas and that of the blood at every point along the capillary. As O_2 is transferred across the alveolocapillary membranes, the capillary Po_2 rises, and the increase in capillary Po_2 narrows the difference between alveolar and

capillary Po_2 (see Fig. 12-1) and slows the rate of diffusion. This means that the blood Po_2 must be known at every moment along the capillary. This information can be obtained by certain measurements and a series of mathematical computations, but this is no longer necessary since the introduction of tests that measure diffusing capacity for CO.

CARBON MONOXIDE DIFFUSING CAPACI- TY (DCO). Carbon monoxide can be deadly if it combines with so much hemoglobin that the amount of O_2 uptake, transport and delivery are decreased to dangerously low levels. But inhalation of a low concentration of CO (0.3%) for a single breath or 1 – 2 minutes is not dangerous. The single-breath test requires only one full inspiration of 0.3% CO. This brings about 10 ml CO into the lungs. If all of it diffused into the blood and were then distributed throughout a 5-L blood volume, 100 ml of blood would contain only 0.2 ml CO. (See Chapter 14 for discussion of CO poisoning.)

The advantages in using CO are: (1) except in heavy smokers, the concentration of CO in mixed venous blood entering the pulmonary capillaries is so close to zero that it need not be measured; (2) CO is a remarkable gas because of its great affinity for hemoglobin (Hb), 210 times that of O_2. Thus a partial pressure of CO of only 0.46 torr (equivalent to 0.065% CO) produces the same percent of saturation of Hb, at equilibrium, as does a partial pressure of 100 torr O_2 (equivalent to 14% O_2). For this reason, any CO in the vicinity of an Hb molecule becomes bound to it, so that the partial pressure of dissolved CO stays at a very low level in the red blood cell. Because Pco in blood is very close to zero even at the end of the pulmonary capillary, CO uptake is never flow-limited (Fig. 12-4). Even if pulmonary blood flow stopped for short periods, transfer of CO could still continue by diffusion.

We can obtain Do_2 by multiplying Dco by 1.23 (a factor derived from Graham's and Henry's laws, p. 159).

At least four technics use CO to measure diffusion. The simplest is a single-breath test developed by Forster and his associates. In this the patient inspires a gas mixture containing a low concentration of CO, then holds his breath for approximately 10 seconds, during which some CO leaves the alveolar gas and enters the blood: the larger the diffusing capacity, the more CO enters the blood during the 10-second period. Since pulmonary diffusing capacity for CO =

$$\frac{\text{ml CO transferred/minute from alveolar gas to blood}}{\text{Mean alveolar CO pressure} - \text{mean capillary CO pressure}}$$

three numbers must be known: (1) milliliters of CO transferred from alveolar gas to blood/minute; (2) the mean alveolar CO pressure; (3) the mean pulmonary capillary CO pressure.

The milliliters of CO transferred can be calculated from measurements of the percent of CO in the alveolar gas at the beginning and at the end of the breath-holding period if the volume of alveolar gas (FRC) is also known. The mean capillary Pco is so small that it can be neglected. In the single-breath test, alveolar Pco is not maintained at a constant concentration because CO is absorbed during breath holding. However, the mean alveolar Pco can be calculated by a special equation.

The single-breath test has the advantages of being quick and requiring little cooperation from the patient, who has only to inhale and hold his breath for 10 seconds. The analyses are performed on gas, and no blood samples are needed. The method has the disadvantages that CO is a nonphysiologic gas, that breath holding is not a normal breathing state and that some dyspneic or exercising patients may find it difficult to hold their breath for 10 seconds.

Normal values for Dco (single-breath test) are 25 ml/minute/torr and for Do_2 by calculation, 31 ml/minute/torr. The term "diffusing *capacity*" is really a misnomer. Webster defines *capacity* as "the ability to contain, absorb or receive" or "the maximal amount of holding space"; this implies a maximal value. Yet Dco, as usually measured, is the value during rest; it rises during exercise when pulmonary blood flow can increase up to 8-fold, probably because area increases as more pulmonary capillaries open, either because pulmonary arterial pressure rises or arterioles, previously constricted, open.

Carbon monoxide diffusing capacity also varies with body size (probably because of change in area available for gas exchange), with position (it is about 25% greater in the supine than in the standing position, probably because more capillaries are open in the upper lobes when the subject is supine) and with alveolar P_{O_2} (it is greater at low P_{O_2}). It is also dependent on the amount of Hb/100 ml of blood in the pulmonary capillaries. Obviously, if there were no hemoglobin, CO could only dissolve in plasma and red cell water (as N_2O does) and could not be used to measure diffusing capacity. Corrections must be made in calculating Dco in patients with severe anemia or polycythemia.

THE MEMBRANE DIFFUSING CAPACITY. If the reaction rates of Hb and O_2 or Hb and CO and certain other data are known, the pulmonary diffusing capacity of man can be separated into its two component parts—the membrane diffusing capacity and the red blood cell and Hb component. The theory is as follows:

If the concentration of O_2 molecules in the alveoli is increased (by breathing 40–100% O_2), there is increased competition between O_2 and CO molecules for the available Hb, and the rate of CO uptake by the red blood cell is decreased, though the transfer characteristics of the alveolocapillary *membranes* remain unaffected. If the concentration of O_2 molecules in alveoli is decreased (by breathing 10–20% O_2), the competition between O_2 and CO is decreased, and therefore the Hb-CO reaction rate is more rapid. By measuring the diffusing capacity of a patient while he is breathing CO in high and again in low concentrations of O_2, Forster has been able to estimate the membrane diffusing capacity. Measurements to date suggest that, in a healthy individual whose pulmonary capacity is about 35 ml O_2/minute/torr, the membrane diffusing capacity is about 70 ml O_2/minute/torr. (The sum of two conductances in series must be calculated as $\frac{1}{sum} = \frac{1}{A} + \frac{1}{B}$; this explains why one com-

ponent [membrane diffusing capacity] appears to be greater than total pulmonary diffusing capacity.)

CLINICAL USE OF DCO AND DO₂

If the physician wants to know whether the lung can no longer transfer O_2 normally, why doesn't he merely measure arterial O_2 content or P_{O_2}? One reason is that Dco may be below normal before the P_{O_2} of arterial blood is decreased. The reserve in the mechanism for transferring O_2 is great enough that blood leaving the alveolar capillaries may be fully oxygenated even though Dco is 50–75% of normal (see Fig. 12-1). Another is that arterial hypoxemia may be caused by many factors, and impairment of diffusion is only one of these; the Dco test therefore provides specificity.

A decrease in Dco may occur clinically in diseases associated with thickening and separation of the capillary and alveolar walls, such as that caused by interstitial or alveolar pulmonary fibrosis. (It is well to remember that the physiologist can diagnose "impairment of diffusion" and can infer that it is caused by fibrous tissue, but only the pathologist can legitimately diagnose "fibrosis.") Carbon monoxide diffusing capacity is decreased for these reasons in patients with sarcoidosis, berylliosis, asbestosis, scleroderma or pulmonary edema. It is decreased in patients with emphysema because of a decrease in surface area for gas exchange owing to destruction of the alveolar and capillary walls. It may be a more sensitive test for early emphysema than tests of mechanical properties of lungs; certainly it should be included in screening tests for early emphysema. Since the diffusing capacity is relatively normal in uncomplicated bronchial asthma, the test can serve on occasion to differentiate asthma from obstructive emphysema.

The pulmonary diffusing capacity is also decreased when the total surface area of the capillaries is decreased, as in pneumonectomy or a space-taking lesion of the lung or in any abnormality that occludes the arterial flow to part of the lung. Pulmonary hypertension need not be accompanied by a reduction in diffusing capacity unless there is obliteration of part of the pulmonary capillary bed. Indeed, pulmonary hypertension, by providing a high enough diastolic pressure to push blood to the top of the lung in erect man, may increase Dco. Pulmonary congestion, such as that associated with mitral stenosis, may cause no reduction in diffusing capacity in early stages of the disease, because the pulmonary capillary bed may be enlarged and apical capillaries, previously closed, may be opened; however, when interstitial or alveolar edema or deposition of fibrous tissue occurs, the diffusing capacity decreases. In conditions associated with increase in blood volume, the pulmonary capillary blood volume may also be increased, with a consequent increase in diffusing capacity.

It is well to remember that impaired diffusion rarely if ever occurs as the sole physiologic abnormality. The pathologic processes that thicken membranes or decrease surface area almost invariably lead to uneven ventilation, uneven capillary blood flow and uneven matching of gas and blood.

EFFECTS OF IMPAIRED DIFFUSION ON ARTERIAL BLOOD

When the diffusing capacity for O_2 is decreased so that equilibrium no longer occurs between gas and capillary blood, arterial Po_2 decreases relative to alveolar Po_2. As further impairment occurs, decrease in arterial O_2 saturation becomes evident and O_2 transport decreases; the hypoxemia becomes more severe during exercise. There is no impairment in outward diffusion of CO_2; if hyperventilation occurs (because of hypoxemia or pulmonary reflexes initiated by pulmonary disease), the Pco_2 of arterial blood will be below normal.

Diffusion of gases from closed spaces into blood is discussed on p. 276; diffusion across the placenta is discussed on p. 242.

13

Matching of Gas and Blood

IN AN IDEAL LUNG, inspiration would draw air of the same composition uniformly to each of the millions of alveoli so that each received a fair share in relation to its prespiratory volume. And the right ventricle would distribute mixed blood of the same composition to capillaries surrounding each alveolus so that each received a fair share of pulmonary blood flow in relation to its ventilation. In this ideal lung (if there were no impairment of diffusion), the P_{O_2} and P_{CO_2} of blood leaving each alveolar capillary would be the same. In the real lung, however, neither alveolar ventilation nor alveolar capillary blood flow is ever distributed perfectly uniformly, even in healthy man, even in the supine posture. And in patients with cardiopulmonary disease the most frequent cause of systemic arterial hypoxemia is not hypoventilation, impairment of diffusion or anatomic right-to-left shunts; it is uneven alveolar ventilation in relation to alveolar blood flow, or more simply, uneven matching of gas and blood. Uneven matching is also an important cause of CO_2 retention.

Let us first discuss nonuniform ventilation, then nonuniform blood flow, and finally what happens when both are present in the same lungs.

NONUNIFORM VENTILATION

Causes

The mechanisms causing uneven ventilation were discussed in Chapter 10; essential-ly these are uneven resistances to air flow and uneven compliances in different parts of the lungs. Figure 10-6 pictured three combinations of uneven compliance and resistance that result in uneven ventilation; you can draw an infinite number of combinations if you wish.

Uneven resistance to air flow may be due to regional obstruction of airways caused by bronchoconstriction (as in asthma or exposure to irritant gases or fumes), collapse of airways (as in emphysema), narrowing (as in bronchitis and bronchiolitis) or compression (by tumors, edema, pleural effusion or forced expiration); it may be due to uneven expansion of the lungs and airways because of the effects of gravity and variations in intrapleural pressure.

Uneven compliance may be due to fibrosis, loss of elastic recoil (as in emphysema), uneven distribution of surfactant, pleural thickening or effusion, pulmonary congestion or edema, compression of lung tissue (by tumors, abscesses or cysts) or uneven intrapleural pressure, as in pneumothorax or surgical opening of one hemithorax.

Tests of Nonuniform Distribution of Gas

Physicians for generations have detected pulmonary disease by noting unequal breath sounds with a stethoscope; radiologists have long observed that lung radiodensity is not uniform because of uneven expansion of lung units; thoracic surgeons for years have directly observed uneven regional expansion of lungs. The pulmonary physiologist has entered on the scene only recently. His contribution has been to devise rapid, simple tests to provide quantitative data on nonuniformity of ventilation. These tests measure the distribution of inspired gas to the alveoli, as though the lungs were an impermeable bag or bellows and the processes of diffusion and gas uptake by flowing blood did not exist. They require the use of gases such as N_2, He or Xe, which are poorly soluble in blood.

The simplest is a single-breath test (Fig. 13-1). The patient expires fully, then inspires O_2 deeply through a mouthpiece and immediately breathes out slowly and completely. Gas is drawn continuously through a fine needle in the mouthpiece to a very rapid N_2 analyzer, which records the N_2 concentration continuously. Assume that the patient's FRC (including his anatomic dead space) is 2,000 ml and the N_2 concentration of this is 80% when he breathes air. If he inspires 2,000 ml of O_2 into his *alveoli* and this O_2 is distributed evenly, each alveolus will now contain 40% N_2. On the other hand, if the 2,000 ml of O_2 are distributed *unevenly*, some alveoli may get less than their share (hypoventilation) and others may get more than their share (hyperventilation); in this case, the composition of alveolar gas will be decidedly *nonuniform* at end-inspiration.

We can determine uneven inspiration by measuring the N_2 concentration of expired alveolar gas after the dead space gas has been washed out. If the inspired O_2 is distributed evenly to all the alveoli so that each now contains 40% N_2 instead of 80%, it is obvious that the first, middle and last parts of expired *alveolar* gas all contain 40% N_2 even if all parts of the lung do not empty synchronously. The N_2 meter record of alveolar gas is shown at the top right of Figure 13-1; i.e., it is a perfectly horizontal record. On the other hand, if the inspired O_2 is distributed unevenly to the various alveoli, end-inspiratory N_2 concentrations vary in different parts of the lungs and the N_2 meter record of al-

veolar gas is far from a horizontal line; the first gas expired usually has a low N_2 concentration (since it ordinarily comes from the hyperventilated parts, which received a larger share of the inspired O_2), and the last gas expired usually has a higher N_2 concentration (since it generally comes from a hypoventilated region that received little O_2, as shown at the bottom right in Fig. 13-1). This rising concentration of N_2 depends both on uneven distribution of the gas *during inspiration* and on unequal rates of gas flow from different regions of the lungs *during expiration*. If all regions emptied synchronously during expiration, the N_2 meter record would still be horizontal even though the concentration of N_2 varied in different parts of the lung at end-inspiration. A special type of uneven emptying was pictured in Figure 10-37.

Another test of distribution requires that the patient breathe O_2 for 7 minutes. Each successive inspiration of O_2 dilutes the nitrogen in the alveoli, and each expiration carries out some alveolar N_2 (N_2 "washout") (Fig. 2-9, p. 18). If all alveoli are uniformly ventilated, the alveolar N_2 concentration will be less than 2.5% at the end of 7 minutes. The rate of elimination of N_2 from a normal lung depends on several factors; it is slower if the FRC is large, the tidal volume is low, the dead space large and the frequency of breathing slow (Fig. 2-8, p. 17). However, if some alveoli are poorly ventilated, they receive less O_2 and their N_2 is not diluted and washed out and may still be quite high at the end of 7 minutes. When these alveoli are emptied by a forced expiration, their contribution to the total expired alveolar gas may result in a N_2 concentration well above 2.5%. However, patients with abnormal distribution demonstrated by the single-breath test may have a normal value for the 7-minute test if they are hyperventilating.

Sometimes alveoli act as though they were *non*ventilated, though in fact they are either very poorly ventilated or intermittently ventilated (completely closed off, nonventilated alveoli lose their gas to blood and collapse; see p. 276). The volume of gas at any mo-

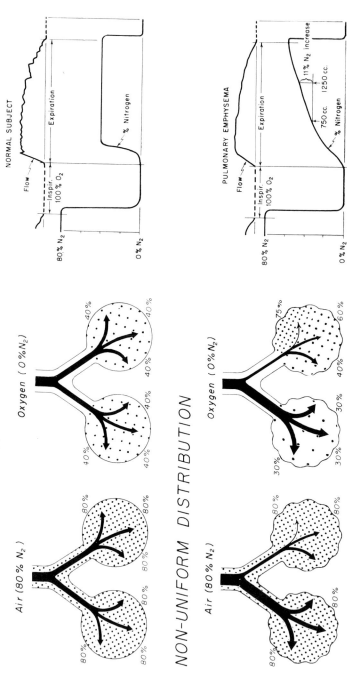

Fig. 13-1.—Distribution of inspired gas. The same volume of gas (air or O_2) is inspired; **above**, distribution is uniform, and **below** it is nonuniform. N_2 molecules are represented by black dots. **Left**, schematic representation of alveolar N_2 during breathing of air; **center**, schematic representation of alveolar N_2 immediately after a single breath of O_2; **right**, records of N_2 concentration and gas flow during the next expiration.

Note: Even when distribution of inspired *air* to the alveoli is nonuniform, it would be undetected, owing to lack of sensitivity of the N_2 meter to small changes in % N_2. In the illustration, both air and alveolar gas (**left**) are pictured as containing 80% N_2. Actually, air contains 79.03% N_2 and alveolar gas about 80–81%. However, even if *all* the air went to half the alveoli, it would lower alveolar N_2 from 80 or 81% to 79.5 or 80.5%, and the N_2 meter would not be able to detect such small changes with accuracy. The breathing of O_2 (**center**) dilutes the N_2, the degree of dilution depending on the fraction of inspired O_2 distributed to the various regions of the lungs. Thus, when there is nonuniform distribution, inhalation of O_2 magnifies the effect of this in the different areas. (From Comroe, J. H., Jr., *et al.: The Lung* [2d ed.]; Chicago: Year Book Medical Publishers, Inc., 1962].)

ment in alveoli, either not ventilated or very poorly ventilated, can be calculated by using the body plethysmograph (p. 000) to measure the total volume of gas in the thorax (whether in free communication with open airways or not) and subtracting from this the lung volume measured by a technic that washes out only alveolar gas in communication with airways. (In using the body plethysmograph to measure total gas volume of the lungs, remember that it actually measures total gas volume within the *thorax*; if there is a pneumothorax, thoracic gas volume exceeds lung volume by the amount of gas in the pleural cavity.)

Another method in use to detect uneven ventilation is the "closing volume" test described on p. 136. This is believed to measure the volume of the lungs at which some airways close toward the end of a full expiration.

The methods described above tell us when there is uneven ventilation and approximately how much, but give no information on the *location* of the poorly ventilated regions (right versus left? upper versus lower lobes?). Such information can be obtained if a patient inhales a single breath of ^{133}Xe and then holds his breath (see Fig. 13-7). Xenon is poorly soluble in blood, so little xenon enters the blood during breath holding. During breath holding, the amount of radioactivity over the right and left upper, middle and lower lung regions is measured by means of external counters, or over the whole lung by means of a scintillation camera. Or ^{133}Xe may be delivered to the alveoli by blood flowing through alveolar capillaries. In this test ^{133}Xe is dissolved in saline and injected intravenously; since xenon is poorly soluble in blood, almost all of it leaves the pulmonary capillary blood to enter alveolar gas. Its rate of washout from different regions can then be measured. (In all tests that use external counters to measure radioactivity in internal organs that are thin in places and thick in others, appropriate control measurements or corrections are required to compare ventilation in one region with that in another.)

NONUNIFORM BLOOD FLOW

Causes

The physiologic mechanisms responsible for nonuniform blood flow in different parts of the lung were discussed in Chapter 11. These were: (1) the effect of gravity on columns of blood in upper and lower parts of the lungs, (2) regional differences in intrapleural pressure, (3) regional changes in alveolar pressure and (4) constriction, obliteration, block or compression of some parts of the pulmonary circulation.

Some specific clinical causes of uneven blood flow are:

1. Regional congestion of vessels such as occurs in some types of heart failure.

2. Closure of some pulmonary vessels due to reduction of circulating blood volume and very low pulmonary vascular pressures, which may occur during severe hypotension and circulatory shock.

3. An open hemithorax, as during thoracic surgical procedures, when one lung is exposed to atmospheric and the other to subatmospheric intrathoracic pressure.

4. Overexpansion of some alveoli and collapse of others.

5. Regional differences in the alveolar pressure transmitted to the pulmonary capillaries because some alveoli are air-filled and some fluid-filled.

6. Tension cysts.

7. Embolization or thrombosis of parts of the pulmonary circulation by blood clots, fat, gas (as in decompression sickness; see p. 249), parasites, oils (used in lymphangiography) or tumor cells.

8. Partial or complete occlusion of one pulmonary artery or some of the arterioles by arteriosclerotic lesions, endarteritis, collagen disease or congenital anomalies.

9. Compression or kinking of large or small pulmonary vessels by masses, pulmonary exudates or pneumo- or hydrothorax.

10. Reduction of part of the pulmonary vascular bed by destruction of lung tissue (as in emphysema) or by fibrotic obliteration of pulmonary vessels.

11. Anatomic venous-to-arterial shunts, as in pulmonary hemangiomas; in such shunts, however, the distribution of blood that is *flowing to capillaries* may be uniform, the abnormality being that some mixed venous blood bypasses capillaries completely to empty directly into pulmonary venules or veins.

Tests of Nonuniform Blood Flow

1. ANGIOGRAM. A nontoxic radiopaque material is injected intravenously or into the pulmonary artery and roentgenograms are made during the moments that the material should be in pulmonary arteries, capillaries and veins; either rapid exposure of serial large films or cineangiography can be used. Figure 1-7, which is an angiogram of a lung outside the thorax, shows uniform distribution of the radiopaque material since there is no obstruction or regional resistance to flow. If there had been regions with no or markedly reduced blood flow, these would have received no or little radiopaque material.

2. LUNG SCANNING AFTER INJECTION OF MACROAGGREGATES OF ALBUMIN. In the conventional angiogram the test substance flows only into regions with a patent circulation. In this test, the test substance is carried only to regions with a patent circulation but blocks some arterioles in these regions. The substance is a macroaggregate of albumin (MAA) labeled with either ^{131}I or technetium, and it is detected by external counters, scanners or camera. [131]Iodinated MAA acts like a relatively stable snowflake; it lodges in a pulmonary arteriole (and so serves as a marker for an *open* vessel) but does not necessarily block flow unless blood cells plug the gaps; in a few hours it is broken up, carried by blood to the liver and metabolized there. The number of particles injected is calculated to block only a very small fraction of the huge number of pulmonary arterioles, but enough to give a picture of the distribution of blood flow.

3. LUNG SCANNING AFTER INTRAVENOUS [133]XE. As mentioned previously, ^{133}Xe dissolves sparingly in saline and quickly comes out of solution when the solution is exposed to alveolar gas. Therefore, if the patient receives ^{133}Xe intravenously or into the right atrium and holds his breath, lung scans show those regions with pulmonary blood flow. Because xenon can enter the lung as a gas only where there is pulmonary capillary blood flow to air-filled alveoli, it provides a means of detecting regions with little or no mechanism for gas exchange.

NONUNIFORM VENTILATION AND BLOOD FLOW

Effects of Uneven Matching

Earlier we said that uneven matching is the most frequent cause of hypoxemia and of CO_2 retention. Now it is important to define matching. A certain volume of alveolar gas is required to arterialize a given volume of mixed venous blood. To simplify the discussion, let us say that blood of healthy man at sea level is arterialized when its Po_2 is about 100 torr and its Pco_2 about 40 torr. The amount of alveolar gas required for this depends on the Po_2 and Pco_2 of mixed venous blood and the rate of blood flow per minute. Again to simplify the discussion, let us say that in a resting healthy adult (O_2 consumption 250 ml/minute and CO_2 production 200 ml/minute) with uniform ventilation and uniform blood flow, 4,000 ml/minute of alveolar ventilation will just arterialize 5,000 ml/minute of mixed venous blood. We say then that proper matching of gas and blood has been achieved. Increasing ventilation further in relation to this pulmonary blood flow will lower arterial Pco_2 below the optimal value; maintaining 4,000 ml/min of alveolar ventilation while decreasing pulmonary blood flow has the same effect. We see, therefore, that it is the optimal *ratio* or matching of gas and blood that produces optimal arterialization of blood. If this ratio of

$$\frac{\text{ventilation}}{\text{blood flow}} = \frac{4,000 \text{ ml/minute}}{5,000 \text{ ml/minute}} = \frac{4}{5} = 0.8 \text{ (de-}$$

termined for the whole lung) also applies

to every region and alveolus of the lung, again arterial blood will be optimally arterialized, and this is true even though one region receives only half of the alveolar ventilation distributed to another region of the same size, as long as the blood flow is also halved. It is for this reason that physiologists emphasize the ventilation: blood flow *ratio* rather than absolute amounts. When the *ratios* are not uniform throughout the lungs, the arterial blood cannot be optimally arterialized. As we shall see, regions with very low ratios (little ventilation relative to blood flow) act as a shunt and interfere mainly with proper oxygenation, and regions with a high ratio act mainly to lower blood CO_2; since lungs that have regions with high ratios also have regions with low ratios, nonuniform ratios always make the lung less effective than an ideal lung both in O_2 uptake and CO_2 elimination.

It is easier to understand the effects of uneven ratios or uneven matching if we first consider two extreme cases: (1) when one lung has no ventilation but normal blood flow and (2) when one lung has normal ventilation and no blood flow. We will then consider the more frequent condition (3) when all alveoli have some ventilation and some blood flow but the *ratios* vary widely.

1. NO VENTILATION; NORMAL BLOOD FLOW. This is pictured schematically in Figure 13-2, *top*. Hypoxemia must result if the patient is breathing air. Mixed venous blood in lung *A* does not come in contact with ventilated alveoli and cannot gain O_2 or lose CO_2. Even if there is *hyper*ventilation of lung *B*, the O_2 content of blood flowing through it will not increase sufficiently to make up for the venous blood pouring through *A*. A few calculations show why this is so. Let us say that mixed venous blood has an O_2 saturation of 60% and that the capacity of hemoglobin for combining with O_2 is 20 ml O_2/100 ml blood. Reference to Figure 14-1 shows that the total O_2 content of 100 ml of this blood is 12.1 ml (12 ml is combined with hemoglobin and 0.1 ml is dis-

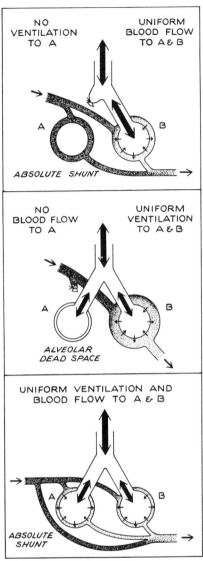

Fig. 13-2.—Uneven ventilation and pulmonary blood flow. The alveoli, where rapid gas exchange occurs, are represented by rounded areas; leading into these are tubes depicting the conducting airways or anatomic dead space in which no effective gas exchange occurs. *Arrows* entering the alveoli show distribution of total inspired gas (*large arrow*) to various alveoli. *Small arrows* crossing alveolar walls show the process of diffusion of O_2 out of the alveoli into the blood and of CO_2 from the blood into the alveoli. The *shaded channel* surrounding the alveoli represents pulmonary blood flow; it enters the capillary bed as mixed venous blood (*dark*) and emerges as arterialized blood (*light*). **Top**, lung *A* has no ventilation but normal blood flow. **Center**, lung *A* has normal ventilation but no blood flow. **Bottom**, a shunt of venous to arterial blood completely bypasses the lung.

solved O_2); that of 1 L is 121 ml. Assume that 2.5 L of this blood flows unaltered through A; this contains 2.5×121 ml, or 302.5 ml of O_2. If alveolar ventilation is normal in B (and there is no impairment of diffusion), blood flowing through it emerges 97.4% saturated with O_2; 100 ml of blood contains 19.8 ml O_2 (19.5 ml is combined with Hb and 0.3 ml is dissolved O_2), and 1 L contains 198 ml O_2. If 2.5 L flows through B per minute, it contains 2.5×198 ml, or 495 ml of O_2. The 5 L of blood contains $302.5 + 495$, or 797.5 ml O_2, 1 L contains 797.5/5, or 159.5, and 100 ml contains 15.95. Hemoglobin is therefore only 79.1% saturated. This represents severe hypoxemia.

Suppose this patient doubled the alveolar ventilation of lung B and his alveolar P_{O_2} rose from 100 to 125 torr. This would increase the dissolved O_2 from 0.3 to 0.375 ml O_2/100 ml blood, but, *because the HbO_2 dissociation curve is almost horizontal between P_{O_2} of 100 and 125, the saturation of hemoglobin with O_2 would rise from 97.4 to only 98.5%.* The O_2 content of 2.5 L of blood flowing through lung B during hyperventilation is now 502 (an increase of 7 ml over 495) and the O_2 saturation of 100 ml of mixed blood from A and B is now 79.8%, an increase of only 0.7%. Even if only 10% instead of 50% of the mixed venous blood flowed unoxygenated into mixed arterial blood, the arterial O_2 saturation would still be low (94% if ventilation of B is normal and 95.2% if it is doubled).

What happens to the P_{CO_2} of arterial blood? Venous blood with a P_{CO_2} of, say, 46 torr passes through A and joins the stream of arterialized blood from B, which has a P_{CO_2} of 40. The P_{CO_2} of arterial blood must therefore rise. It has been widely taught that a shunt such as this ($\dot{V}_A/\dot{Q}c = 0/2.5$) causes hypoxemia without CO_2 retention. This is true only when the respiratory centers, in response to an immediate increase in arterial P_{CO_2}, initiate impulses to the respiratory muscles calling for increased ventilation and the muscles, thorax and lungs can respond with hyperventilation. Therefore,

hyperventilation of lung B can decrease the CO_2 content of blood flowing through it. When blood from B, low in CO_2, mixes with blood from A, high in CO_2, the mixture (systemic arterial blood) may have a normal CO_2 content (see p. 195). As pointed out earlier, the shape of the HbO_2 dissociation curve prevents similar correction of hypoxemia in this case.

This condition, in which mixed venous blood flows unaltered into the systemic arterial blood, is called an absolute *venous-to-arterial shunt*. Pulmonary arterial blood flows to the systemic circulation without any effective contact between blood and alveolar gas; the shunt may be between large vessels (pulmonary hemangioma) or through alveolar capillaries if these alveoli receive no ventilation (e.g., are collapsed or are filled with fluid or exudate). We differentiate these from regions with a very low $\dot{V}_A/\dot{Q}c$ ratio because, in an absolute shunt, venous blood bypasses ventilated alveoli so that it cannot be oxygenated no matter how high the P_{O_2} in the nearest alveoli; because of this, the diagnosis of the presence and magnitude of an absolute shunt can be made by measuring arterial blood O_2 during the inhalation of O_2.

Let us start with the previous example, in which lung A had normal blood flow but no ventilation. The patient now breathes O_2. The 2.5 L of blood flowing through A contains, as before, 302.5 ml O_2. The 2.5 L flowing through B contains 500 ml O_2 combined with hemoglobin (now 100% saturated), but also contains 50 ml of dissolved O_2 (because of the high alveolar P_{O_2}, 670 torr). Five L of mixed venous blood now contains 852.5 ml O_2, and its saturation is 84.5%. Note that inhalation of O_2 has increased the arterial O_2, *but not to maximal values*. An absolute shunt is the only clinical condition known in which inhalation of O_2 does not increase arterial O_2 to maximal levels. Inhalation of O_2 increases arterial O_2 to maximal values in a patient with poorly ventilated alveoli, because if he breathes O_2 long enough (10–20 minutes), N_2 will be eliminated and the alveolar O_2 concentration will rise maximally even in these. This is also true in patients with impairment of diffusion of O_2 across alveolocapillary membranes; the partial pressure of O_2 rises to maximal values in arterial blood because of the very large initial alveolar-to-arterial O_2 difference (see Fig. 12-1). Therefore, when breathing O_2, only a patient with an absolute shunt has *systemic arterial blood that is not oxygenated maximally*; this is because a stream of mixed venous (poorly oxygenated) shunted blood merges in the pulmonary veins with a stream of fully oxygenated blood from the alveolar capillaries.

If all alveoli receive 100% O_2 and there is *no* absolute shunt, arterial Po_2 should rise to 670 torr. With small absolute shunts, inhalation of O_2 may increase the *Hb saturation* to 100% but it *cannot raise the dissolved O_2 or Po_2 to maximal levels.*

Let us calculate arterial O_2 when there is a 10% absolute shunt. If mixed venous O_2 saturation and cardiac output are the same as in the previous example, the shunt will be 500 ml and will contribute 5×12.1, or 60.5, ml O_2 to mixed arterial blood. The 4,500 ml that passes through alveolar capillaries will contribute 45×22, or 990 ml O_2 (each 100 ml of blood contains 20 ml O_2 combined with fully saturated Hb and 2 ml of dissolved O_2, owing to the high alveolar Po_2, 670 torr; see p. 183). The total 5,000 ml, contains $60.5 + 990$, (1050.5) ml of O_2, and 100 ml of mixed arterial blood contains $\frac{1,050}{50}$, or 21 ml. Since fully saturated Hb can contain only 20 ml O_2, *Hb* is maximally *saturated*. But the blood does not contain maximal *amounts* of O_2 because it has only 1.0 ml of dissolved O_2 instead of 2.0 ml/100 ml, and the Po_2 is only 385 instead of 670 torr. This emphasizes the necessity for measuring arterial Po_2 instead of HbO_2 saturation to detect small shunts (20% or less of the cardiac output). It also emphasizes the need to think in terms of maximal *oxygenation* of arterial blood (hemoglobin O_2 + *dissolved* O_2) instead of maximal *saturation of hemoglobin.*

2. NORMAL VENTILATION; NO BLOOD FLOW. This is pictured schematically in Figure 13-2, *center.* This situation occurs clinically when a balloon is inflated to occlude the pulmonary artery to lung *A* or when a large embolus blocks it and there is no change in ventilation or airway resistance. Let us assume that before the occlusion, half of the total pulmonary blood flow (5 L/minute) and half of the total alveolar ventilation went to each lung. Immediately after the occlusion, all of the blood flow must go to lung *B*, but half of the ventilation still goes to lung *A* (Table 13-1). The ventilation to lung *A* is wasted because it is ineffective in arterializing mixed venous blood. It is, therefore, equivalent to ventilation of the conducting airway—it is "dead space ventilation." Since it is located anatomically in alveoli, it has been called "alveolar dead space." (The alveolar dead space is not the *volume of the alveolar gas* but the *volume of gas entering it* per breath or per minute). Ventilation of alveolar dead space requires work of the respiratory muscles without serving any useful function.

Immediately after the occlusion, lung *B* must arterialize 5 L of blood but still receives only 2 L of alveolar ventilation/minute. Since this amount of ventilation had been just enough to maintain alveolar Po_2 and arterialize 2.5 L of mixed venous blood, it cannot arterialize twice as much; hypoxemia and CO_2 retention must occur. If compensatory mechanisms double alveolar ventilation, then arterial O_2 and CO_2 will return to normal. However, this requires 8 L of alveolar ventilation instead of 5. The lung has two compensatory mechanisms that at least partially restore the normal relation between ventilation and blood flow: (1) low alveolar Po_2 (and probably high alveolar Pco_2) in poorly ventilated alveoli cause local pulmonary arteriolar constriction that increases resistance to blood flow and redistributes blood to favor well-ventilated alveoli; (2) low alveolar Pco_2 in alveoli with no pulmonary blood flow constricts alveolar ducts locally, decreases compliance of these alveoli and re-

TABLE 13-1.—Effects of Occlusion of Pulmonary Artery to One Lung

| | Lung A | | Lung B | |
	Ventilation	Blood Flow	Ventilation	Blood Flow
Before occlusion	2.0	2.5	2.0	2.5
Immediately after occlusion	2.0	0	2.0	5.0
1 minute later	4.0	0	4.0	5.0
After compensation	1.0	0	4.0	5.0

distributes gas to favor alveoli with good blood flow. If the second of these operates, then, after compensation (Table 13-1), lung *A* receives less ventilation, so that total ventilation can return to 5 L/minute. If there is a "purpose" to the location of smooth muscle in pulmonary arterioles and alveolar ducts, it may well be to keep $\dot{V}_A/\dot{Q}_C$ ratios uniform throughout the lungs.

In the case of the absolute shunt, one stream of unaltered venous blood merges with a stream of arterialized blood to form mixed arterial blood. In the case of alveolar dead space, there is a shunt of air instead of blood—one stream of unaltered air (from alveoli with no blood flow) merges in the trachea with a stream of alveolar gas to form mixed alveolar gas. Just as the blood shunt changes the composition of arterial blood toward that of venous blood, so the air shunt changes the composition of mixed alveolar gas toward that of inspired air.

In an "ideal" lung with uniform alveolar ventilation and capillary blood flow, equal volumes of alveolar gas from the two lungs, each with the same P_{O_2} and P_{CO_2}, meet in the trachea and emerge as alveolar gas with a P_{O_2} of 100 and a P_{CO_2} of 40 torr. In this case of complete occlusion of the pulmonary artery to lung *A*, equal *volumes* of gas will mix in the trachea, but the P_{O_2} of gas from the alveolar dead space (lung *A*) will be 149 and its P_{CO_2} zero (Fig. 13-3), whereas the P_{O_2} of gas from fully functioning lung *B* will be 100 and its P_{CO_2} 40. The P_{CO_2} of mixed alveolar gas will be $\frac{40+0}{2}=20$, and its P_{O_2} will be $\frac{149+100}{2}=125$ torr. These values of expired alveolar gas are not in themselves diagnostic of pulmonary vascular occlusion, since they could be due to overall hyperventilation of normal lungs; however, if the P_{O_2} of arterial blood is 100 and its P_{CO_2} is 40, then the differences between arterial blood and expired alveolar gas tensions *are* diagnostic. Such differences in P_{CO_2} are more useful diagnostically than differences in P_{O_2} because impairment of diffusion can cause large differences of P_{O_2} between alveolar gas and arterial blood but not between the two CO_2 tensions.

3. NONUNIFORM VENTILATION AND NONUNIFORM BLOOD FLOW. We have been discussing two extreme cases of uneven matching of gas and blood. Physiologists speak in terms of ratios of gas to blood and call these "alveolar ventilation-blood flow ratios" or "ventilation-perfusion ratios." They use the symbol V for ventilation, V_A for alveolar ventilation and $\dot{V}_A$ for alveolar ventilation/

Fig. 13-3.—Washout of CO_2 from lungs with no pulmonary blood flow. The heart of an experimental animal is stopped (*vertical arrow*) while constant artificial ventilation continues ($\dot{V}_A/\dot{Q}_C = 1/0$). A CO_2 meter records the breath-to-breath concentration of CO_2 in expired air. The % CO_2 in end-expired (alveolar) gas falls breath by breath (since no CO_2 can be added to alveolar gas) and it approaches that of moist inspired gas. Alveolar O_2 concentration (not shown) rises simultaneously to that of moist inspired gas.

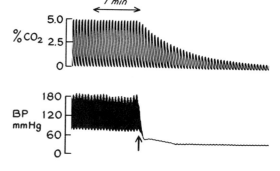

minute. Similarly, Q is blood flow, Qc is pulmonary capillary blood flow and $\dot{Q}c$ is pulmonary capillary blood flow/minute. The ventilation-blood flow ratio in symbols is $\dot{V}A/\dot{Q}c$. In the first, extreme case, $\dot{V}A/\dot{Q}c$ for lung *A* was 0/4, or zero; in the second, $\dot{V}A/\dot{Q}c$ for *A* was 4/0, or infinity.

Just as there is a ventilation-blood flow ratio for these whole lungs, so there can be a ventilation-blood flow ratio for each of 300 million alveoli in our two lungs. In the "ideal" lung, the ratios are the same throughout. But even lungs of healthy man are not "ideal"; when man stands, the lower lobes get more

Fig. 13-4. — Ventilation-blood flow ratios ($\dot{V}A/\dot{Q}c$). The conventional coordinates (Pco_2 vs. Po_2) are the same as in the O_2-CO_2 diagram (Fig. 14-7), and again lines of equal O_2 saturation of HbO_2 have been placed on the graph; however, the latter are incomplete, and the CO_2 isopleths are deleted so that additional lines may be clearly visible. The latter include:

1. A group of lines of equal R (respiratory exchange ratio) radiating from the moist inspired gas point ($Po_2 = 149$ and $Pco_2 = 0$ torr). These are analogous to lines of equal barometric pressure on a weather map. They were calculated from the alveolar air equation (see p. 11). Every point on any one of these lines could represent an alveolus which is exchanging O_2 and CO_2 in the same *ratio*, though the absolute quantities may be different. Thus an alveolus at *A* on the 0.5 R line might have a Po_2 of 110 and a Pco_2 of 22 torr, whereas another alveolus at *B* on the same 0.5 R line might have a Po_2 or 80 and a Pco_2 of 39. In both, the ratio is the same. These R lines permit ready determination of PA_{CO_2}, PA_{O_2} or R if 2 of the 3 values are known. If $PA_{O_2} = 110$ and $R = 0.7$, PA_{CO_2} must be 30 torr. If PA_{CO_2} is 40 and $R = 0.8$, PA_{O_2} must be 102 torr.

2. A series of parallel lines of alveolar ventilation expressed as L/minute of alveolar ventilation for every 100 ml of O_2 consumed.

3. A curved "distribution line" ($\dot{V}A/\dot{Q}c$), which represents all possible combinations of Po_2 and Pco_2 that could occur in alveolar gas and pulmonary capillary blood after mixed venous blood has equilibrated with alveolar gas at all possible ventilation/blood flow ratios. This particular line applies only when venous blood and inspired air have the composition indicated at the 2 extremes of the line. Mixed venous blood to all pulmonary capillaries is assumed to have the same composition; this is not true in those pulmonary diseases in which bronchial arterial blood flows through some alveolar capillaries. (From Rahn, H., and Fenn, W. O.: *A Graphical Analysis of the Respiratory Gas Exchange* [Washington: American Physiological Society, 1955].)

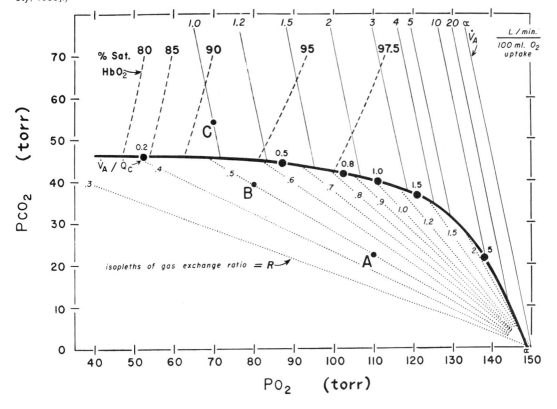

blood flow and the upper lobes less (p. 151). Since gravity does not directly change the distribution of air, the ratio decreases in the lower lobes and increases in the upper lobes. In healthy man under basal conditions (O_2 consumption 250 ml/minute; arterial O_2 20 ml/100 ml; mixed venous O_2 15 ml/100 ml; 4 L/minute of alveolar ventilation and 5 L/minute of capillary blood flow), there may be a few alveoli with ratios of zero or infinity, but the great majority will be close to 4/5, or 0.8. (This assumes that the mixed venous O_2 saturation is that of a normal resting man. During exercise, $\dot{V}_A$ may increase 4-fold and $\dot{Q}_c$ only 2-fold; the extra O_2 is supplied to the tissues by increased removal of O_2 from each unit of blood and the arterial-venous O_2 difference doubles.)

Patients with pulmonary disease have more alveoli with a ratio of zero or infinity and many more that deviate markedly from the overall ratio of 0.8. They may have a continuous spectrum of alveoli between the two extremes. (Fig. 13-4). Alveoli with ratios greater than 0.8 have too much ventilation for their blood flow; those with ratios less than 0.8 have too little ventilation for their blood flow. Those with large ratios behave like alveolar dead space; those with low ratios behave like shunts.

Uneven ventilation with uniform blood flow causes hypoxemia; nonuniform blood flow with uniform ventilation also causes hypoxemia. When both are nonuniform, more severe hypoxemia results, unless compensatory mechanisms match poor ventilation with poor blood flow and increased perfusion with increased ventilation.

What about arterial CO_2? Examination of the CO_2 dissociation curve (p. 195) shows that when alveolar ventilation is doubled (and P_{CO_2} falls from 40 to 20 torr), blood CO_2 content decreases by 12.1 ml/100 ml (from 48.4 to 36.3), but when alveolar ventilation is halved (and P_{CO_2} rises from 40 to 80 torr), blood CO_2 content increases by 15.2 ml CO_2/100 ml blood. Therefore, even when lungs have as many regions with $\dot{V}_A/\dot{Q}_c$ ratios of 2 as with 0.5, the CO_2 of arterial blood will rise. Further, regions with more blood flow contribute more to pulmonary venous blood (and therefore to systemic arterial) than do those with poor blood flow; this also increases arterial blood CO_2. The reason why some patients with uneven matching appear not to have CO_2 retention (at a time when they have hypoxemia) is that these patients have increased their ventilation in response to increased CO_2 or hypoxemia or both, and the increased ventilation lowers arterial CO_2, just as does hyperventilation of normal lungs. If alveolar ventilation were deliberately held to a normal value, CO_2 retention would then be apparent. This is obvious in patients with severe emphysema in whom the hypoxic drive to breathing is suddenly removed by giving them O_2 to breathe; when ventilation decreases, arterial P_{CO_2} rises abruptly, sometimes to dangerous levels.

Tests of Uneven Matching

1. CALCULATIONS OF TOTAL DEAD SPACE AND TOTAL SHUNT. The classic tests for diagnosing and characterizing uneven distribution of gas and blood measure total venous-to-arterial shunt and total dead space ventilation. If there are many alveoli with large ratios, the total dead space ventilation should be greater than normal; if there are many alveoli with low ratios, the total shunt should be greater than normal.

The concept of dead space is easy to grasp when dealing with a conducting tube (all of which is dead space) or with alveoli with *no* blood flow (all of the tidal volume entering and leaving these is dead space ventilation). The concept of dead space is harder to understand when there is *some* blood flow but not enough to match the ventilation (blood flow may be less than normal or ventilation greater than normal). Here *some* of the ventilation is "wasted" as far as further oxygenation of the blood is concerned because there is an upper limit to the amount of O_2 carried by Hb and little dissolved O_2 is added by raising alveolar P_{O_2} from 100 to 140 torr. What the physiologist does is to pretend that an alveolus with a high ventilation-blood flow ratio is two alveoli (Fig. 13-5, *bottom*). The

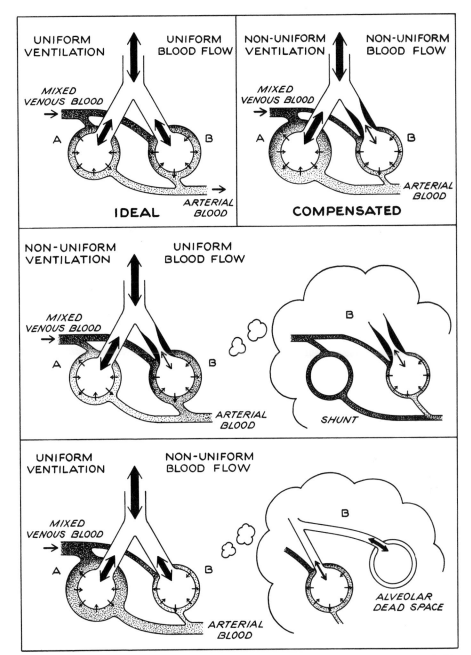

Fig. 13-5.—Uneven alveolar ventilation in relation to capillary blood flow. Symbols same as in Figure 13-2. **Top left**, ideal relationship. Uniform ventilation and uniform capillary blood flow to alveoli A and B. Arterial blood is normal if amount of alveolar ventilation is properly matched to metabolic rate. **Top right**, uneven ventilation and uneven blood flow but properly matched; A has increased ventilation and increased blood flow; B has decreased ventilation and decreased blood flow. **Center**, nonuniform ventilation. Alveolus B, with inadequate ventilation to match its blood flow, is divided on the right into 2 "pretend" alveoli: 1 with enough blood flow to match its ventilation and the other with the remaining blood flow and no ventilation. **Bottom**, nonuniform blood flow. Alveolus B, with inadequate blood flow to match its ventilation is divided on the right into 2 "pretend" alveoli: 1 with just enough ventilation to match its blood flow and the other with the remaining ventilation and no blood flow.

Note: Alveolus A (**center**) has too much ventilation for its blood flow and alveolus A (**bottom**) has too much blood flow for its ventilation; these too can be divided into "pretend" alveoli.

first "pretend" alveolus is an "ideal" one in which ventilation just matches blood flow. The second is all alveolar dead space; it has no blood flow but receives the excess ventilation. After certain measurements, one can calculate the total dead space ventilation for the lungs, then measure the volume of the conducting airway (by a technic based on a single-breath test; see Fig. 13-1) and, by subtraction, compute the volume of alveolar dead space.[1]

If the tidal volume in a healthy man is 450 ml and his anatomic dead space is 150 ml, 150/450, or 33%, of his tidal volume is wasted, ineffective or dead space ventilation. If a patient's anatomic dead space is 150 ml and total dead space is 300 ml, 300/450, or 66%, of his tidal volume is wasted, of which half is ineffective ventilation of alveoli that have too much ventilation for their blood flow.

You will often see the term *physiologic dead space* used to describe what I call *total* dead space. In supine man, total dead space is just about equal to the volume of the conducting airway measured by an independent method; this is the irreducible dead space under physiologic conditions. When total dead space exceeds the volume of the conducting airway (in supine man), the excess is always *pathologic* and should not be called physiologic dead space. The term "physiologic dead space" is a misnomer because it includes the pathologic alveolar dead space

resulting from disease as well as the physiologic alveolar dead space of upright man and the volume of the conducting airway.

The concept of shunt is easy to understand when the shunt is *absolute* and there is no contact between alveolar gas and blood. It is harder to grasp when there is some ventilation but not enough to match the blood flow (Fig. 13-5, *center*). In these cases the physiologist pretends that there are two bloodstreams to each alveolus that has a low ventilation-blood flow ratio. The first carries just enough blood to match the ventilation of the alveolus, and the second carries the rest. The first "pretend" capillary has an ideal relationship with the alveolus; the second has no alveolus and carries shunted blood. By certain measurements, assumptions and calculations, one can measure the total shunt and determine if it is greater than normal. By use of the O_2 test (p. 175), one can measure *absolute* shunt. The difference between total and absolute shunt is the excess blood flow to poorly ventilated alveoli. It is better to call this *relative* shunt than physiologic shunt; it is always pathologic except in upright man.

2. SINGLE-BREATH CO_2 TEST. The procedures just mentioned serve to characterize the physiologic disturbance and determine the amount of poorly matched gas and blood. If we are content merely to know that a patient *has* uneven ventilation in relation to blood flow (without a quantitative analysis of the $\dot{V}A/\dot{Q}c$ ratios), we can use a single-breath CO_2 test in the same way that we use the single-breath N_2 test to detect uneven distribution of inspired gas. A rapid CO_2 analyzer continuously measures the CO_2 tension of the gas leaving the mouth during a single expiration. The early portion of the expired breath comes from well-ventilated regions of the lung, the later portions from poorly ventilated regions. If the last part of the expired alveolar gas contains only a slightly greater concentration of CO_2 than the first, the ratios of alveolar ventilation to blood flow must be very similar in both regions of the lung. If

---

[1]The calculations are based on Bohr's equation:

$$\text{Volume of alveolar ventilation (ml)} = \frac{\text{Amount of } CO_2 \text{ (ml) in expired gas}}{\% \text{ alveolar } CO_2} \times 100$$

Expired gas is a mixture of alveolar gas and dead space gas. Because inspired air contains practically no CO_2 (0.04%), all of the CO_2 in expired gas must come from alveolar gas. Further, the CO_2 cannot come from alveoli with no capillary blood flow (alveolar dead space) or from the "pretend" alveoli, which have ventilation but no blood flow. If we know the *per cent* of CO_2 in our "pretend" ideal alveoli and the *amount* of CO_2 in *expired* gas, we can calculate the volume of alveolar ventilation (from ideal alveoli) and the rest is dead space ventilation (conducting airway + alveolar dead space).

ventilation is *un*even, but blood flow matches it, the P_{CO_2} will be similar in all alveoli and all the expired alveolar gas will have the same CO_2 concentration. If the last part of the expired alveolar gas is much higher in CO_2 than the first, ventilation/blood flow must vary (the first part coming from a region with an increased ratio, and the last part from a region with a decreased ratio). This, of course, holds only if the various regions of the lungs empty asynchronously; if all alveoli empty evenly throughout the entire expiration, streams of gas of both high and low CO_2 concentration will merge in constant proportions, and the CO_2 concentration in the mixed alveolar gas will be about the same throughout expiration. Thus, in Figure 13-2, *center*, continuous, rapid CO_2 analysis of expired alveolar gas would show 20 torr in the first, middle and last gas expired, since ventilation is uniform, even though the alveolar ventilation/blood flow is grossly different in the two lungs. The single-breath CO_2 test for uneven ventilation/blood flow would give a falsely normal result, but if the difference between the CO_2 tensions of arterial blood and expired alveolar gas was also measured, the abnormality would be demonstrated clearly.

3. DIFFERENCE IN P_{N_2} BETWEEN AL-VEOLAR GAS AND ARTERIAL BLOOD. We are accustomed to think of gas exchange in terms of P_{O_2} and P_{CO_2}, and we forget about P_{N_2}. However, Rahn and his associates have pointed out that because $P_{O_2}+P_{CO_2}+P_{N_2}+P_{H_2O}$ must equal 760 torr in alveolar gas at sea level, whenever the sum of $P_{O_2}+P_{CO_2}$ rises, P_{N_2} must fall, and whenever the sum of $P_{O_2}+P_{CO_2}$ falls, P_{N_2} must rise. Normally the body uses more O_2/minute than it forms CO_2 (respiratory quotient [RQ] less than 1.0), and this accounts for the fact that the alveolar gas P_{N_2} exceeds the P_{N_2} in inspired air. When alveoli have a high $\dot{V}_A/\dot{Q}_c$, their P_{O_2} rises more than P_{CO_2} falls (see Fig. 13-4), and their P_{N_2} must be less than inspired P_{N_2}. When alveoli have a low $\dot{V}_A/\dot{Q}_c$, their P_{O_2} falls far more than their P_{CO_2} rises, and their

P_{N_2} must be more than inspired P_{N_2}. Because alveoli with a high ratio have more influence on mixed expired alveolar gas than alveoli with a low ratio and alveoli with a low ratio have more influence on mixed arterial blood than those with a high ratio, the P_{N_2} in arterial blood is always greater than that in mixed alveolar gas (Fig. 13-6). And the difference between P_{N_2} in arterial blood and alveolar gas is an index of uneven matching (particularly of shuntlike $\dot{V}_A/\dot{Q}_c$ abnormalities) because it is affected neither by absolute right-to-left shunts (the P_{N_2} of mixed venous and systemic arterial blood are identical, since tissues do not metabolize N_2) nor by impaired diffusion (the P_{N_2} in alveolar gas and in end-pulmonary capillary blood is practically the same).

We learned earlier that there is always a difference between the P_{O_2} of mixed alveolar gas and of arterial blood when there is uneven matching. However, because anatomic shunts and impairment of diffusion also produce P_{O_2} differences, the P_{O_2} test is not specific in detecting uneven matching. The P_{N_2} test is not limited in this way.

The P_{N_2} of arterial blood can be measured by gas chromatography. Rahn has proposed that the P_{N_2} of anaerobically collected urine is the same as that of arterial blood and that this urine may be used instead of blood to simplify the test.

Fig. 13-6.—Effect of uneven ventilation and blood flow on mixed expired P_{N_2} and blood P_{N_2}. See text. (Redrawn from Canfield, R. E., and Rahn, H.: J. Appl. Physiol. 10:165, 1957.)

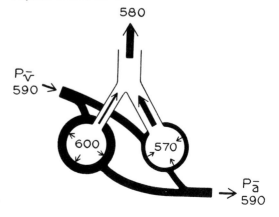

Locating Regions with Uneven Matching

The tests mentioned so far provide overall measurements for the two lungs as a whole. One can locate the disturbance (right vs. left lung) by separating the air flow to the two lungs by a double-lumen tube (technic of bronchospirometry) and measuring ventilation and O_2 uptake of each lung separately. One can block blood flow to one lung by inflating a balloon at the tip of a catheter in the right or left pulmonary artery and determine whether there is a shunt (absolute or relative) in the other lung. One can sample gas from different lobes of the lung and see if blood is flowing equally to all lobes by determining O_2 loss and CO_2 gain in relation to ventilation.

A method introduced of Hugh-Jones and his associates measures the relative dilution in different regions of inspired insoluble radioactive gases and the disappearance rates of inspired soluble radioactive gases. They determine relative rates of ventilation and blood flow to upper, middle and lower lobes of both right and left lungs by using a battery of detectors at the desired location on the

surface of the chest. Bates and his associates have shown that radioactive xenon dissolved in saline can also be given intravenously and its appearance and disappearance measured over various lung areas (Fig. 13-7). The use of the Anger scintillation camera permits serial pictures of the location and intensity of radioactivity following intravenous injection of ^{133}Xe. The first picture after the ^{133}Xe reaches the lung is taken while the patient holds his breath; this indicates the distribution of ^{133}Xe throughout the pulmonary circulation. When blood containing ^{133}Xe flows past airless alveoli or other solid tissue, it cannot release its xenon; in the first picture, such regions appear bloodless, just as do those with lung tissue that is normal except for having no blood flow. Subsequent photographs taken during regular breathing measure the rate of washout of xenon from ventilated parts of the lung and therefore can detect different regional rates of alveolar ventilation if they exist. It may be difficult to distinguish between emphysematous areas with poor blood flow and regions with little or no blood flow because of pulmonary emboli.

Fig. 13-7.—Measurement of regional ventilation and blood flow by means of ^{133}Xe and external counters. If a relatively insoluble gas such as ^{133}xenon is inhaled, a high immediate concentration indicates good alveolar ventilation in relation to the lung volume of that region. If radioactive xenon is dissolved in saline and given rapidly intravenously, a high local concentration in any lung region indicates good pulmonary capillary blood flow to ventilated alveoli, since xenon leaves the blood in the pulmonary capillaries; the curves on the *right* show that there is much less blood flow to the upper lobe than to the lower lobe and that ventilation of the lower lobe is good (the xenon excreted into the alveolar gas is rapidly washed out by ventilation). When ^{133}Xe is inhaled, the initial heights of the 2 records (*1* and *3* on left) indicate the relative volumes of alveolar ventilation of the 2 regions. When the breath is held, little Xe leaves the alveolar gas because it is sparingly soluble in blood; when breathing resumes, Xe is washed out at rates depending on the alveolar volume and alveolar ventilation of each region.

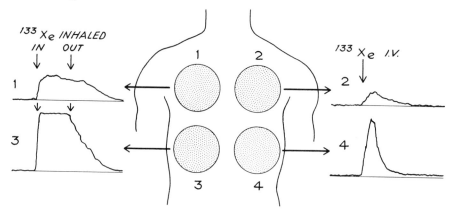

14

The Transport of Oxygen by Blood

THE MAIN FUNCTION of respiration is to arterialize mixed venous blood. However, blood leaving pulmonary capillaries must then transport O_2 to tissues throughout the body, and blood leaving tissue capillaries must transport CO_2 to the pulmonary capillaries. This chapter deals with the transport of O_2 by blood; the next two chapters will deal with the exchange of O_2 and CO_2 across tissue capillaries and the transport of CO_2 by blood.

The needs of tissues for O_2 can be met by loading more O_2 into each unit of arterial blood, by unloading more O_2 from each unit of blood in tissue capillaries, by increasing the number of units of blood flowing to tissues or by a combination of these.

HEMOGLOBIN AND OXYGEN

Blood can carry any gas in solution; the amount is governed by Henry's law, which states that the amount dissolved is directly proportional to the partial pressure of the gas. The amount of O_2 dissolved in blood is small. Figure 14-1 shows that 1 ml of plasma at 37 C takes up 0.00003 ml of O_2 for each 1.0 torr increase in Po_2. Good numbers to remember are that 100 ml of plasma takes up 0.3 ml of O_2 when equilibrated with gas with a Po_2 of 100 torr (the average Po_2 of alveolar gas and arterial blood of man at sea level). If pure plasma containing no O_2 flowed through the pulmonary capillaries and there were no barrier to diffusion, each 100 ml would take up 0.03 ml of O_2 when the alveolar Po_2 was 10 torr; 0.06 ml when alveolar Po_2 was 20; 0.15 ml when it was 50; 0.3 ml when it was 100 and 2.0 ml when it was 673. The last value is the alveolar Po_2 when a normal man breathes pure O_2 at sea level long enough to wash out all of the N_2 in his lungs so that his alveolar gas contains only CO_2 (40 torr Pco_2), water vapor (47 torr PH_2O) and O_2 $(673 + 40 + 47 = 760)$.

The tissues of resting man use about 250 ml O_2/minute. If blood were plasma and man breathed air, his heart would have to pump 83 L/minute to satisfy the tissue demand for O_2, assuming that every molecule of O_2 was removed from plasma as it flowed through the tissue capillaries. And if he exercised and doubled his O_2 requirements, his cardiac output would have to double (to 166 L/minute), for there would be no reserve supply of O_2 in plasma.

Fortunately, blood is far more than plasma. It contains a chemical substance, hemoglobin, that permits whole blood to take up 65 times as much O_2 as plasma at a Po_2 of 100 torr; if tissues extracted *all* of the O_2 from *whole blood* passing through systemic capillaries, resting man would need a cardiac output of only 1.3 L/minute, instead of 83 L/minute if man had only plasma.

Hemoglobin (Hb) is one of the most remarkable biochemical substances known because it is essential for the transport of both O_2 and CO_2 by blood. Its name "hemoglobin" indicates that it is a combination

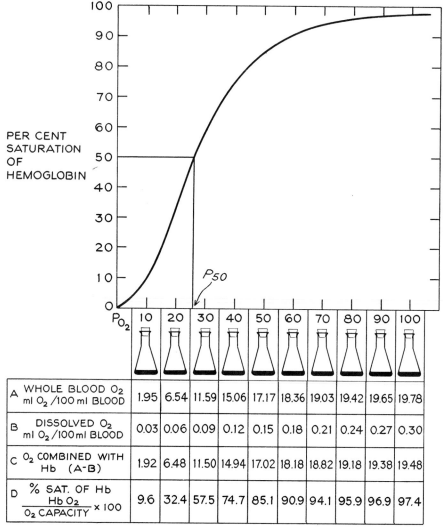

Fig. 14-1.—"Standard" HbO_2 dissociation (and association) curve. For normal man with hemoglobin A, blood pH 7.40 and body temperature 37 C. (Data of J. W. Severinghaus: J. Appl. Physiol. 21:1108, 1966.) P_{50} = blood Po_2 required for 50% saturation of hemoglobin with O_2 at 37 C and pH 7.4.

	Po_2	10	20	30	40	50	60	70	80	90	100
A	WHOLE BLOOD O_2 ml O_2/100 ml BLOOD	1.95	6.54	11.59	15.06	17.17	18.36	19.03	19.42	19.65	19.78
B	DISSOLVED O_2 ml O_2/100ml BLOOD	0.03	0.06	0.09	0.12	0.15	0.18	0.21	0.24	0.27	0.30
C	O_2 COMBINED WITH Hb (A-B)	1.92	6.48	11.50	14.94	17.02	18.18	18.82	19.18	19.38	19.48
D	% SAT. OF Hb $\frac{Hb\,O_2}{O_2\,CAPACITY} \times 100$	9.6	32.4	57.5	74.7	85.1	90.9	94.1	95.9	96.9	97.4

of heme (a pigment) and globin (a protein).

Much attention has been given to the structure of the Hb molecule. The molecular weight is 66,700. The globin molecule consists of four chains: two of these are identical α chains, each with 141 amino acids; two are identical β chains, each with 146 amino acids. The precise amino acids, the sequence in which they are arranged and their spatial relationships are known for the usual type of human hemoglobin (A); the changes in amino acids that characterize more than

120 variants have also been determined.

Hemoglobin also contains four heme groups, each enfolded in one of the four chains that collectively constitute globin. An iron molecule lies at the center of each heme group; each can take up one molecule of O_2. Neither heme alone, iron alone nor globin alone can take up O_2; only the three together, in their proper spatial relationship, can do this.

There are three special properties of the chemical reaction of hemoglobin with O_2:

(1) Hemoglobin combines rapidly and reversibly with O_2. The oxygenated form, HbO_2, is oxyhemoglobin (not *oxidized* hemoglobin). Strictly, since each hemoglobin molecule combines with 4 O_2 molecules, we should use the symbol Hb_4O_8; for convenience we use HbO_2. The unoxygenated or deoxygenated form, Hb, is deoxyhemoglobin (formerly incorrectly called reduced hemoglobin). In each form, iron is in the ferrous state. (2) Each of the four chains, acting separately, combines with O_2 in a hyperbolic curve (Fig. 14-2) similar to that of O_2 plus myoglobin, a hemoglobin-like compound in muscle that has a molecular weight $1/4$ that of hemoglobin (its globin has only one chain). This relationship, as we shall see later, is un-

suited for unloading of O_2 to tissues. However, when the four chains act together as part of the hemoglobin molecule, the curve of O_2 uptake is S-shaped (see Fig. 14-1) and uniquely suited for both loading of O_2 in the lungs and unloading in tissue capillaries. The interaction of the chains, during which successive oxygenation of the iron atoms facilitates further oxygenation, means that a combination of any three iron atoms and O_2 will accelerate greatly the combination of O_2 with the fourth iron atom. Similarly, release of O_2 by any three iron atoms makes the fourth release its O_2 molecule more rapidly. This interaction tends to make each hemoglobin molecule carry either four molecules of O_2 or none and insures effective uptake and re-

Fig. 14-2.—Variations in the HbO_2 dissociation curve. **A**, effect of changes in temperature; **B**, effect of changes in blood pH; **C**, hyperbolic curve of "purified" hemoglobin A (dialyzed to be salt-free) is similar to curve of myoglobin (Mb); **D**, the dissociation curve of fetal blood (but not pure HbF) is to the left of adult blood containing HbA; addition of diphosphoglycerate (DPG) shifts curve of blood with HbA to the right and increases P_{50} (decreases affinity of O_2 for Hb and facilitates unloading of O_2 in tissues).

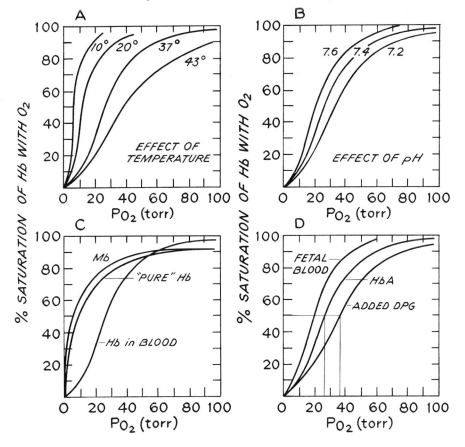

lease of O_2. (3) The rate of reaction of Hb + O_2 and hence the shape of the O_2 uptake curve depends in part on the pH (see Fig. 14-2). The Bohr shift, which occurs when $HbO_2 \rightleftharpoons Hb + O_2$, releases or binds protons (H ions) at the imidazole group of the histidine residues of the peptide chains and makes the intra-erythrocyte environment more or less acid. Presumably, interaction between α and β chains is necessary for the Bohr effect.

The Hb and O_2 Curve

Under specified physical and chemical conditions, the Po_2 of plasma determines the amount of O_2 that combines with hemoglobin in red cells. The relationship between Po_2 and HbO_2 is, however, not a straight line but an S-shaped curve; the slope is steep when Po_2 is low and practically level when Po_2 is high.

You can construct such a curve by placing a small amount of whole blood (which in this case contains 15 gm Hb/100 ml blood) in each of 10 flasks with gas mixtures that have the same Pco_2 of 40 torr but differing Po_2 of 10, 20, 30, 40, 50, 60, 70, 80, 90 or 100 torr (see Fig. 14-1). Mix the blood and gas by swirling the flask (at 37 C) until the blood takes up as much O_2 as it can, and then measure this amount and express it as ml O_2/100 ml blood. Some of this O_2 is dissolved in plasma and the watery components of the red cells; calculate this amount for each pressure and subtract it from the total O_2 for each flask. You now know the O_2 combined chemically with Hb at each Po_2, and can graph the amount of O_2 on the ordinate and the corresponding Po_2 on the abscissa. Usually we graph % saturation rather than ml of O_2 on the ordinate. Percent of saturation of Hb

with $O_2 = \dfrac{O_2 \text{ combined with Hb}}{O_2 \text{ capacity of Hb}} \times 100$. The

O_2 capacity is the *maximal amount* of O_2 that will combine with Hb at a high Po_2. The capacity varies with the number of grams of Hb/100 ml of blood; 1 gm fully loaded with

O_2 combines with 1.34 ml of O_2, and 15 gm combines with 15×1.34, or 20.1 ml of O_2. We use *% saturation* to take account of the varying Hb concentration of anemic, normal and polycythemic persons.

The upper, relatively flat part may be considered the *as*sociation part of the curve because (except when arterial Po_2 is very low) it is the part concerned with O_2 uptake; the lower part of the curve may be considered the *dis*sociation part of the curve because (except when arterial Po_2 is very high, as during inhalation of O_2 at high pressure) it is the part concerned with release of O_2 from HbO_2 for use by tissues. Though this is an artificial division, it is instructive to consider these parts separately.

THE ASSOCIATION PART OF THE CURVE (LOADING OF O_2). This has several remarkable features. First, when exposed to a relatively low Po_2, 100 torr (the Po_2 of alveolar gas of man breathing air at sea level), the hemoglobin in 100 ml of blood combines with almost 20 ml O_2 and is 97.4% saturated.

Second, when exposed to a Po_2 greater than 100 torr, Hb cannot accept much more O_2; it is probably fully saturated when the Po_2 is about 250. Therefore, the saturation can increase only 2.6% and the O_2 associated with Hb can increase only 0.5 ml/100 ml blood, no matter how high the Po_2 of alveolar gas or plasma is raised. Since maximal hyperventilation with air rarely raises alveolar and arterial Po_2 to more than 130 torr, it cannot add more than a total of 0.3 ml of O_2 (dissolved plus combined) to each 100 ml of blood of a healthy man whose ventilation was previously normal (Table 14-1). (This is not true for removal of CO_2; see p. 195).

Third, between O_2 tensions of 100 and 70 torr there is very little change in the amount of O_2 associated with Hb. This is called the flat or almost horizontal part of the curve. A decrease from 100 to 90 decreases the saturation to only 96.9%; from 100 to 80, to 95.9%; from 100 to 70, to 94.1%. This means that man can live at reasonably high altitudes — where the inspired, alveolar and arte-

TABLE 14-1.— MEAN VALUES FOR BLOOD O_2, CO_2 AND pH IN
HEALTHY RESTING YOUNG MEN*

	ARTERIAL BLOOD	MIXED VENOUS BLOOD
1. O_2 pressure (torr)	100	40
2. Dissolved O_2 (ml O_2/100 ml W.B.†)	0.3	0.12
3. O_2 content (ml O_2/100 ml W.B.)	20.3	15.5
4. O_2 combined with Hb (ml O_2/100 ml W.B.)	20.0	15.4
5. O_2 capacity of Hb (ml O_2/100 ml W.B.)	20.6	20.6
6. % saturation of Hb with O_2	97.1	75.0
7. Total CO_2 (ml CO_2/100 ml W.B.)	49.0	53.1
(mmoles CO_2/L)	21.9	23.8
8. Plasma CO_2 (ml CO_2/100 ml plasma)	59.6	63.8
a. Dissolved CO_2 (ml CO_2/100 ml)	2.84	3.2
b. Combined CO_2 (ml CO_2/100 ml)	56.8	60.5
c. Combined CO_2/dissolved CO_2	20/1	18.9/1
d. CO_2 pressure (torr)	40	46.5
9. Plasma pH	7.40	7.376

*Modified from Albritton, E. C. (ed.): *Standard Values in Blood* (Philadelphia: W. B. Saunders Company, 1952).
†W.B. = whole blood.

rial Po_2 are lower than at sea level — without much reduction in the uptake of O_2 by Hb. It means also that the Hb of a patient with respiratory or pulmonary disease and an arterial O_2 tension of 70 torr will still be 94.1% saturated with O_2, a decrease of only 3.3%. It is true that this very small change in O_2 content makes it more difficult at sea level to diagnose hypoxemia if one measures O_2 content or saturation of Hb, but the change in Po_2 is large and easy to measure with an O_2 electrode; this is not true at high altitudes because the HbO_2 saturation and arterial O_2 tension of a healthy man are lower and close to the steep slope of the dissociation curve.

Fourth, the association part of the curve is not a fixed line determined only by the Po_2 of arterial blood. The height of the curve and its slope also vary with change in blood temperature and blood pH (see Fig. 14-2, *A* and *B*). This means that even when lungs, respiration and hemoglobin molecules of a patient with acidosis are all completely normal and his arterial Po_2 is 100 torr, the saturation of Hb with O_2 must still be less than 97.4% and, if he has fever as well, even lower. Because hemoglobin is almost maximally loaded with O_2 at a Po_2 of 100 torr and a temperature of 37 C, one might think that cold could not improve oxygenation. But it does. Figure 14-2,

A, shows the dramatic effect of cold: if the temperature of blood is 10 instead of 37 C, Hb will be fully saturated with O_2 at a Po_2 of 30 instead of 250 torr; at 20 degrees it will be fully saturated at a Po_2 of 60 torr. A surgeon needs to know this when he deliberately makes a patient hypothermic during open heart surgery; this information is also helpful when using artificial oxygenators to insure maximal uptake of O_2 by Hb. However, the effect of cold on release of O_2 to tissues (O_2 dissociation) must also be considered.

Fifth, there are several conditions in which Hb cannot take up O_2 normally. One is when CO is inhaled. Because Hb has a much greater affinity for CO than for O_2 (see p. 192), low concentrations of CO may lead to severe hypoxemia. This is particularly dangerous because the Po_2 of arterial blood remains normal and neither circulation nor respiration is stimulated (see p. 40). Another is the formation of methemoglobin from hemoglobin by the action of agents that oxidize the Fe^{2+} ion of Hb to Fe^{3+}. Among these are drugs or chemicals, including nitrites, aniline, sulfonamides, acetanilid, pamaquine, primaquine and phenylhydrazine. Methemoglobinemia also occurs when Hb is normal when methemoglobin reductase in erythrocytes is deficient; some Hb is oxidized slowly to methemoglobin in healthy man, but the met-hemoglobin is promptly reduced back to Hb by DPNH with the aid of a special reduc-tase. A third type of Hb that is inactive for O_2 transport is sulfhemoglobin.

Sixth, several of the abnormal hemoglo-bins do not take up normal amounts of O_2 when arterial blood Po_2 is normal, and pa-tients with these hemoglobins are hypoxemic despite normal lungs.

THE DISSOCIATION PART OF THE CURVE (UNLOADING OF O_2). The release of O_2 from HbO_2 is just as essential to life as the loading of Hb with O_2. Like the association portion of the curve, the dissociation portion has several remarkable features.

First, at low Po_2, between 10 and 40 torr, the curve is very steep. The Po_2 of metaboli-cally active tissues is in this range. Because the Po_2 determines the amount of O_2 that Hb can hold, other factors being constant, HbO_2 in capillary blood supplying active cells dis-sociates and releases O_2. Figure 14-1 shows that if the Po_2 is 40 torr, Hb can hold only 75% of its O_2; if 20, only 32%, and if 10, only 9.6%. The flat upper part of the curve pro-tects the body by enabling blood to load O_2 despite a large decrease in Po_2; the steep middle and lower parts protect the tissues by enabling them to withdraw large amounts of O_2 from blood for relatively small decreases in Po_2.

Second, nice as this unloading mechanism is, active tissues have means of improving on it. The shape of the association part of the curve changes with increased blood tempera-ture and decreased pH, but the lower or dis-sociation portion changes even more. Figure 14-2 shows that if the pH decreases to 7.20, as a result of the addition either of lac-tic acid or of CO_2, the curve shifts to the right. And it shifts far more in the dissocia-tion part than in the association part of the curve. This means that more acid blood in the pulmonary capillaries still takes up near-normal amounts of O_2, but that the acidifica-tion of blood in the tissue unloads much more O_2 than normal. At a blood Po_2 of 30

torr and a pH of 7.4, Hb holds 57% of its O_2; at the same Po_2 but a pH of 7.2, Hb can hold only 45%; the difference between 57 and 45% represents extra O_2 set free for use by tissue cells. The effect of Pco_2 or pH on the HbO_2 curve is known as the Bohr effect.

High temperatures have an influence simi-lar to low pH (see Fig. 14-2). An increase in blood temperature from 38 to 43 C interferes a little with the association of O_2 with Hb in the pulmonary capillaries but makes much more O_2 dissociate from Hb in the tissue capillaries. Since active tissues, which need more O_2, have a higher Pco_2, lower pH and higher temperature, they have a built-in mechanism for releasing more O_2 from HbO_2 when it is needed most. On the other hand, cold, which enables Hb to join fully with O_2 at relatively low Po_2, prevents dissociation of HbO_2 until tissue and capillary blood Po_2 are very low. Blood at 10 C may give up no O_2 even at a Po_2 as low as 25 torr; the bright red color of capillary and venous blood is apt to be misleading, since tissues are receiving no O_2. Very cold ears become bright red (not blue) because, when cold, HbO_2 cannot dis-sociate to yield O_2.

Third, a specific chemical, present in high concentrations in red blood cells and only in trace amounts in other cells, regulates the release of O_2 from HbO_2. This substance is 2,3 diphosphoglycerate (2,3 DPG, or simply DPG), formed during anaerobic glycolysis in red cells. Tissues other than red cells convert their 1,3 diphosphoglycerate (1,3 DPG) almost completely to 3 phosphogly-cerate, with the formation of 1 mole of adenosine triphosphate (ATP). Red cells, however, convert much of their 1,3 DPG to 2,3 DPG (DPG) and then back to 3 phos-phoglycerate (Fig. 14-3); in this shunt process, no ATP is formed. For decades, biochemists thought it uneconomical that red cells should make use of this reaction, which produces no high-energy phosphate, unless they gain some advantage from it; we know now that the advantage is the produc-tion of a substance to regulate O_2 release.

In 1967, Benesch and Benesch and Chan-

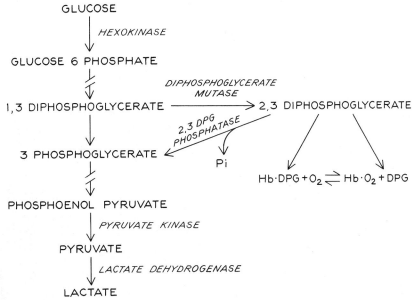

Fig. 14-3. — Formation of 2, 3 diphosphoglycerate in erythrocytes. The vertical chain at the left shows the glycolytic path in cells other than erythrocytes. In red blood cells, the enzyme diphosphoglycerate mutase catalyzes the conversion of much of 1, 3 diphosphoglycerate to 2, 3 diphosphoglycerate. That not bound by deoxygenated Hb is converted to 3 phosphoglycerate without the formation of ATP. The enzyme catalyzing the formation of 2, 3 DPG is strongly inhibited by free 2, 3 DPG; thus the level of free 2, 3 DPG can control its own production, i.e., when more DPG is bound by deoxygenated Hb, DPG decreases and its formation is increased. (Redrawn from Mulhausen, R. O.: Circulation 42:195–198, 1970.)

utin and Curnish found that DPG, when added to red cells in amounts comparable to those normally present, had a profound effect on the affinity of Hb for O_2 and therefore on the shape of the dissociation curve and on release of O_2 to tissues. The effect of DPG on the dissociation curve can be measured by constructing the entire curve (see Fig. 14-2) or by determining the Po_2 required to produce 50% saturation of Hb with O_2; the latter, determined at 37 C and pH 7.4, is called the P_{50}. The P_{50} of blood containing normal adult hemoglobin is about 26 torr. Diphosphoglycerate is normally present in red cells in a concentration of about 15 μmoles/gm of Hb. Higher concentrations shift the dissociation curve to the right and the P_{50} to a higher value; this makes more O_2 available to tissues. Lower concentrations shift the curve to the left and lower the P_{50}; this means that less HbO_2 dissociates at a given Po_2 and less O_2 is available to tissues. Since the effect of added DPG is similar to the

effect of acid, it is logical to consider that DPG acts through the same mechanism that acid does. Further, increased amounts of DPG do make the interior of the red cell somewhat more acid. However, DPG must act differently from acid, since acidosis for more than a few hours actually diminishes the amount of DPG in red cells (by inhibiting the activity of phosphofructokinase and the rate of glycolysis).

Granted that the concentration of free DPG within the red blood cell influences O_2 release from hemoglobin, what determines the rate of formation of DPG? Some possible factors are:

1. Active tissues generate more heat; increased temperature of capillary blood may accelerate glycolysis in red cells.

2. 2,3 Diphosphoglycerate affects O_2 release only when it binds to Hb (especially deoxyhemoglobin), presumably on a site or sites on β chains. When more deoxygenated Hb is present, it can bind more DPG and

less DPG is free; glycolysis may then be stimulated by low levels of unbound DPG in the cell. Increase in deoxyhemoglobin also increases the pH of the red cell by the Bohr effect, and this in turn increases the rate of glycolysis.

3. Hormones may increase anaerobic glycolysis in the red cell. Some believe that thyroid, testosterone and growth hormone increase the intra-erythrocytic concentration of DPG.

4. Catecholamines that stimulate β receptors may influence some aspect of red cell metabolism, since propranolol, which blocks β receptors, decreases the affinity of blood for O_2. Since propranolol has no effect on dialyzed hemoglobin solutions, its effect could be mediated by decreased binding of DPG to red cell membranes, or to leak of K^+ from red cells with a consequent increase in H^+ activity within the red cell.

Fourth, the discovery of the regulatory effect of DPG does not mean that there are no other, as yet undiscovered, factors that may also facilitate O_2 release; Shappell and his associates have reported that blood drawn from the coronary sinus of patients during an attack of angina pectoris had a higher P_{50} (and therefore decreased affinity for O_2) even though they found no change from control values of pH or erythrocytic

concentrations of DPG or ATP. Such rapid changes might be due to changes in inorganic ions, such as chloride.

Conditions known to raise P_{50} and favor release of O_2 from HbO_2 are:

1. Residence at high altitude, hypoxia resulting from cardiopulmonary disease, and anemia; in each of these there is more deoxygenated Hb and more binding of DPG to Hb than normal, and in each the shift of the curve to the right is a useful compensatory mechanism.

2. Sickle cell anemia. The affinity of pure hemoglobin S for O_2 is the same as that of normal cells with hemoglobin A, but sickle cells contain more DPG than do normal cells.

3. Exercise.

4. Deficiency of pyruvate kinase in red cells (Fig. 14-4). This leads to a great increase in DPG (probably because of an increase in organic phosphate) and a shift of the dissociation curve to the right. (In one patient with this disorder, the P_{50} was 38.)

5. Administration of thyroid hormone, testosterone and growth hormone.

Conditions known to lower P_{50} and hinder dissociation of HbO_2 are:

1. Storage of blood in banks. The level of DPG is greatly decreased after 1 week in storage, and the HbO_2 curve shifts to the left.

Fig. 14-4.—Dissociation curves of abnormal blood or Hb. **A**, blood with hexokinase deficiency and with pyruvate kinase deficiency in red cells. (Data of Oski, F.: Science 165:601, 1969.) **B**, blood containing abnormal hemoglobins compared to blood with HbA. Arrows point to P_{50} of each. Note that Hb Kansas is poorly saturated even at normal arterial blood Po_2. (Redrawn from Stamatoyannopoulous G., *et al.*: Annu. Rev. Med. 22:221–234, 1971.)

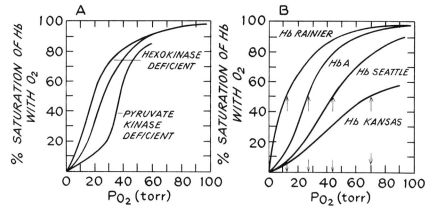

Because it takes 24 hours for bank blood cells to regain a normal level of DPG, it is best not to use bank blood for very ill patients in whom O_2 delivery to tissues is critical. This is particularly true in patients subjected to open heart surgery, who might receive large quantities of stored blood during cardiopulmonary bypass.

2. Deficiency of hexokinase in red cells (see Fig. 14-4). This blocks glycolysis at the initial step of the phosphorylation of glucose and decreases DPG formation. In one patient with this deficiency, the P_{50} was 19.

3. High-affinity variants of hemoglobin. Increased affinity blocks release of adequate O_2 tissues, and tissue hypoxia in turn generates secondary polycythemia.

4. Carbon monoxide poisoning (see p. 192).

ABNORMAL HEMOGLOBINS

Modern technics for separating and analyzing proteins and amino acids have permitted detection of more than 120 variants of normal adult hemoglobin. When the first variants were discovered, they were designated by letters of the alphabet: A for normal adult hemoglobin, F for fetal hemoglobin, S for sickle cell hemoglobin, etc. Because there are not enough letters in the alphabet, new variants now bear the name of the city or location where they were first described, e.g., Hb Seattle, Hb Kansas.

The abnormality is usually a substitution of one amino acid for another in α or β chains; for example, valine replaces glutamic acid at position 6 in the β chains of hemoglobin S. Or the abnormality may be a substitution of γ or Δ chains for β chains; in some forms of Hb, the chains are all β or γ. In only one, hemoglobin M, is the structural change in, or immediately associated with, the heme group. The abnormality does not necessarily produce any obvious physiologic disturbance or even any change in the dissociation curve. When it does affect the Hb + O_2 reaction, its effect is usually most marked in the *un*loading of O_2 from Hb, either favoring or

interfering with release. However, in at least 1 type of abnormal Hb (Hb Kansas — see Fig. 14-4), there is marked change in the association part of the curve; Hb Kansas, which has variant β chains, is only 70–75% saturated with O_2 at the Po_2 normally present in arterial blood.

Abnormal hemoglobin may affect the dissociation curve only slightly but produce profound effects in other properties of the Hb molecules. Thus, the unique feature of hemoglobin S is that it is much less soluble when deoxygenated than is hemoglobin A, and it then crystallizes within the erythrocyte. This changes the shape of the cell from a biconcave to a crescent or "sickle" cell. This cell is mechanically more fragile and apt to rupture; also, because of its shape, it tangles with other sickle cells and so increases blood viscosity, reduces blood flow through fine vessels and favors blockage or thrombosis.

The changes in the dissociation curve of abnormal hemoglobins may be due to an intrinsic change in the Hb molecule per se so that the effect still occurs when Hb is purified and completely separated from its usual chemical environment (including DPG), or it could be due to an altered response of Hb to DPG or to both. A full characterization of an abnormal hemoglobin, therefore, requires that its combination with O_2 be studied both when hemoglobin is pure and when it is within its normal environment — in red cells in whole blood.

For example, Hb Chesapeake increases O_2 affinity and Hb Seattle decreases O_2 affinity by direct action on pure Hb. And young, newly formed red cells with HbA have a decreased affinity for O_2 that may have physiologic value, for example, in increasing O_2 delivery to tissues during a patient's recovery from hemorrhage; since this effect cannot be explained by changes in the environment of Hb, it is probably an intrinsic change in Hb. However, Hb Hiroshima, Rainier and Bethesda interfere largely with the binding of DPG by deoxyhemoglobin; the substituted amino acids in these three hemoglobins are very near the end of the β chains and at, or close to, the location believed to be the main binding site of DPG.

Fetal hemoglobin (F), which differs from adult Hb (A) in that two γ chains replace the β chains, differs in two other ways: (1) Pure HbF has slightly less affinity for O_2 than does HbA, and (2) HbF within fetal red cells has greater affinity for O_2, probably because DPG does not bind normally to HbF and has relatively little effect on O_2 release. Hemoglobin F enables fetal red cells to accept more O_2 as they flow through the umbilical placental capillaries, where blood Po_2 is much lower than in postnatal pulmonary capillary blood; shortly after birth HbF begins to disappear from the circulation and is normally present in only small amounts after a few months.

Hemoglobin H consists of two pairs of β chains (instead of 1 pair of α and 1 pair of β chains). Biologically, it has 12 times the affinity for O_2 that normal adult hemoglobin A has. Life would be impossible if all Hb were of the H type because H does not give up its O_2 at the Po_2 of active tissues; patients whose blood contains hemoglobin H do not have large amounts of it.

In hemoglobin M, a histidine residue normally linked to a heme group at position 63 in the β chain is replaced by a tyrosine residue; the Hb molecule so altered binds O_2, but Fe^{2+} is rapidly *oxidized* (not *oxygenated*) to Fe^{3+} and methemoglobin is formed. Since the Fe^{2+} form of Hb combines rapidly and reversibly with O_2 and the Fe^{3+} form does not, a large percentage of hemoglobin M is incompatible with life. Patients with HbM must, therefore, have an additional type of Hb; sometimes the latter has an abnormality which favors increased or decreased affinity.

CARBON MONOXIDE AND HEMOGLOBIN

Oxygen is not the only gas that combines with hemoglobin. So does carbon monoxide. And it has an affinity for hemoglobin that is about 210 times that of O_2 for Hb. This means that O_2, to compete with CO on even terms for Hb, must be present in 210 times the concentration of CO. Since O_2 is almost 21% of air, it is easy to remember that blood equilibrated with air +0.1% CO (a 210:1 ratio of O_2:CO) will contain 50% HbO_2 and 50% HbCO; so will blood equilibrated with alveolar gas (14% O_2) containing 0.066% CO. But the inhalation of 0.1% CO in air does not instantly raise HbCO from 0 to 50%. A simple calculation shows why. If a man's blood volume is 6 L and each liter can, when fully saturated, combine with 200 ml of CO (just as it can combine with 200 ml of O_2), each liter must contain 100 ml of CO to be *half* saturated, and for this his total blood volume must contain 600 ml of CO. But if he inspires 6 L of air/minute containing 0.1% CO, and all inspired air becomes alveolar gas, the maximal amount of CO reaching the alveolo-capillary membranes per minute is 6 ml. And if all alveolar CO diffused into capillary blood and joined with Hb, it would require 100 minutes to transfer enough CO from air to blood to produce 50% HbCO. The actual time to reach 50% HbCO for any constant concentration of CO in inspired air depends on the tidal volume and frequency of ventilation, diffusing capacity for CO, pulmonary blood flow and O_2 concentration of inspired gas. CO is a dangerous gas because it gives no warning (it is colorless, odorless, tasteless and nonirritant and causes no increase in ventilation, no dyspnea and no cyanosis) and so can be inhaled for periods long enough to cause severe tissue hypoxia and death.

If CO did nothing but exclude O_2 from some or much of the available hemoglobin, it would have the same effect as severe anemia; when there is 50% HbCO, each liter of blood has half its usual HbO_2, and if each liter gives up the usual amount of O_2 to tissues, the saturation of mixed venous blood will be quite low, which of course means that tissue Po_2 will be low. But CO does more than this; by its presence, it shifts to the left the dissociation curve of the Hb combined with O_2. This means that, although this Hb takes on a normal load of O_2 in pulmonary capillaries, it releases O_2 to tissues only when exposed to a low Po_2. Therefore less O_2 is available to tissues, or is available only when tissue Po_2 is very low. This is particularly dangerous in the heart muscle since 60–70% of O_2 in arterial blood is normally extracted from blood flowing through the coronary circulation (instead of 25% average value for all organs and tissues); HbCO may therefore prevent unloading of the amount of O_2 needed by the myocardium. Figure 14-5 shows the $O_2 + Hb$ curves for blood containing no HbCO and for blood containing 20–60% HbCO and, for comparison with the latter, a curve for anemic blood containing 40% of the normal amount of Hb but no HbCO. These curves were deliberately constructed differently from that in Figure 14-1 (where the ordinate was percent saturation of Hb with O_2) to show the absolute amount of O_2 bound to Hb and so make it easier to see how low the O_2 is in venous blood when 100 ml of arterial blood has given up 5 ml of O_2 to tissues. Large amounts of HbCO are a serious matter. However, the effect on O_2 delivery to tissues of small amounts of HbCO (5–8%, such as might be present in the arterial blood of heavy smokers), though greater than a loss of 5–8% of Hb by bleeding or decreased red cell formation, is not serious in otherwise healthy man; it would decrease average tissue Po_2 from 40 to about 35 torr. This is of little consequence except in patients who have ischemic disease of some organs (such as coronary insufficiency) and borderline O_2 supply on that account, and who do not increase local blood flow to supply more O_2/minute.

TOTAL OXYGEN TRANSPORT

Pulmonary ventilation and diffusion play a vital role in oxygen transport by providing a proper alveolar and arterial Po_2 and Pco_2 for loading O_2 into mixed venous blood in the pulmonary capillaries. But a proper type and quantity of hemoglobin are also necessary for optimal loading and unloading of O_2, and the heart and vessels are necessary to deliver the proper amount of oxygenated blood to all tissues in proportion to their need. The total O_2 delivered to body tissues each minute equals (cardiac output in L/minute) × (ml of O_2 contained in 1 L of arterial blood). At

Fig. 14-5.—Calculated O_2 dissociation curves of human blood containing varying amounts of HbCO. Absolute amounts of bound O_2 are plotted instead of % HbO_2 saturation. Note that blood with 60% of its Hb as HbCO and 40% as HbO_2 has a greater affinity for O_2 than blood with only 40% of normal Hb value but no HbCO. (Redrawn from Roughton, F. J. W., and Darling, R. C.: Am. J. Physiol. 141:17–31, 1944.)

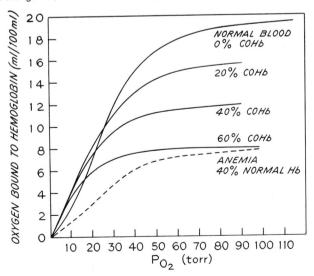

rest, this is about 5×200, or 1,000 ml O_2/minute; only about ¼ of this is used by the tissues, and ¾ returns to the heart in mixed venous blood. During maximal exercise, the milliliters of O_2 contained in 1 L of arterial blood do not increase, but cardiac output does. If cardiac output increases to 24 L/minute, the total O_2 delivered is now 24 $\times 200$, or 4,800 ml/minute; now, however, the tissues use about ¾ of this, and only about ¼ returns to the heart in mixed venous blood. This means that both loading and unloading mechanisms are working well;

the tissues (by changes in temperature, acidity, P_{O_2} and P_{CO_2}) have extracted 3 times as much O_2 from each liter of blood as they did at rest, and the lungs (by greatly increased frequency and tidal volume of breathing) have added 3 times as much O_2 to each liter and almost 15 times as much O_2 to blood per minute as they did at rest.

We shall not discuss here the mechanisms that regulate the output of the heart to meet overall needs for blood and that regulate blood vessel caliber to distribute this output to meet the separate requirements of individ-

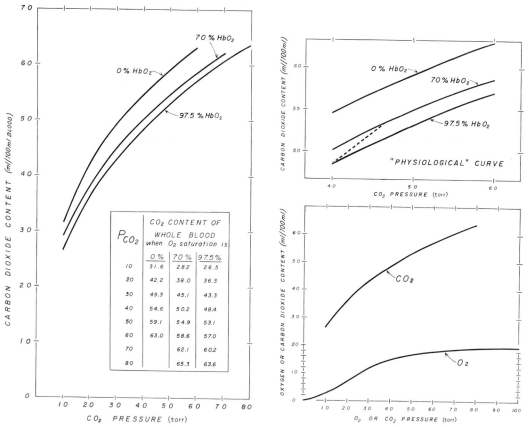

CARBON DIOXIDE DISSOCIATION CURVES FOR WHOLE BLOOD

Fig. 14-6.—CO_2 dissociation curves. The large graph shows the relationship between P_{CO_2} and CO_2 content of whole blood; this varies with changes in saturation of Hb with O_2. Thus, P_{CO_2} of the blood influences O_2 saturation (Bohr effect), and O_2 saturation of the blood influences CO_2 content (Haldane effect). The O_2-CO_2 diagram (see Fig. 14-7), by combining much of Figures 14-1 and 14-6 into one, gives the correct figure for both CO_2 and O_2 at every P_{O_2} and P_{CO_2}. **Above right,** greatly magnified portion of the large graph to show the change that occurs as mixed venous blood (70% HbO_2, P_{CO_2} 46 torr) passes through the pulmonary capillaries and becomes arterial blood (97.5% HbO_2, P_{CO_2} 40 torr). *Dashed line* is a hypothetical transition between the two curves. **Below right,** O_2 and CO_2 dissociation curves plotted on same scale to show the important point that the O_2 curve has a very steep and a very flat portion and the CO_2 curve does not. (From Comroe, J. H., Jr., *et al.*: *The Lung* [Chicago: Year Book Medical Publishers, Inc., 1962].)

ual organs and tissues. Nor shall we discuss the mechanisms that regulate red blood cell and hemoglobin formation, except to mention that the levels of erythropoietin (a hormone, formed largely in the kidneys, that regulates hemoglobin concentration) appears to be regulated by tissue P_{O_2} and thus, at least in part, by the affinity of O_2 for hemoglobin. When the affinity is great, tissues must operate at a low P_{O_2} to release O_2 from HbO_2, and this generates more erythropoietin and thus, in turn, more hemoglobin; when the affinity is normal or low, HbO_2 releases O_2 at a higher P_{O_2}, tissue P_{O_2} is higher and less hemoglobin is formed. Patients who have "high-affinity" hemoglobin develop polycythemia, and it is this that often gives the first clue to the hemoglobin abnormality.

THE CARBON DIOXIDE DISSOCIATION CURVE

Just as the amount of O_2 carried by the blood is related to the P_{O_2} to which the blood is exposed, so the amount of CO_2 in blood is related to the P_{CO_2} of blood. The CO_2 dissociation curve is pictured in Figure 14-6. The mechanisms by which CO_2 is transported in plasma and erythrocytes are discussed in Chapter 16. Here it is sufficient to note that there is no steep portion followed by a flat or nearly horizontal portion, as with the HbO_2 curve, and in the physiologic range of CO_2 content and tension, the relation between the two is almost linear. This means that if man hypoventilates and alveolar P_{CO_2} rises, then arterial, capillary, tissue and venous CO_2 rise. If he hyperventilates and alveolar P_{CO_2} falls, then arterial, capillary, tissue and venous CO_2 fall. Doubling alveolar ventilation halves alveolar P_{CO_2} (from 40 to 20 torr); halving alveolar ventilation doubles alveolar P_{CO_2} (from 40 to 80 torr). At 40 torr, the CO_2 content in Figure 14-6 is 48.4 ml/100 ml; at 80 it is 63.6; at 20 it is 36.3. This means that hyperventilation of some regions can compensate for hypoventilation of others as far as CO_2 removal is concerned.

Fig. 14-7.—The O_2-CO_2 diagram of Rahn and Fenn. (Redrawn from *A Graphical Analysis of the Respiratory Gas Exchange: The O_2-CO_2 Diagram* [Washington: American Physiological Society, 1955].) See text. Note: Values in this diagram for % saturation HbO_2 at different P_{O_2} differ slightly from Severinghaus' recent and more precise data used in Figure 14-1.

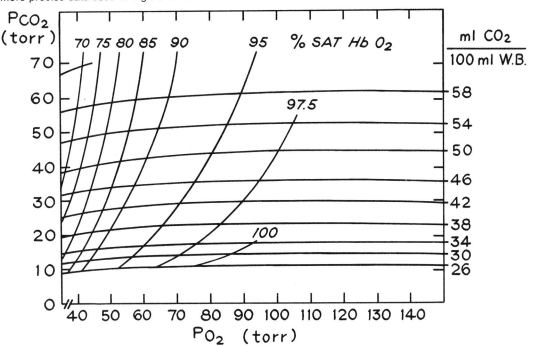

Hyperventilation of one region cannot compensate for hypoventilation of another as far as the uptake of O_2 by Hb is concerned *unless* the patient is hypoxemic and the % HbO_2 saturation is on the steep part of the curve.

THE OXYGEN-CARBON DIOXIDE DIAGRAM

Although O_2 and CO_2 dissociation curves are usually pictured separately to demonstrate their different shapes, it is equally instructive to put them together so that one can easily determine the O_2 saturation at any given Po_2 *and* Pco_2. The O_2-CO_2 diagram of Rahn and Fenn does this (Fig. 14-7). Here Po_2 is the abscissa and Pco_2 the ordinate. There are 7 lines of % saturation of HbO_2 varying from 70 to 100% (these are called isopleths because each represents equal volumes of O_2 combined with Hb) and 9 lines that are isopleths of CO_2 in ml/100 ml. If you want to identify the HbO_2 dissociation curve pictured in Figure 14-1, follow the 40 torr Pco_2 line from left to right and note the HbO_2 saturation at each Po_2. However, the diagram is used most to obtain the HbO_2 saturation of Hb when Pco_2 deviates from 40 torr. For example, if Po_2 is 93 torr and Pco_2 is 70 torr, the O_2 saturation of Hb is only 95% (it would be 97% if Pco_2 were 40 torr).

15

Blood-Tissue Gas Exchange

THE LOADING OF O_2 in pulmonary capillaries depends on the diffusing capacity of lung tissues that separate air and blood, the partial pressure of O_2 in the gas and blood and the

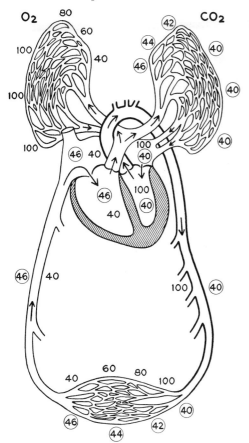

Fig. 15-1.—O_2 and CO_2 tensions in pulmonary and systemic blood. Figures in *circles* are CO_2 tensions; others are O_2 tensions.

chemical environment of Hb. Very much the same factors determine the unloading of O_2 in the tissue capillaries. Arterial blood at a high O_2 saturation and tension flows into the tissue capillaries (Fig. 15-1). The tissue cells continuously use O_2 and lower the Po_2 in and immediately around the cell below the Po_2 of capillary blood. Oxygen in the plasma, at a tension of approximately 100 torr, diffuses across the capillary wall into extracellular fluid and into cells. This lowers plasma Po_2, causes HbO_2 to dissociate and frees more O_2 for tissue utilization.

FACTORS DETERMINING TISSUE Po_2

Figure 15-2 pictures tissue supplied by a capillary network. The Po_2 at any point in the tissue depends on several factors: (1) the distance from the point to the nearest capillary with flowing blood; in Figure 15-2, cell *1* is relatively far from the nearest capillary, and cell *3* is very close but its nearest capillary is closed; (2) the intercapillary distance; cell *2* is in intimate contact with capillaries on all sides; (3) the radius of the capillary; (4) the metabolism and rate of O_2 consumption of the tissue; (5) the rate of diffusion of O_2 through the capillary and the tissue, and (6) the rate of blood flow through the capillary. Davies has shown that the tissue Po_2 is high in the immediate vicinity of a small arteriole but much lower midway between two arterioles. He placed a very fine O_2 electrode (14 μ diameter) on the surface of the brain

197

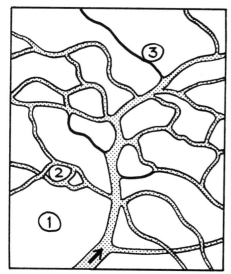

Fig. 15-2.—Schema showing intercapillary distances. Oxygen from blood flowing through tissue capillaries must diffuse over a longer path to reach cell *1* than cell *2*. Oxygen has a short path to cell *3* when its capillary is open and a much longer one when it is closed.

of a cat and measured tissue Po_2 at 25 μ intervals. In one experiment, his electrode first rested directly on an arteriole, then on brain tissue, a second arteriole, brain tissue and then a venule (Fig. 15-3). His records clearly show a small decrease in tissue Po_2 midway between two arterioles 100 μ apart but a very great decrease in brain Po_2 100 μ away

Fig. 15-3.—Tissue Po_2. Relative Po_2 of cerebral cortex of cat measured at various distances from two arterioles and a venule. (Redrawn from Davies, P., and Brink, F.: Fed. Proc. 16:690, 1957.)

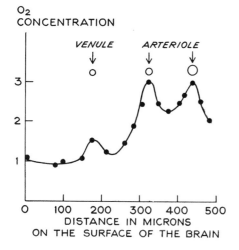

from the nearest arteriole. Note that the venule supplies O_2 to tissue cells if the Po_2 of its blood is higher than that of the brain tissue. The concept that O_2 exchange occurs only through *capillary* walls must be revised; diffusion of O_2 is not limited to specific vessels but occurs whenever the vessel wall is thin enough and the O_2 gradients across it are great enough.

The distance beween a cell and its nearest capillary may change in two ways: (1) arterioles may open or close, thereby increasing or decreasing the number of open capillaries with flowing blood. We have already stated that the number of open capillaries in the pulmonary circulation may increase or decrease; the tissue capillaries of the systemic circulation behave similarly. Krogh demonstrated that actively contracting muscle has 10 times as many open capillaries as resting muscle. Active tissues have a lower Po_2, higher Pco_2, lower pH, higher temperature and a higher concentration of certain metabolic products—all of which dilate arterioles locally by direct action, increase the number of open capillaries, decrease intercapillary distance and increase blood flow. The process of opening additional capillaries is far more efficient than widening those already open because the latter would increase the capillary diameter and would not decrease the distance for diffusion. The radius of the capillary is usually not greater than 2–3 μ (just wide enough for red cells to pass through in single file) unless there is a high hydrostatic pressure and tissue hypoxia with capillary dilation. (2) With increased transmural pressure or change in capillary permeability, tissue edema may occur. This increases the distance for diffusion just as alveolocapillary block does in the lung. Further, if edema increases tissue pressure sufficiently, it may compress some capillaries and further impede O_2 transfer.

Tissue metabolism influences tissue Po_2 in two ways: (1) the more active the tissue, the higher the local Pco_2, (H^+) and temperature and the lower the Po_2, and all of these factors favor local vasodilation, increase in blood flow and dissociation of O_2 from HbO_2 in capillary blood; and (2) the greater the use of O_2, the lower the tissue Po_2 and the steeper the concentration gradient for diffusion. The net effect of these on tissue Po_2 depends on how much blood flow changes and the HbO_2 curve shifts in relation to the increased O_2 use.

If tissue metabolism is zero, then the Po_2 of capillary and venous blood equals arterial Po_2; this occurs with cyanide poisoning, which prevents the use of O_2 by cytochrome oxidase. Tissue metabolism is decreased by cold; whether tissue Po_2 falls depends on the concomitant change in capillary blood flow and shift of the HbO_2 curve.

Increase in blood flow has the effect of supplying more O_2 molecules and maintaining a high capillary blood Po_2. The blood flow that is important for gas exchange is that through small, thin-walled vessels; the blood flowing through physiologic or pathologic artery-to-vein or arteriole-to-venule shunts does not supply O_2 to tissue cells. If capillary blood flow were infinitely rapid, capillary Po_2 would equal arterial Po_2. If capillary blood flow were to stop, tissue Po_2 would fall to zero in a very short time—depending on tissue metabolic rate (Fig. 15-4).

Two frequent questions are: (1) Which is more important for tissues—O_2 content or O_2 tension? (2) How high must tissue Po_2 be for O_2 to enter into chemical reactions? The answer to the first is that both are important: the tension must be high enough to permit diffusion from the capillary to its most remote cell; the content (number of molecules of O_2 per unit of blood) must be large enough so that the O_2 needs of all cells, near and remote, are met. As an extreme example, it is possible to equilibrate blood with a low concentration of CO in air so that its O_2 saturation is practically zero but its Po_2 almost normal. However, 100 ml of this blood can supply no more than 0.3 ml of O_2 (all dissolved); if the tissues need 4.5 ml, the Po_2 falls to zero at the very beginning of the capillary.

The answer to the second question is that chemical reactions proceed at a normal rate even though the Po_2 is very low ($4\,\mu$ moles/L or 3 torr Po_2) if the O_2 molecules are in close contact with the active enzymes (Fig. 15-5). The respiratory enzymes that use O_2 are the cytochromes, flavoproteins and pyridine nucleotides, which are the principal components of mitochondria; O_2 molecules must diffuse to them to be used. There is no evidence that oxidative metabolism proceeds at a higher rate if the Po_2 is raised to very high levels; the role of O_2 *tension* is to insure diffusion and delivery of O_2 molecules to the precise point of use.

ARTERY-TO-VEIN DIFFERENCE FOR O_2

We know that some tissues characteristically have a high blood flow relative to O_2 need and a small artery-to-vein O_2 difference and that others have a low blood flow rela-

Fig. 15-4 (left)—Po_2 of brain tissue during occlusion of the local circulation; Po_2 is measured on a small pial vein. Note the rapid decrease in Po_2 when the circulation is stopped. (Redrawn from Davies, P., and Brink, F.: Fed. Proc. 16:690, 1957.)

Fig. 15-5 (right).—Rate of O_2 use in a cytochrome-oxidase system. The O_2 used by the in vitro enzyme system remains constant (*straight line*) until a very low Po_2 is reached. (Redrawn from Chance, B.: Fed. Proc. 16:672, 1957.)

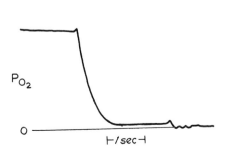

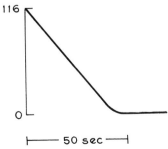

TABLE 15-1. — DIFFERENCES IN BLOOD FLOW, O_2 USED AND VENOUS Po_2 OF SELECTED ORGANS AND TISSUES*

TISSUE OR ORGAN	BLOOD FLOW ML/Minute	BLOOD FLOW % of CO	O_2 USED ML/Minute	O_2 USED % of total	A-V O_2 ML O_2/100 ML BLOOD	Po_2 VENOUS BLOOD TORR
Heart	250	4	26.4	11	11.4	23
Skeletal muscle	1,200	21	72.0	30	8.4	34
Brain	750	13	48.0	20	6.3	33
Splanchnic (liver)	1,400	24	60.0	25	4.1	43
Kidneys	1,100	19	16.8	7	1.3	56
Skin	500	9	4.8	2	1.0	60
Other	600	10	12.0	5	--	--
	5,800	100	240.0	100	4.1 (av.)	46 (av.)

*Modified from Finch, C. A., and Lenfant, C.: N. Engl. J. Med. 286:407, 1972. CO = cardiac output.

tive to O_2 used and a large A-V O_2 difference (Table 15-1). The A-V O_2 difference of mixed venous blood (average of blood from all organs and tissues) is 4.1 in this example. Organs or tissues with a high flow and a low A-V O_2 difference use the extra blood for nonmetabolic purposes (glomerular filtration in the kidney and heat loss in the skin). What sets the actual limit to O_2 extraction by different tissues is not known. For example, heart muscle of resting man uses more than half of the O_2 in its capillary blood; venous blood from the heart has a low Po_2. Skeletal muscle, which normally extracts less at rest, can extract all of the O_2 from its capillary blood during maximal exercise, and the Po_2 of venous blood from these muscles is zero; heart muscle does not do this with increasing cardiac work and elects to get its additional O_2 largely by increasing coronary arterial blood flow. How these decisions are made is not known.

O_2 STORES: TISSUE SURVIVAL

The body has essentially no stores of O_2 to use during complete anoxia or asphyxia.

Farhi and Rahn estimate that a 70-kg man has only about 1,550 ml of O_2 in his body at any moment, enough to maintain life for about 6 minutes if it could be properly distributed; 370 ml is in alveolar gas, about 280 ml in arterial blood, about 600 ml is in capillary and venous blood, 60 ml is dissolved in body tissues and 240 ml is bound to muscle myoglobin. Cells do not necessarily die when they have used the last O_2 available to them if they have mechanisms for anaerobic metabolism and a supply of substrate that can be used to provide energy. Some turtles, for example, can live for as long as 17 hours in complete absence of O_2 (atmosphere of N_2), because of their reserves of glycogen and anaerobic metabolic processes. The newborn of many species survive complete ischemia longer than adults of the same species. Different organs and tissues of mammals have different survival times if made completely ischemic, and regulatory mechanisms manage to redistribute blood in emergencies to favor those with the shortest survival times (these are usually vital organs such as cerebral cortex and heart).

16

Transport and Elimination of Carbon Dioxide

THE MAIN FUNCTION of the cardiovascular-pulmonary system is to supply each cell with an adequate flow of arterial blood so that each can live in its optimal environment. But blood flow has a dual function: it supplies essential materials and removes waste products. One of the products of cell metabolism is CO_2. It is carried by venous blood to the lungs, where excess CO_2 is eliminated in expired gas. Because $CO_2 + H_2O \rightleftharpoons H_2CO_3$, or carbonic *acid*, CO_2 transport and elimination are important in acid-base chemistry as well as in respiratory physiology. Actually, the lungs are the most important organ in the body for acid excretion; ordinarily, the kidneys of a healthy, resting man excrete 40–80 mEq/day and the lungs excrete about 13,000 mEq/day. The lungs excrete volatile acid (the CO_2 of carbonic acid); the kidneys excrete nonvolatile acids.

HYDROGEN IONS, ACIDS AND BASES

For excellent and complete discussions of acid-base chemistry, read Davenport, Pitts or Christensen. What follows here is brief background information necessary to understand CO_2 transport and elimination.

An atom, electrically neutral, consists of a positively charged nucleus surrounded by one or more electrons. When an atom of one species donates the electrons of its outer valence shell to the atom of another species, the donor becomes a *positively* charged ion

(cation, because it migrates to the cathode) and the recipient becomes a *negatively* charged ion (anion, because it moves to the anode). The hydrogen atom has only one electron in its single shell; the chloride atom has seven in its outer shell. When the hydrogen atom donates its electron to the chloride atom, these become the hydrogen ion, H^+ and the chloride ion, Cl^-. The hydrogen ion is also known as a proton.

When molecules, such as sodium chloride, dissolve in water, their ions, Na^+ and Cl^-, become relatively independent in their behavior—they dissociate. Substances that dissociate into electrically charged ions are capable of carrying electrical currents and are called *electrolytes*. *Strong* electrolytes dissociate almost completely; *weak* electrolytes ionize only partially in solution. Hydrochloric acid in aqueous solution dissociates almost completely to form H^+ and Cl^- ions and is therefore a strong electrolyte or a strong acid.

An *acid* (defined chemically; Brønsted classification) is any compound capable of donating a proton (or hydrogen ion) to a base; the general equation is $HX \rightleftharpoons H^+ + X^-$. A *base* is any compound capable of accepting a proton; the general equation is $X^- + H^+ \rightleftharpoons HX$. Substances that neither donate nor accept protons are neither acids nor bases. Thus, N^+ and K^+ are not bases (as many clinicians believe) because they do not accept protons, and Cl^- and SO_4^{2-} are not

201

acids, since they have no H ions to donate.

The H ion or proton may come from dissociation of electrically neutral molecules:

$$HCl \rightleftharpoons H^+ + Cl^-$$
$$H_2CO_3 \rightleftharpoons H^+ + HCO_3^-$$

or from further dissociation of an anion:

$$H_2PO_4^- \rightleftharpoons H^+ + HPO_4^=$$

or from dissociation of a cation:

$$NH_4^+ \rightleftharpoons H^+ + NH_3$$

Some anions, such as $H_2PO_4^-$, can act either as acids and donate an H ion ($H_2PO_4^- \rightleftharpoons H^+ + HPO_4^=$) or as bases and accept an H ion ($H_2PO_4^- + H^+ \rightleftharpoons H_3PO_4$).

For many years clinicians have used confusing jargon according to which all *cations* (except for H^+) are bases and all *anions* (except for OH^-) are acids. Use of the Brønsted definition permits sharp distinction between a disturbance in acid-base balance and a disturbance in electrolyte balance without acidosis or alkalosis; these sharp distinctions, in turn, permit precise and correct treatment of each disturbance.

H ION CONCENTRATION; pH

Blood and other body fluids are acid or alkaline because they have an excess or deficiency of free H ions. The actual concentration of free H ions in blood is very low—about 40×10^{-9} Eq/L; this might also be expressed as 40 μmEq or 40 nanoEq/L. In 1909 Sorenson proposed the expression pH; the symbol p in pH should not be confused with another symbol, capital P, as used in P_{O_2}, P_{CO_2} or P_{N_2} to express the partial pressure of a gas. Sorenson defined pH as the negative logarithm to the base of 10 of the hydrogen ion concentration:[1]

---

[1]Recently there have been many suggestions that we abandon the term pH and talk directly in terms of (H^+). There are good arguments for and against these proposals. The glass electrode in theory measures the active concentration rather than the total concentration of H ions (although in the biologic range the two are regarded as identical); pH is a measure of availability, or escaping tendency, of hydrogen ions and not of (H^+) itself.

$$pH = -\log (H^+)$$

If the (H^+) is 40×10^{-9} Eq/L,

$$
\begin{aligned}
\text{then pH} &= -\log (40 \times 10^{-9}) \\
&= -\log 40 - \log 10^{-9} \\
&= -1.6 - (-9) \\
&= -1.6 + 9 \\
&= 7.4
\end{aligned}
$$

The molecules of pure distilled water dissociate to yield a very small number of H ions and an equally small number of OH ions; the concentration of each is 10^{-7} Eq/L. Water is neutral and has a pH of 7.0. If additional free H ions are added, the (H^+) of the solution becomes greater than 10^{-7} and its pH becomes less than 7.0. If the H ions are removed (by adding a proton acceptor), the (H^+) decreases and the pH increases to more than 7.0. The pH scale ranges from 0 to 14 (from 1.0 Eq of H^+/L to 10^{-14} Eq H^+/L). Because the scale is logarithmic, a decrease of 1 pH unit represents a 10-fold increase in H ion concentration.

Clinically, (H^+) or pH is measured by an electrode made of a thin glass membrane that is freely permeable only to H ions. Although pH can be measured in any body fluid (such as cerebrospinal fluid; see p. 60), blood pH is usually measured because it is representative of the various extracellular fluid compartments that, in turn, are in dynamic equilibrium with intracellular buffers. Although whole blood is usually used, the glass electrode measures pH of the plasma and ignores that of the red blood cells. A competent laboratory technician can perform duplicate determinations on a blood sample in 5–10 minutes.

Hydrogen ions are formed continuously in the body. Aerobic metabolism (oxidative phosphorylation) produces CO_2 and H_2O, which is converted to H_2CO_3 and then dissociates to $H^+ + HCO_3^-$. Hydrogen ions are also formed as sulfuric acid and phosphoric acid from metabolism of sulfur-containing amino acids and of phospholipids. Incomplete or anaerobic metabolism of fat and carbohydrate can yield lactic acid, pyruvic acid, acetoacetic acid or βOH butyric acid. The total amount of H$^+$ produced daily in the form of nonvolatile acids in a healthy man on a normal meat diet is 50–70 mEq. Why, then, are there so few free H ions? The reason is that the body has both chemical and physiologic ways of reducing the number of free H ions. *Chemically*, blood and tissues contain buffers that "soak up" H ions so that a single injection of even large amounts of acid produces only a small increase in (H$^+$). *Physiologically*, healthy lungs and kidneys eliminate the acid end products of tissue metabolism almost as fast as they are formed.

BUFFERS

Buffers are solutions that have the capacity to resist changes in pH when either acids or bases are added to them. The classic example of a buffer is a weak acid (or a weak base) that dissociates only slightly into its ions and its highly ionized salt. Why does this mixture resist change in pH? Suppose that HCl is added to a mixture of acetic acid (a weak acid) and sodium acetate (its salt). The HCl will react with the highly ionized sodium acetate to form sodium chloride and additional acetic acid. However, acetic acid is only slightly ionized or dissociated into

hydrogen and acetate ions. The decrease in HCl and the increase in acetic acid does not reduce the total amount of *acid* present, but it does decrease the concentration of *free* H ions in solution. Because a buffer binds, "soaks up" or takes free H ions out of circulation, its pH changes far less on addition of acid than that of an unbuffered substance. If 1 ml of 0.1 N HCl is added to 99 ml of pure water, the pH will decrease from 7.0 to 3.0; if the same amount of HCl is added to a buffer mixture of 0.1 N acetic acid and 0.1 M sodium acetate, the pH will change only from 4.73 to 4.72.

Different buffers have different buffering powers. The action of a buffer can be demonstrated by constructing its titration curve. This is done as follows: Measure a known amount of a buffer, dissolve it in water and measure the pH of the solution. Add a known small amount of a strong acid and measure the pH of this mixture. Repeat the process over and over, adding equal increments of acid each time. Then plot the amount of acid added (ordinate) vs. the pH (abscissa). The pH changes rapidly at first, then much more slowly and finally, as the titration nears completion, very rapidly again. The pH change per unit of added acid is least at the pH corresponding to half neutraliza-

Fig. 16-1.—Titration curve for the buffer system HCO$_3^-$/H$_2$CO$_3$. The pK is 6.1; the change in pH is least at pK when a given amount of acid or base is added. The buffer value is the quantity of H$^+$ that can be added to or removed from the solution with a pH change of 1.0, on the steep slope of the curve, between pH 5.6 to 6.6 (*stippled zone*). Far fewer H$^+$ are required to change pH in the physiologic or pathologic range for blood, 6.9 to 7.9 (*hatched zone*). The pK is the pH corresponding to half neutralization of the weak acid; this follows since, when (HCO$_3^-$) = (H$_2$CO$_3$),

$$pH = pK + \log \frac{1}{1}$$
$$= pK + 0$$
$$= pK$$

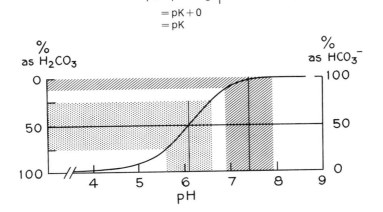

tion, at which point the buffer is half dissociated; this is called the pK value. The buffer value is the quantity of H ions that can be added to (or removed from) a solution (in its most effective range) with a change of one pH unit. As a rule, buffers are reasonably effective over a range of 1.0 pH unit on each side of the optimal or halfway point (Fig. 16-1). If a buffer has a pK value of 5.3, it is most effective in body fluids whose pH range is 4.3 to 6.3; it is a poor buffer in blood whose pH is 7.4.

The Henderson-Hasselbalch Equation

The Henderson-Hasselbalch equation is a special form of the law of mass action, which states that the velocity of a reaction is proportional to the product of the molar concentrations of the reactants. In the case of a reversible chemical reaction:

$$(A) + (B) \underset{V_2}{\overset{V_1}{\rightleftharpoons}} (C) + (D) \qquad (1)$$

velocity 1 is proportional to $(A) \times (B)$ and velocity 2 is proportional to $(C) \times (D)$. At equilibrium, when the two velocities are equal and no further change occurs in the concentration of A, B, C or D, then

$$\frac{(C) \times (D)}{(A) \times (B)} = K \qquad (2)$$

The constant, K, at equilibrium is always the same for A + B regardless of the proportions or concentration of A and B initially present. The stronger the acid, the more it is dissociated into ions, the greater is the ratio of ions to undissociated molecules and the larger is the value of K_A.

Let us apply the law of mass action to the ionization of a weak acid, such as H_2CO_3. The reaction is

$$H_2CO_3 \rightleftharpoons H^+ + HCO_3^- \qquad (3)$$

The law of mass action states that

$$\frac{(H^+) \times (HCO_3^-)}{(H_2CO_3)} = K_A \qquad (4)$$

where K_A is the ionization or dissociation constant of the weak acid, H_2CO_3. The Henderson-Hasselbalch equation rearranges this in several ways.

First, to express (H^+) in terms of pH, the equation is changed into its logarithmic form. In the case of the buffer pair HCO_3^-/H_2CO_3 this becomes,

$$\log \frac{(H^+)(HCO_3^-)}{(H_2CO_3)} = \log K_A \qquad (5)$$

or

$$\log (H^+) + \log \frac{(HCO_3^-)}{(H_2CO_3)} = \log K_A \qquad (6)$$

Transposing,

$$\log (H^+) = \log K_A - \log \frac{(HCO_3^-)}{(H_2CO_3)} \qquad (7)$$

Changing both sides of the equation,

$$-\log (H^+) = -\log K_A + \log \frac{(HCO_3^-)}{(H_2CO_3)} \qquad (8)$$

Substituting pH and pK for the negative logarithms of (H^+) and K_A, respectively, the equation becomes

$$pH = pK + \log \frac{(HCO_3^-)}{(H_2CO_3)} \qquad (9)$$

Second, the Henderson-Hasselbalch equation substitutes *dissolved* CO_2 for H_2CO_3. This is possible because the concentration of dissolved CO_2 vastly exceeds that of H_2CO_3 at equilibrium (809 times as much). And it is convenient in the practice of medicine because clinically it is easy to measure P_{CO_2} of blood and then calculate dissolved CO_2 by multiplying P_{CO_2} (in torr) by the solubility of CO_2 (in mmoles CO_2/L/torr P_{CO_2}); thus, when Pa_{CO_2} is 40 torr, dissolved CO_2 is 40×0.0301, or 1.2 mmoles/L.

The final equation then becomes

$$pH = pK' + \log \frac{(HCO_3^-)}{(CO_2)} \qquad (10)$$

Since the pK for the HCO_3^-/CO_2 system in blood (pK') is 6.1,

$$pH = 6.1 + \log \frac{(HCO_3^-)}{(CO_2)} \qquad (11)$$

Figure 16-1 shows the titration curve for HCO_3^-/CO_2; the point of maximal buffering is at the pK' value of 6.1. Since the pH of man's blood is 7.4 (and it rarely falls below 6.9 or exceeds 7.9), the HCO_3^-/CO_2 system cannot be very effective in blood. Furthermore, this system is not an effective buffer against CO_2, because the reaction ($CO_2 + H_2O \rightleftharpoons H_2CO_3 \rightleftharpoons H^+ + HCO_3^-$) forms a H ion and a HCO_3^- ion, leaving the H ion to be buffered by other mechanisms. It *is* an effective buffer against fixed acids since

$$H^+ + Cl^- + Na^+ + HCO_3^- \rightleftharpoons NaCl + H_2CO_3$$

In this case a highly dissociated, strong acid is converted into a poorly dissociated, weak acid, leaving NaCl as a neutral salt.

Why do we consider the HCO_3^-/CO_2 system essential in the elimination of CO_2 and of the H_2CO_3 that forms when CO_2 reacts with water? It is because managing CO_2 formed in tissue metabolism requires not only chemical buffering but also transport of CO_2 from its site of formation to its site of elimination and then eliminating all of the CO_2 that is formed. The HCO_3^-/CO_2 system is an extremely effective way to *transport* CO_2 in blood (see p. 208) to the lungs, where the body has remarkable physiologic mechanisms for eliminating (or retaining) CO_2 through pulmonary ventilation. The body also has effective ways of eliminating (or retaining) HCO_3^- by glomerular filtration and tubular reabsorption. Buffering is limited in a closed system (blood without lungs or kidneys) because accumulation of a weak acid slows the reaction. However, when the system is an open one (e.g., lungs with pulmonary ventilation to remove CO_2), these limitations do not exist. Another unique feature of the system is that it is subject to precise physiologic regulation.

To make the point, Gilman has rewritten the Henderson-Hasselbalch equation as

$$pH = constant + \frac{kidneys}{lungs}$$

The Blood Buffers

Since HCO_3^-/CO_2 is not optimally effective as a buffer system at pH 7.4 and is not a buffer against CO_2, we must look for other blood buffers that *do* operate chemically in the physiologic range and permit the transport of CO_2 to organs of elimination without wide swings in blood pH.

Blood contains a number of buffers; these include the HCO_3^-/CO_2 system already discussed, a $HPO_4^{2-}/H_2PO_4^-$ system, which is relatively unimportant, and numerous protein buffers, grouped together as Pr^-/HPr, which are very effective. A protein is a buffer because its molecule contains a large number of acidic and basic groups. Proteins are built of amino acids, which are amphoteric electrolytes (ampholytes) — i.e., they act as acids and as bases, since they contain at least one carboxyl group and one amino group. For example, glycine, which is usually written as NH_2—CH_2—COOH, exists in solution as H_3N^+—CH_2—COO^-, in which both the acidic and basic groups are ionized. This is called a zwitterion, since it is formed by the internal wandering of an H ion in the molecule. In this form, it is electrically neutral (isoelectric) since it has one positive and one negative charge. A basic group acts as a buffer by taking up H ions in acid solution and forming cations (—H_3N^+). An acidic group acts as a buffer by giving up H ions in alkaline solution and forming anions (—COO^-).

Proteins, constructed from amino acids via the peptide linkage, still retain many free —NH_2 and —COOH groups and, like amino acids, have an isoelectric point. Figure 16-2 shows the isoelectric point of a protein with 4 H_3N^+ and 4 COO^- groups. When 4 H ions are added to the solution, 3 combine with COO^- groups, suppress their ionization and form undissociated COOH groups. One H ion remains free in solution, making it more acid, but far less acid than if all 4 H ions were free. The strength of a protein buffer is measured by determining its pK.

The imidazole group (Fig. 16-2) of the

amino acid histidine is of special physiologic importance for two reasons: (1) Hb is rich in histidine and (2) the pK of imidazole is 7.0, which is in the physiologic range for blood.

The buffer capacity of red cell protein (Hb) is far greater than that of plasma proteins. This is partly because the buffer value of Hb is greater (1 gm of HbO_2 binds 0.183 mEq of H ions for a change in pH from 7.5 to 6.5; 1 gm of plasma proteins binds only 0.11 mEq). More important, there is much more Hb; 1 L of blood contains 150 gm of Hb and 38.5 gm of plasma protein. From these figures we can calculate that the HbO_2 contained in 1 L of blood binds more than 6 times as many H ions as its plasma proteins (150 × 0.183 or *27.5* vs. 38.5 × 0.110 or *4.24*).

BUFFERING POWER OF HB VS. THAT OF HBO_2. The titration curve of Hb is parallel

Fig. 16-2.—**A**, schematic representation of the buffering action of a protein. **B**, buffering action of hemoglobin in the physiologic range. Much of this is accomplished by the imidazole groups of histidine (pK = 7.1). (Figs. 16-2 through 16-4 from Davenport, H. W.: *The ABC of Acid Base Chemistry* [5th ed.; Chicago: University of Chicago Press, 1969.])

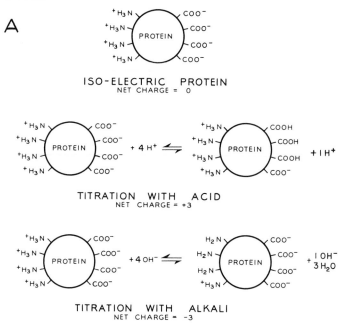

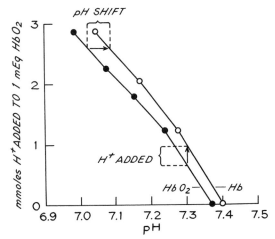

Fig. 16-3.—Titration curves of oxyhemoglobin (*filled circles*) and of reduced hemoglobin (*open circles*) at 37 C in the presence of carbon dioxide at a partial pressure of 39 torr. The horizontal arrow shows the shift in pH that occurs when Hb is deoxygenated without any change in the amount of acid added or removed by external means; the increase in pH is caused by removal of H⁺ from solution as Hb becomes a weaker acid. The vertical arrow shows the extra H⁺ that can be added without change in pH. (Adapted from the data of Rossi and Roughton, J. Physiol. 189:1, 1967.)

with that of HbO_2 over the physiologic range (Fig. 16-3); however, HbO_2 is a stronger acid than deoxygenated Hb. When 1 mEq of HbO_2 is deoxygenated to Hb, the pH shifts about 0.048 units (*horizontal arrow*, Fig. 16-3); if one now titrates Hb back to the original pH, about 0.3 mmoles H⁺ ions can be added. This means that the two important chemical changes that occur in the tissue capillaries—the delivery of O_2 and uptake of CO_2—are mutually helpful. We have already noted (p. 188) that the addition of acid to blood shifts the HbO_2 dissociation curve so that more O_2 is freed from HbO_2 (the Bohr effect). We now see that the loss of O_2 from HbO_2 produces Hb, a weaker acid, which is capable of accepting a large number of H⁺ *without any change in pH* (the Haldane effect; the equal hydrogen ion, or isohydric change). This property of blood—being able to take up an appreciable number of H ions without changing its pH—is of unique and extraordinary value in maintaining blood neutrality while transporting CO_2 from tis-

sues to lungs. Davenport has calculated that if R = 0.7 (CO_2 produced/O_2 consumed = 0.7), then, for every mmole of O_2 used, 0.7 mmole of CO_2 is produced; this amount of CO_2, converted to H_2CO_3, yields 0.7 mmole of H ions, and all of the H ions produced under these conditions could be taken up by the Hb formed by the dissociation of HbO_2, with no change in blood pH. Others have calculated that if there were no Hb and CO_2 had to be transported only in plasma, the venous blood would be 800 times more acid than arterial blood (pH 4.5 vs. 7.4); with hemoglobin, the pH of venous blood is 7.37. It is of interest that strenuous muscular exercise results not only in a great increase in CO_2 production but also in more complete dissociation of HbO_2 to Hb, which has greater capacity to soak up H ions and so minimizes change in blood pH (p. 188).

CARBAMINO COMPOUNDS. We have said that amino acids can act as buffers and mop up H⁺. Carbon dioxide can also react directly with amino groups of proteins to form carbamino compounds.

$$R—NH_2 + CO_2 \rightleftharpoons R—NHCOO^- + H^+$$

This is a mechanism by which CO_2 may be *carried* in the blood but is not a buffering mechanism, since it produces H ions, which must either be mopped up by buffers or decrease the pH (just as the reaction $CO_2 + H_2O \rightleftharpoons H_2CO_3 \rightleftharpoons H^+ + HCO_3^-$ produces H ions, which must then be buffered).

The amount of carbamino compounds formed with Hb is greater than with HbO_2, so that the capacity of blood to carry CO_2 increases as more HbO_2 dissociates in the capillaries of active tissues.

CARBON DIOXIDE TRANSPORT AND ELIMINATION

Transport of Carbon Dioxide from Tissues to Lungs

We have mentioned the important ways in which blood combines with CO_2 and the buffering mechanisms in blood. All that remains is to describe the actual processes and assign quantitative values to each.

The process starts with formation of CO_2 by active cells. This increases local tissue tension of CO_2 above that of arterial blood, and CO_2 molecules diffuse from the tissue into the plasma of capillary blood. Most of the CO_2 so added to plasma diffuses into the red blood cells, but some does enter into three reactions in the plasma (Fig. 16-4). The first is simple solution in plasma as dissolved CO_2. Like dissolved O_2, this amount depends entirely on the partial pressure and solubility coefficient of the gas. If arterial blood P_{CO_2} is 40 torr and end-capillary blood P_{CO_2} is 46, the additional dissolved CO_2 is 6×0.0301, or 0.18 mmoles/L. The second reaction is the hydration of CO_2:

$$CO_2 + H_2O \rightleftharpoons H_2CO_3 \rightleftharpoons H^+ + HCO_3^-$$

Very little CO_2 is so hydrated in plasma because the chemical reaction is a very slow one (there is no enzyme in plasma to catalyze the reaction) and accumulation of H_2CO_3 stops the reaction. The H ions formed are buffered by the weak systems in plasma. A third reaction is formation of some carbamino compounds with plasma proteins; H ions so formed are buffered in the plasma.

The major buffering of CO_2 occurs within red blood cells (see Fig. 16-4.) Five reactions occur in red cells; three of these are mechanisms for transporting CO_2, and two are buffering mechanisms. First, as in the plasma, a small amount of CO_2 dissolves in the fluid of the erythrocyte as a function of

Fig. 16-4.—Schematic representation of the processes when CO_2 passes from the tissues into the plasma and into the erythrocytes. The main body of the HbO_2 and of the Hb molecule is indicated but not drawn structurally. The buffering of hydrogen ions is emphasized by circling the H^+ that are released and buffered. (Redrawn from Davenport.)

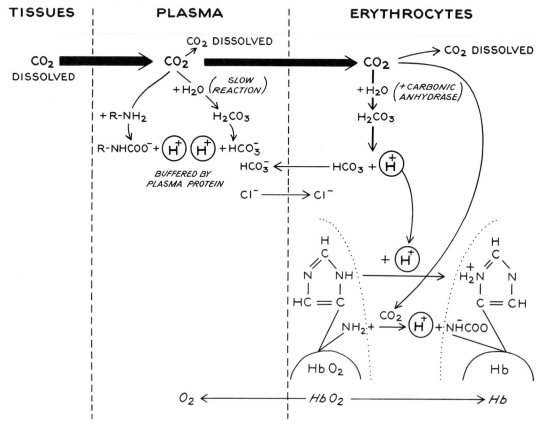

the P_{CO_2}. The second reaction, hydration of CO_2,

$$CO_2 + H_2O \rightleftharpoons H_2CO_3 \rightleftharpoons H^+ + HCO_3^-$$

proceeds far more rapidly in red cells than in plasma for two reasons: (1) a special enzyme, carbonic anhydrase, exists in high concentration in red blood cells (there is none in plasma), and this makes the reaction $CO_2 + H_2O \rightleftharpoons H_2CO_3$ go 13,000 times as fast; (2) the products of the reaction, H^+ and HCO_3^-, do not accumulate in red cells as they do in plasma and therefore do not slow or stop the reaction going to the right. Hydrogen ions are mopped up by the Hb buffers; HCO_3^- ions leave the red cell because a concentration difference builds up between the red cell and the plasma. The red cell membrane is readily permeable to negatively charged ions such as HCO_3^- or Cl^- but less permeable, under normal conditions, to cations such as Na^+ or K^+. When the HCO_3^- ions diffuse outward, they are therefore unaccompanied by cations, and the red cell is left with a net positive electric charge. This tends to bring negatively charged ions of any kind into the cell from the plasma; Cl^- ions, the most abundant plasma anions, migrate inward ("chloride shift," first described by Hamburger). The exchange of HCO_3^- ions formed in red cells with Cl^- ions from plasma increases the CO_2 carrying power of plasma, though the buffering occurred in red cells.

Some movement of water inward occurs simultaneously to maintain osmotic equilibrium; this results in a slight swelling of erythrocytes in the venous blood, relative to those in arterial blood. Normal biconcave red cells permit this change in volume without rupture.

The third reaction is combination of CO_2 with Hb to form carbamino compounds; this is a rapid reaction that requires no special enzyme. The reaction is $Hb\ NH_2 + CO_2 \rightleftharpoons Hb\ NHCOOH \rightleftharpoons Hb\ NHCOO^- + H^+$. The

TABLE 16-1.—Transport and Buffering of CO_2 in Blood*

Transport

	ARTERIAL BLOOD	VENOUS BLOOD	VENOUS MINUS ARTERIAL
Whole blood (1,000 ml)			
Total CO_2	21.53	23.21	1.68
Plasma (600 ml)			
Total CO_2	15.94	16.99	1.05
As dissolved CO_2	0.71	0.80	0.09
As bicarbonate ions	15.23	16.19	0.96
Red blood cells (400 ml)			
Total CO_2	5.59	6.22	0.63
As dissolved CO_2	0.34	0.39	0.05
As carbamino CO_2	0.97	1.42	0.45
As bicarbonate ions	4.28	4.41	0.13

Buffering

	ARTERIAL BLOOD	VENOUS BLOOD	VENOUS MINUS ARTERIAL
Plasma (600 ml)			
Net negative charge on proteins	7.89	7.80	−0.09
Bicarbonate ions	15.23	16.19	+0.96
Chloride ions	59.59	58.72	−0.87
Red blood cells (400 ml)			
Net negative charge on hemoglobin	22.60	21.15	−1.45
Bicarbonate ions	4.28	4.41	+0.13
Chloride ions	18.11	18.98	+0.87
Carbamino CO_2	0.97	1.42	+0.45

*From Davenport, H. W.: *The ABC of Acid-Base Chemistry* (4th ed.; Chicago: University of Chicago Press, 1958). All values are mmoles/L and measured in whole blood and in the 600 ml of plasma and 400 ml of red cells separated from 1 L of whole blood containing 8.93 mmoles Hb/L.

pK of Hb NHCOOH is below 6.0, so that at physiologic pH, it is almost completely ionized. Therefore, in both this reaction and in the second reaction (hydration of CO_2), the H ions produced must be buffered if a large change in pH is to be prevented.

The fourth reaction is the actual buffering of these H ions by the buffering groups of the protein part of the Hb molecule. The fifth is the acceptance of H ions by the Hb formed when O_2 is dissociated from HbO_2.

If, for arterial and for venous blood, one measures the CO_2 in red blood cells and in plasma (quickly separated from each other under physiologic conditions), one obtains data like those in Table 16-1. Whole venous blood contains, in this case, 1.68 mmoles more CO_2 than arterial; 1.05 mmoles of this is in the plasma and only 0.63 in the red cells. From this it is obvious that about $\frac{2}{3}$ of the CO_2 added to capillary blood is *carried* in the plasma to the lungs. However, Table 16-1 shows that most of the *buffering* occurred in the red cells. There is a decrease of only 0.09 mmoles in the net anionic charge on the plasma proteins while the net anionic charge on Hb decreased by 1.45 mmoles. Of the CO_2 buffered within the red cells, 0.45 mmoles was formed as carbamino compound and 1.00 mmoles as bicarbonate; 0.87 mmoles of the HCO_3^- shifted to the plasma. Since the total increase in plasma HCO_3^- was 0.96 mmoles, only 0.09 mmoles (0.96 − 0.87) was due to primary chemical buffering in the plasma.

The Elimination of Carbon Dioxide in the Lungs

In the lungs, the alveolar P_{CO_2} (40 torr) is lower than the P_{CO_2} of mixed venous blood flowing into the pulmonary capillaries (46 torr, in a resting man), and the CO_2 reactions described before go to the left because some CO_2 leaves the blood. At the same time, reduced Hb becomes HbO_2, which is a stronger acid; this also drives CO_2 from the red blood cell. We learned earlier that when tis-

sue CO_2 enters systemic capillary blood, it shifts the HbO_2 dissociation curve to the right and so facilitates unloading of O_2 from HbO_2. Now we see that when O_2 enters the blood in the pulmonary capillaries, it facilitates unloading of CO_2 from mixed venous blood. Further, the carbamino groups of HbO_2 can hold less CO_2 than those of Hb, and this results in a further loss of CO_2. It is important to remember that most of the bicarbonate shifts back into the red cell and forms H_2CO_3 there; the carbonic anhydrase in the red cell speeds the breakdown of H_2CO_3 to CO_2 and H_2O. The CO_2 then diffuses across the red cell membrane into the plasma and then across the alveolocapillary membranes into alveolar gas.

Factors That Influence Carbon Dioxide Transport and Elimination

INHALATION OF O_2. When O_2 instead of air is breathed at sea level, the amount of dissolved O_2 in arterial blood increases from 0.3 to 2.0 ml/100 ml of blood and, since most of this dissolved O_2 diffuses from blood to tissues before HbO_2 dissociates into Hb and O_2, less HbO_2 changes to Hb in capillary blood. This interferes with the uptake and buffering of CO_2 in blood and raises venous blood and tissue P_{CO_2} slightly. When man breathes O_2 at 3 atmospheres pressure (see p. 280), all of his tissue needs can be met without *any* dissociation of HbO_2 and there is a greater rise in tissue P_{CO_2}. Lambertsen has concluded, however, that the increase in brain P_{CO_2} is far less than required to explain the convulsions that occur under these conditions (p. 282).

SEVERE ANEMIA. This could interfere with CO_2 transport because fewer red blood cells means less carbonic anhydrase and less Hb. Carbonic anhydrase deficiency is not a problem because normally this enzyme is present in very great excess. A lack of Hb available to accept H^+ ions could result in a rise in the P_{CO_2} and (H^+) of venous blood and tissues but, as a rule, the cardiac output increases enough so that active tissues receive more blood per unit of time and therefore enough Hb buffer.

INHIBITORS OF CARBONIC ANHYDRASE. There is no naturally occurring disorder in which this enzyme is absent or inactive, but it can be inhibited by certain chemicals. The most potent and specific of these are acetazolamide (Diamox), ethoxzolamide (Ethamide), dichlorphenamide (Daranide) and thiazides, which, in large amounts in vitro, can almost completely inhibit the activity of blood carbonic anhydrase. However, far more carbonic anhydrase is usually present than needed, and almost 99% of it must be inhibited to produce physiologic effects.

It is important to remember that, in the absence of carbonic anhydrase, the reaction $CO_2 + H_2O \rightleftarrows H_2CO_3$ still goes to the same equilibrium value; only the velocity of the reaction is changed. However, if CO_2 entering red cells from tissues is not quickly converted to H_2CO_3, CO_2 piles up in plasma and then in tissues, and Pco_2 rises in systemic capillary blood and tissues. In the venous blood, hydration of CO_2 continues and Pco_2 decreases; the reaction may be complete by the time venous blood reaches the pulmonary capillaries. But blood of resting man spends only about ¾ second in the pulmonary capillary, and this is inadequate time for the second of the reverse reactions, which are

$$HCO_3^- + H^+ \rightleftarrows H_2CO_3$$

$$H_2CO_3 \rightleftarrows H_2O + CO_2$$

In the absence of carbonic anhydrase, H_2CO_3 changes very slowly to $H_2O + CO_2$. Therefore, loss of CO_2 to alveolar gas is incomplete, alveolar Pco_2 decreases and the quantity of CO_2 eliminated is less. Since CO_2 cannot escape from blood between the time blood leaves the pulmonary capillaries and the time it reaches systemic capillaries, and since conversion to H_2CO_3 to CO_2 continues during this time, arterial blood Pco_2 continuously rises, and consequently Pco_2 in systemic capillary blood and in tissues must rise; this is an unusual situation in which arterial Pco_2 exceeds pulmonary capillary and alveolar Pco_2. The precise time course of the noncatalyzed reaction is unknown because there is no instantaneous method for measuring blood Pco_2. The decreased elimination of CO_2 is transient; when a new steady state is established with higher tissue Pco_2, normal elimination of CO_2 resumes.

Carbonic anhydrase inhibitors, given therapeutically to man, appear to affect renal mechanisms for acidification of the urine (which also depend on the enzyme to accelerate the conversion of $CO_2 + H_2O$ to H_2CO_3 and provide H ions) in lower dosage than required to affect CO_2 transport in blood; consequently *nonrespiratory* acidosis may occur rather than *respiratory* acidosis.

RED BLOOD CELL HEMOLYSIS. Hemolysis obviously decreases the number of circulating red blood cells, but it does more than this. It spills their contents into the plasma; these include Hb (a protein with osmotic properties similar to albumin), potassium, carbonic anhydrase and other enzymes. There have been no measurements of CO_2 transport and elimination under these conditions.

IMPAIRMENT OF DIFFUSION. As mentioned elsewhere, CO_2 diffuses through watery fluids 20 times faster than O_2. Impaired diffusion for O_2, even if severe but still compatible with life, does not prevent CO_2 elimination. Retention of CO_2 caused by longer distances for gas diffusion or by decreased area for gas exchange probably occurs only in patients with very severe pulmonary disease kept alive by inhalation or insufflation (see p. 159) of high concentrations of O_2.

ACID-BASE DISORDERS

Respiratory and Nonrespiratory Acidosis and Alkalosis

1. IF THE Pco_2 OF BLOOD IS HIGH AND THE pH LOW, the patient obviously has

acidosis, and it must be respiratory acidosis, caused by the inability of the lungs to eliminate CO_2 as rapidly as it forms. Only two measurements are necessary: pH of arterial blood using a glass electrode and P_{CO_2} of the same blood using the Severinghaus CO_2 electrode (Fig. 2-2). The apparatus is available in any hospital; the measurements take less than 10 minutes. In an adult or neonatal intensive-respiratory-care unit, blood samples can be taken as often as needed through an indwelling plastic tube in an artery and the measurements used at once as a guide to treatment.

2. IF THE P_{CO_2} IS LOW AND THE pH IS HIGH, the patient has alkalosis, and it must be respiratory alkalosis caused by primary hyperventilation. Hyperventilation (alveolar ventilation in excess of production of CO_2 by metabolism) lowers arterial P_{CO_2}, increases the ratio of $\dfrac{HCO_3^-}{CO_2}$ to > 20:1 and increases blood pH.

3. IF THE P_{CO_2} IS LOW AND THE pH IS ALSO LOW, the patient has acidosis, and it must be nonrespiratory acidosis. Nonrespiratory acidosis may be caused by (a) renal failure and inability of the kidney to excrete enough H ions, (b) severe diabetes, with nonvolatile acids instead of CO_2 as the end products of metabolism, (c) ingestion of excess acid or loss of large amounts of base (as when large amounts of pancreatic juice are lost in diarrhea) or (d) tissue hypoxia or ischemia, which leads to incomplete oxidation of carbohydrate to lactic acid. These are sometimes called "metabolic" acidosis, which is utterly confusing, first because respiratory acidosis is itself due to *metabolically produced* CO_2, and second, because the extra acid that causes metabolic acidosis may be ingested (not metabolically produced) acid such as salicylic acid. (Scientists who introduce new terminology should, by law, be required to post a $1,000 bond, to be forfeited if the terminology is both misleading and used!)

4. IF THE P_{CO_2} IS HIGH AND THE pH IS ALSO HIGH, the patient has alkalosis, and it must be nonrespiratory alkalosis. Nonrespiratory alkalosis may follow the ingestion of too much sodium bicarbonate or other alkali or the loss of large amounts of acid by vomiting of acid gastric juice. This is often called "metabolic" alkalosis; again, this is confusing, because neither of these types is caused by normal or abnormal metabolic processes. The terms "metabolic acidosis" and "metabolic alkalosis" should be banned and replaced with "nonrespiratory" acidosis or alkalosis. The primary event in *non*respiratory acidosis or alkalosis is an excess or deficit of H ions that is *not* caused by retention or elimination of CO_2.

Difficulties in Diagnosis

The description of these four acid-base disturbances seems to indicate that recognition of acid-base disturbances is easy, yet the general belief is that it is difficult. Why? There are three main reasons:

1. More than one acid-base disturbance may occur at the same time. For example, a patient with pulmonary emphysema having alveolar hypoventilation and CO_2 retention (respiratory acidosis) may also be hypoxemic and have nonrespiratory acidosis from anaerobic metabolism and accumulation of lactic acid. Or a patient with primary hyperventilation (respiratory alkalosis) may also have a peptic ulcer and ingest large amounts of bicarbonate to control his gastric acidity (nonrespiratory alkalosis).

2. Pure disturbances of acid-base balance occur only briefly. The body has compensatory mechanisms that try hard to restore a normal environment; these mechanisms produce changes that may make the diagnosis less obvious. Two organs attempt compensation—the kidneys and the lungs. Because a respiratory disorder—too little or too much alveolar ventilation—causes *respiratory* acidosis or alkalosis, it is the kidneys that must compensate in these conditions; they

TABLE 16-2.—CHANGES IN BLOOD P_{CO_2}, HCO_3^- AND pH DURING RESPIRATORY ACIDOSIS

STATE	BLOOD P_{CO_2} TORR	DISSOLVED CO_2 MMOLE/L	TOTAL CO_2 MMOLE/L	*HCO_3^-	$\dfrac{HCO_3^-}{CO_2}$	pH = $6.1 + LOG \dfrac{HCO_3}{CO_2}$	STANDARD HCO_3 MMOLE/L
1. Control	40	1.2	25.2	24.0	$\dfrac{24.0}{1.2} = 20$	$6.1 + 1.3 = 7.40$	25.2
2. Acute respiratory acidosis; no compensation	53.2	1.6	28.8	27.2	$\dfrac{27.2}{1.6} = 17$	$6.1 + 1.23 = 7.34$	25.2
3. Respiratory acidosis; partial compensation	53.2	1.6	30.4	28.8	$\dfrac{28.8}{1.6} = 18$	$6.1 + 1.26 = 7.36$	26.8
4. Chronic respiratory acidosis; complete compensation	53.2	1.6	33.6	32.0	$\dfrac{32.0}{1.6} = 20$	$6.1 + 1.3 = 7.40$	30.2

*HCO_3^- = Total CO_2 − dissolved CO_2

do so by excreting additional H ions or bicarbonate ions.

Let us consider acute respiratory acidosis as an example. There is an immediate increase in blood P_{CO_2} that causes a decrease in blood pH. When there is a stimulus to renal mechanisms and time for them to be effective, the tubular cells secrete a more acid urine by exchanging H ions for Na ions; the H ions are excreted as HCl or NH_4Cl (the tubular cells can form NH_3^+) and the HCO_3^- ions are reabsorbed. Sodium normally combined with chloride in the blood as neutral NaCl is now combined as $NaHCO_3$; the plasma (Na^+) does not change, but the plasma Cl^- combined with it decreases by the same number of mEq/L that plasma (HCO_3^-) increases. Increased tubular reabsorption of bicarbonate begins in a few hours but is not maximal for several days. If renal compensation is complete, blood pH will return to normal as a result of increase in (HCO_3^-) even though P_{CO_2} is still greater than normal; this is called "compensated respiratory acidosis." The respiratory insufficiency is still present, the blood P_{CO_2} remains elevated, but the acidosis is compensated (it is unlikely in practice that compensation will be complete because some deviation from normal values must occur to start compensation and presumably to keep it operating).

The sequence of events in terms of the Henderson-Hasselbalch equation is shown in Table 16-2. The immediate effect of respiratory insufficiency is inability to eliminate all of the CO_2 formed in metabolism: P_{CO_2} rises from 40 to 53.2 torr, and pH decreases to 7.34 (acute respiratory acidosis, 2); total blood CO_2 increases not because of renal compensation (HCO_3^- retention does not occur immediately) but because of chemical buffering of the added CO_2 by blood proteins (p. 215). When renal mechanisms lead to reabsorption of HCO_3^-, blood HCO_3^- rises further and there is partial compensation for the low pH (3); when enough HCO_3^- is retained to restore HCO_3^-/CO_2 to 20/1, pH returns to control values (4), although respiratory insufficiency and high Pa_{CO_2} still exist.

Compensation can also occur for respiratory alkalosis and for nonrespiratory acidosis or alkalosis. In the first, the kidneys eliminate additional HCO_3^- ions. In the second, respiration and alveolar ventilation increase and lower alveolar and arterial blood P_{CO_2}; in the third, respiration and alveolar ventilation decrease and increase alveolar and arterial blood P_{CO_2}. This explains why blood CO_2 is decreased in nonrespiratory acidosis and increased in nonrespiratory alkalosis.

Each of the four major types of acid-base disturbances may occur with or without compensation: (1) respiratory acidosis with or without renal compensation; (2) respiratory alkalosis with or without renal compensation; (3) nonrespiratory acidosis with or without respiratory compensation; (4) nonrespiratory alkalosis with or without respiratory compensation.

3. The third reason for some difficulties in diagnosis of acid-base disorders is that the clinical laboratory measurement of blood (or plasma) CO_2 long preceded the measurement of blood pH by the glass electrode, and this in turn preceded the direct measurement of blood Pco_2 by the CO_2 electrode of Severinghaus (Fig. 2-2). And the study of acid-base disturbances in patients with vomiting, diarrhea and renal failure long preceded similar studies in patients with primary respiratory disorders of hypoventilation or hyperventilation.

Before measurements of pH and Pco_2 of arterial blood became routine, a physician sent a sample of blood to the laboratory for determination of venous CO_2 content and guessed at the diagnosis on the basis of the value reported. On the basis of his knowledge of nonrespiratory acidosis and alkalosis, he (and his clinical laboratory) came to believe that high blood CO_2 (as in nonrespiratory alkalosis) was diagnostic of *all* types of alkalosis and that low blood CO_2 (as in diabetic or renal nonrespiratory acidosis) was diagnostic of *all* types of acidosis. Some physicians and laboratories still make this dangerous error. Respiratory physiologists well know that total blood CO_2 can be *high or low* in *either acidosis or alkalosis*. In respiratory insufficiency, an *increase* in blood CO_2 is not only associated with acidosis—it is the *cause* of it; in hyperventilation syndromes, a *decrease* in blood CO_2 is not only associated with alkalosis—it is the *cause* of it.

If the physician knew only that his patient's blood CO_2 *content* was increased, he would not know whether the patient had CO_2 retention caused by pulmonary insufficiency (respiratory acidosis) or had ingested too much bicarbonate (nonrespiratory alkalosis).

Diagnostic Tests

Some clinicians believe that analysis of acid-base disorders requires no more than measurement of blood pH, Pco_2, and total CO_2 and familiarity with the changes that occur in blood bicarbonate solely because of increase or decrease in Pco_2 (see Fig. 14-6, the CO_2 dissociation curve). Others believe that more quantitative approaches help in diagnosis of acid-base disturbances.

1. MEASUREMENT OF STANDARD BICARBONATE. This measures the CO_2 content of whole blood as it would be if arterial Pco_2 were 40 torr and there were *neither* hyperventilation nor hypoventilation. Part of the blood sample is used to measure actual blood CO_2, pH and Pco_2; the remainder is equilibrated under *standard conditions* (at 37 C in a tonometer with a gas whose Pco_2 is 40 torr and Po_2 is high enough to saturate hemoglobin fully) and "standard bicarbonate" measured. In a healthy man who has no acidosis or alkalosis, compensated or uncompensated, total blood CO_2 and standard bicarbonate are the same (see Table 16-2, *1*). Standard bicarbonate is also normal in a patient with acute uncompensated respiratory acidosis (or alkalosis) (see Table 16-2, *2*) even when CO_2 content is increased (owing to CO_2 retention); this is because the kidneys have not had time to retain bicarbonate. In this instance, equilibration of the patient's blood with a gas whose Pco_2 is 40 torr has eliminated completely the chemical change in blood produced by respiratory acidosis, and the normal standard bicarbonate tells the physician that the process was an acute one (no time for renal compensation) and that the acid-base disturbance was not a complex, mixed disturbance but was due to a single cause (CO_2 retention). However, once compensation has occurred, the standard bicarbonate increases (*3* and *4*) and the amount of the increase reflects the amount of renal compensation; in *4*, the standard bicarbonate remains 5 mmole/L above normal even when the blood is equilibrated with a gas whose

Pco_2 (40 torr) is that of normal alveolar air (rather than 53.2 torr as a result of ventilatory insufficiency). The standard bicarbonate test, in this case, has eliminated the change in blood due to insufficient pulmonary ventilation (CO_2 retention) but has not eliminated the compensatory increase in blood bicarbonate due to reabsorption of bicarbonate by renal mechanisms. Astrup has stated that the standard bicarbonate expresses "only the nonrespiratory side of acid-base metabolism . . . so that the influence of respiration on the base content of the blood is eliminated"; this is true only if one considers that *compensation* for pure respiratory acidosis is not part of the respiratory acidosis.

2. WHOLE-BLOOD BUFFER BASE. This is defined by Singer and Hastings as the sum of the concentrations of buffer anions (in mEq/L) contained in whole blood. The buffer anions are the bicarbonate in plasma and in red cells; hemoglobin; plasma proteins, and the phosphate in plasma and red cells. The total quantity of buffer anions in normal blood, as determined by the titration of whole blood with strong acid, is about 45 – 50 mEq/L. The total buffer base is therefore about twice the concentration of bicarbonate; the additional is largely anions associated with hemoglobin.

When whole blood is exposed in vitro to varying concentrations of carbon dioxide, the carbonic acid formed is buffered by hemoglobin (and to a much lesser extent by the small quantity of other nonbicarbonate buffer anions), and bicarbonate ion will thus be generated. The increase in the concentration of bicarbonate ions will be exactly balanced by the reduction in the number of negative charges on hemoglobin and other buffers, as shown by the following reaction:

$$H_2CO_3 + Na\ Proteinate \rightleftharpoons H\ Proteinate + NaHCO_3$$

Because of these reciprocal changes, the *total* buffer anion content of whole blood (Proteinate + HCO_3^-) will not be altered by changes in Pco_2. Whole-blood buffer base has been used as the critical index of metabolic changes in acid-base balance, since in vitro this variable changes only when blood gains or loses fixed acid. To calculate whole-blood buffer base, one needs only to determine any two of the three variables included in the Henderson-Hasselbalch equation (pH, Pco_2 and bicarbonate concentration) and the hematocrit value or the hemoglobin concentration. With the use of a nomogram constructed by Singer and Hastings, whole-blood buffer base can then easily be calculated, as well as the buffer base *excess* or *deficit* relative to normal values.

It should be pointed out, however, that the base excess tells only the amount of acid that must be added to a liter of *blood* to bring its base excess to zero. In addition to blood, body fluids and cells are involved in acid-base disturbances, and each has different concentration of proteins, bicarbonate and other buffers and different CO_2 titration curves. Indeed, Pitts estimates that 97% of buffering in the body is by *intra*cellular fluids.

Clinicians must use measurements on blood (easy to obtain) as a guide to disturbances that affect the whole body but must remember that corrective therapy must be designed for the whole body and not only for the circulating blood.

Two convenient methods of calculating base excess and buffer base excess (or deficit) are the Siggaard-Andersen alignment nomogram (Fig. 16-5) and a convenient slide rule devised by Severinghaus. based on the nomogram.

Acid-Base Diagrams

Many diagrams have been constructed to help the clinician separate respiratory and nonrespiratory components of acid-base disturbances and to supply quantitative data for the deviation from normal. All are linked by the Henderson-Hasselbalch equation and in a sense contain the same fundamental information. Some of the most widely used of these diagrams are:

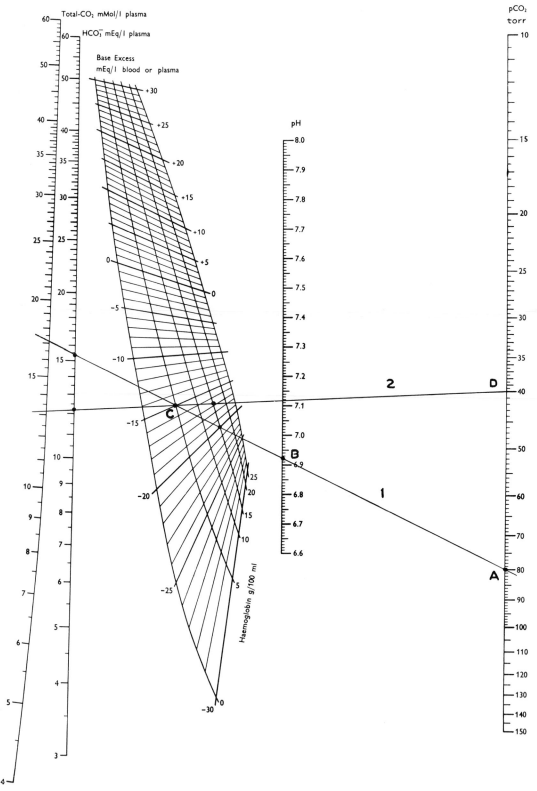

Fig. 16-5.—See legend on facing page.

1. The pH/bicarbonate graph (Davenport, 1958).

2. The standard bicarbonate diagram (Jergensen and Astrup, 1957).

3. The log P_{CO_2}-log CO_2 content graph (Peters and Van Slyke, 1931).

4. The pH-log P_{CO_2} graph (Astrup, 1956).

5. The buffer base-P_{CO_2} graph (Singer, 1951).

6. The pH-log P_{CO_2} graph (Siggaard-Andersen, 1962).

The two diagrams most commonly used are Davenport's pH/bicarbonate graph and Siggaard-Andersen's pH-log P_{CO_2} graph, which provide values for standard bicarbonate base excess (Astrup) and buffer-base (Singer).

THE pH VERSUS BICARBONATE GRAPH (DAVENPORT) (FIG. 16-6). This is a graph of plasma (HCO_3^-) vs. plasma pH. Because (HCO_3^-), pH and P_{CO_2} are related by the Henderson-Hasselbalch equation, the intersection of any vertical with any horizontal line corresponds to a value for P_{CO_2}. All points with a P_{CO_2} of 40 torr are linked by one curved line (the P_{CO_2} 40 isobar); similarly, isobars are constructed for P_{CO_2} 10, 15, 20, 30, 60, 80, 120, and 160 (Fig. 16-6, A). The buffer line for "normal" plasma (CAB) is then constructed; this is really the dissociation curve for plasma, but with additional information on pH; it describes what happens if blood is equilibrated with gases with a wide variety of CO_2 tensions (the line is straight over the physiologic range included in this graph). The actual data obtained from analysis of the patient's blood are now plotted. If his acid-base status is normal, the point falls on or near A, i.e., his P_{CO_2} is 40, pH is 7.40 and his plasma bicarbonate is 24.5 mEq/L. If he has uncompensated respiratory acidosis or alkalosis, the point will move to the right or left of A, along line CAB. If he has severe acute uncompensated respiratory acidosis and a P_{CO_2} of 80 the point falls on C (pH = 7.19 and (HCO_3^-) = 30.0 mEq/L). If he has severe respiratory alkalosis and a P_{CO_2} of 20 torr, the point falls on B (pH = 7.59 and (HCO_3^-) = 19.5 mEq/L). Blood from patients with nonrespiratory acidosis falls below the normal buffer line, and blood from patients with nonrespiratory alkalosis lies above the normal buffer line. If these nonrespiratory changes are uncompensated, they move up and down the P_{CO_2} isobar. Compensatory changes strive to bring the blood pH back to the pH 7.4 line.

One can also read the "standard" bicarbonate from this graph. The patient's blood has a buffer curve which will be parallel to the curve CAB; from the single graphed point derived from the patient's blood, his buffer curve can be drawn. FDE (Fig. 16-6, B) is such a curve drawn from the values at point D; the (HCO_3^-) at the point of intersection of FDE and the isobar for P_{CO_2} 40

Fig. 16-5.—Siggaard-Andersen alignment nomogram. A straight line joining any 2 known points (total CO_2, base excess at a known Hb, pH and P_{CO_2}) may be used to compute the other variables at its intersection with their lines. Straight line 1 drawn through values for blood P_{CO_2} (point A) and pH (point B) measured at 37 C gives values for base excess (where the line crosses the appropriate Hb concentration) and for total CO_2 and plasma HCO_3^-.

This nomogram may also be used to predict the buffer base of the blood which would exist in vivo if P_{CO_2} were altered and, especially, restored to a normal value of 40 torr. When P_{CO_2} is altered in vivo by ventilatory changes, the base of the blood exchanges with extracellular fluid. Since extracellular fluid lacks protein buffers (in particular, hemoglobin), the blood in vivo behaves in the same manner as blood in vitro diluted to about one-fourth to one-third of its actual hemoglobin concentration. As P_{CO_2} is changed in vivo, straight lines through values for simultaneously sampled pH and P_{CO_2} all pivot, or intersect, on a hemoglobin line of $1/4$ or $1/3$ the actual blood hemoglobin value approximately at point C. To estimate base excess which would be found in vivo after correcting P_{CO_2} to 40 torr, draw straight line 2 from C to $P_{CO_2} = 40$ torr and read the base excess where this new line intersects the actual hemoglobin value. (From Siggaard-Andersen, O.: Scand. J. Clin. Lab. Invest. 15:211, 1963, and Severinghaus, J. W., in Altman, P. L. and Dittmer, D. S. [eds.]: *Respiration and Circulation* [Bethesda, Md.: Federation of American Societies for Experimental Biology, 1971], p. 222.)

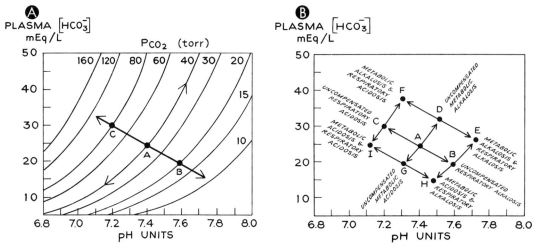

Fig. 16-6.—The pH vs. bicarbonate diagram of Davenport. **A (left)**, isobars for P_{CO_2} (lines of equal P_{CO_2} are from 10 to 160 torr). *CAB* is the buffer curve for normal plasma. **B (right)**, line *FDE* represents "metabolic" (nonrespiratory) alkalosis; line *IGH* represents "metabolic" (nonrespiratory) acidosis; *AB* is uncompensated respiratory alkalosis, and *AC*, uncompensated respiratory acidosis. (Redrawn from Davenport, H. W.: *The ABC of Acid-Base Chemistry* [5th ed.; Chicago: University of Chicago Press, 1969].)

is the "standard" bicarbonate. The difference between the patient's actual and standard bicarbonate is then obtained by subtraction. Alternatively, the vertical displacement of the patient's buffer line from the normal buffer line is the extra base ("base excess") or extra acid ("acid excess").

THE pH-LOG P_{CO_2} GRAPH (SIGGAARD-ANDERSEN). To use this graph one must obtain arterial blood (as little as 150 μL, using microtechnics). One part of the blood is equilibrated with gas that has a low P_{CO_2}, the second with a gas with high P_{CO_2} and the third is not equilibrated. The pH of all three is then measured. From these three values, and the hemoglobin concentration, one can derive values for actual plasma bicarbonate, actual Pa_{CO_2}, standard bicarbonate, total CO_2 content, buffer base and base excess or base deficit. Apparatus for equilibration and microanalysis and charts for graphing are commercially available; microanalysis is particularly useful when only very small amounts of blood are available.

Diagrams such as Davenport's and Sig-

gaard-Andersen's identify clearly any primary, uncompensated, single disturbance of blood acid-base chemistry, and they give quantitative information on the amount of change in blood buffers produced in single disturbances by renal or pulmonary compensation. Unfortunately, as stated previously, acid-base disturbances do not always occur singly and in pure form. No acid-base method can distinguish between a primary accumulation of base resulting from overdose of sodium bicarbonate (nonrespiratory alkalosis) and secondary accumulation of base resulting from renal tubular reabsorption of bicarbonate compensating for primary respiratory acidosis. However, if a patient has a P_{CO_2} of 80 torr with a *normal* pH but a base excess of 23 mEq/L, the experienced clinician at once knows that two acid-base disturbances are present—one being respiratory acidosis and the other nonrespiratory alkalosis. (The *expert* clinician who knows the change in blood bicarbonate to be expected for a given change in P_{CO_2} could make the same diagnosis from measurement of pH, P_{CO_2} and blood CO_2 content.)

Mixed types of acid-base disturbances often occur in sick people. In differentiating these, there is at the moment no solution for the physician except to evaluate all information (laboratory and clinical), to understand the pathophysiologic mechanisms involved in acid-base disturbances and, so informed, to act intelligently.

17

Defense Mechanisms of the Lungs

THE AIR PASSAGES from the nose and mouth to the alveolar membranes are often regarded only as conducting tubes. After reading Chapter 10, one might think that the airways are lined with mathematical equations; actually they are lined with glandular, epithelial and ciliated cells, capillaries and nerve endings, and have elegant built-in air-conditioning and cleansing mechanisms and warning devices. And they also serve other functions not directly related to the process of pulmonary ventilation.

SMELL AND TASTE

The sensory receptors for these are located in the nose, mouth and pharynx. In animals, the odor receptors serve to locate food and identify special friends (usually of the opposite sex) or enemies. Taste receptors often help in the selection of essential foods and minerals. In man, these receptors serve esthetic values more and survival less; indeed, the main thrust of television advertising today is complete elimination of human scent.

Taste and smell are in the domain of the neurophysiologist, but two points pertain to the inhalation of gases: (1) the sense of taste is really a blending of sensation from taste buds and olfactory receptors; complete nasal obstruction alters or dulls the taste of many foods because their volatile components cannot reach and stimulate receptors for smell during either inspiration or expiration.

(2) Receptors for smell are in the posterior nasal cavity and not in the trachea, bronchi or alveoli; a person who uses inhalers containing volatile vasoconstrictor agents destined for the nose or who wishes to detect the presence of potentially dangerous gases (such as cyanide, phosgene or oxides of nitrogen) should *sniff*. Sniffing brings small amounts of ambient gases to the olfactory receptors in the posterior nasal passages and not much further; *deep breathing* carries these gases into the lungs, where they may damage airways or alveoli or be absorbed into the pulmonary capillary blood. A reflex initiated in nasal receptors by irritants can cause apnea and so prevent further inhalation.

AIR CONDITIONING

The upper respiratory tract is a remarkable organ for conditioning inspired air so that, regardless of its initial composition or character, it is warm and moist and almost free of particles when it reaches the alveoli. The mucosa of the nose, mouth and pharynx has a large surface area and a rich blood supply that serves to add heat to cold air or remove heat from hot air; in all likelihood the countercurrent system is utilized in the nasal turbinates to equalize air and blood temperatures. Walker and Wells have nicely described the exchanges of heat and water during one respiratory cycle. During inspiration in temperate or cold climates, heat and water are transferred from the respiratory tract mucosa to the inspired air (heat by turbulent convection and water by evaporation); these transfers cool the mucosa. During expiration, some of the heat and water vapor return to the mucosa from the alveolar gas. Thus the respiratory tract conditions inspired air to protect the lung and then conserves body heat and water by regaining some of these during expiration. Under average conditions, an adult male at rest loses 250 ml of water and 350 kilocalories of heat daily in his expired air. If he breathes air saturated with water vapor at body temperature, he, of course, loses none; if he breathes very cold, dry air, he loses much more and may suffer some dehydration of the respiratory tract and even tracheobronchitis on this account.

If he breathes air saturated with water vapor at temperatures greater than his body temperature, his body will gain heat. This may occur during inhalation anesthesia delivered through a mask and a closed circuit with CO_2 absorbent; the gas temperature in this system may rise to as much as 47 C because of the chemical reaction between CO_2 and the soda lime used to absorb it. Even under extreme conditions, however, the upper respiratory tract protects the alveoli. Moritz and his associates have shown that when hot, dry air up to 500 C or cold air at −100 C is inhaled by anesthetized animals, it is cooled or warmed almost to body temperature by the time it reaches the lower trachea. The capacity of the heat-exchange system of the upper respiratory tract is adequate unless too many calories are involved. Hot *dry* air has few calories because of its low heat capacity (0.24 calories/gm) and its low weight (1 L of dry air at 0 C weighs only 1.3 gm); when 500 ml of dry air at 100 C above the body temperature becomes dry air at 37 C, it provides only 10.5 calories of heat energy. Theoretically, this should raise the temperature of 1 gm of tissue 10.5 C. However, dry air quickly becomes saturated with water vapor; 22 mg of water is added to 500 ml of dry air at 37 C. This water is evaporated from the surface of the mucosa, and the process releases

12 calories. The tissue temperature will rise if the person exposed to hot air hyperventilates, because more calories are presented to the tissues each minute, or if steam is inhaled, because water droplets have a greater heat capacity (1.0 calorie/gm) and also prevent evaporation of water from the mucosa. Except during marked hyperventilation with cold dry air, the inspired gas becomes saturated with water vapor at 37 C (100% relative humidity) before it reaches the alveoli.

The mouth and pharynx can perform these air-conditioning functions almost as well as the nose and pharynx. The trachea and bronchi cannot because blood flow to them is quite low compared to the high blood flow to tissues of the mouth, nose and pharynx; a patient breathing through an endotracheal or tracheotomy tube may have problems of air conditioning when ambient conditions are extreme (if the air is very hot or cold and very dry) or during hyperventilation; for such a patient, the physician should supply moist air (or moist O_2) to prevent local drying and damage to respiratory epithelium, cilia and glands.

Very hot air or steam that reaches alveolar ducts and alveoli is apt to produce little heat damage there (because the huge flow of pulmonary capillary blood at 37 C limits the increase in temperature of these tissues) even though it causes burns of the conducting airway.

FILTRATION AND CLEANSING MECHANISMS

The upper respiratory tract also filters air. Hairs at the inlet block the passage of gross objects. Beyond this, the contours of the nasal turbinates force the inspired air to pass in numerous narrow streams so that solid particles must pass fairly close to either the nasal septum or mucosa of the turbinates. Many particles simply impinge directly on the mucosa or settle by gravity; possibly electrostatic precipitation plays some role in their deposition. Particles with a diameter larger than 10 μ are almost completely removed from the air in the nose, along with some of the smaller, even submicronic ones (diameter less than 1 μ). Particles not removed in the nose may impinge on the walls of the nasopharynx and larynx. Particles between 2 and 10 μ usually settle on the walls of the trachea, bronchi and bronchioles; particles between 0.3 and 2.0 μ in diameter and all foreign gases and vapors reach the alveolar ducts and alveoli. Particles smaller than 0.3 μ are apt to act as vapors and remain as aerosols in the expired gas.

The filtration mechanism of the upper respiratory tract is important for several reasons: it removes foreign particles, such as silica (which can cause pulmonary fibrosis), asbestos fibers (which can provoke pleural mesothelioma) or inert dusts (which can cause bronchoconstriction and excessive secretion of mucus); it removes bacteria suspended in air; it removes other bacteria, viruses and some irritant or toxic gases or vapors (including carcinogens) that are adsorbed onto larger particles. Unless overloaded, the filtration mechanism keeps alveoli practically sterile.

How are these particles removed once they have settled on the walls of the nose, pharynx, trachea, bronchi or bronchioles? Partly by explosive blasts of air generated by sneezing or by coughing (see p. 230) but largely by an upward-moving layer of mucus (secreted by nasal, pharyngeal and tracheobronchial gland cells) inched along by a remarkable wave created by beating cilia.

Cilia

Cilia are very primitive structures, found in many forms of animal life—from unicellular organisms to man. No matter where found, the fine structure of each cilium as seen by electronmicroscopy has an invariable pattern of two central filaments surrounded by a circle of nine. In man, there are ciliated epithelial cells in the paranasal sinuses, the eustachian tubes and the whole respiratory tract (except part of the pharynx,

the anterior third of the nose and the terminal respiratory units).

Cilia are powered by a contractile mechanism and beat in strokes like oars of a boat (Fig. 17-1); each cilium makes a forceful, fast, effective stroke forward followed by a less forceful, slower stroke backward to get into working position again. There is precise timing and coordination of the strokes of a row of cilia so that together they move as a wave. The cilia of the respiratory tract do not beat in air but in a sheet of mucus; the effect of the wave is to move the whole mucus sheet (and anything trapped on it) up the respiratory tract. The speed of this upward movement depends on the length and frequency of beating of the cilia. If a cilium is 10 μ long and if it moves through 90 degrees of a circle during each cycle, each stroke can cause a maximal travel of the mucus sheet of 16 μ; if it beats 20 times per second, it can move the sheet 320 μ/second or 19.2 mm/minute. Experimentally, the effective velocity has been measured by timing the movement of carbon or other fine particles placed on the mucus-cilia apparatus; speeds of 16 mm/minute have been observed.

Cilia also have considerable power. Hilding placed a plug of mucus in an excised closed trachea and found that the cilia moved it toward the larynx even though the movement developed a subatmospheric pressure of 40 mm H_2O behind it and a pressure of 55 mm H_2O ahead of it.

Cilia move the mucus sheet and entrapped particles to the pharynx where they can be swallowed or expectorated. The ciliary escalator is in constant operation: it provides a quiet, unobtrusive, round-the-clock mechanism for removal of foreign particles, in contrast to the periodic, explosive and tiring cough mechanism.

We know little of the physiologic mechanisms regulating the activity of cilia. Nerves are not necessary for their motion. Electrical stimulation of nerves to airways produces no striking or consistent effect. However, after a lung has been removed from an animal (to be sure that all nerves are severed) and then

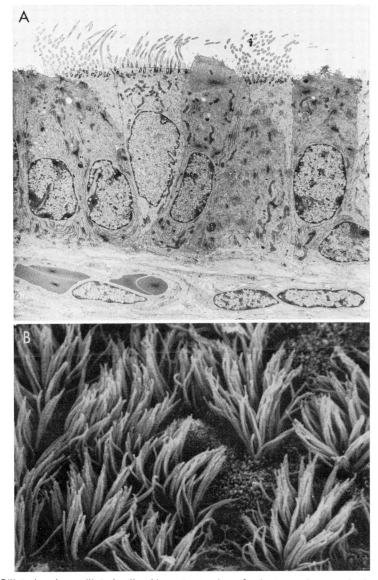

Fig. 17-1.—Ciliated and nonciliated cells of hamster trachea. **A**, electron micrograph of section of trachea containing goblet, ciliated and brush cells. **B**, scanning electron micrograph showing surface characteristics of cilia (projecting into the lumen of the airway) and nonciliated brush cells. (Courtesy of Dr. Ellen Dirksen and Maria Maglio.)

reimplanted, the rate at which cilia propel foreign particles upward is slowed for several months. Drugs that stimulate or block parasympathetic and sympathetic nervous systems do little to change their pattern. Some viruses can grow in ciliated cells without impairing ciliary beating, but drying is reported to damage cilia irreversibly. Inhaled irritants, such as sulfur dioxide and the oxides of nitrogen, seem to slow their beat, after an initial brief period of acceleration. Major surgical operations disrupt the process of cleansing by cilia and lead to the accumulation of mucus plugs and atelectasis. If an irritant settles on an epithelial cell and paralyzes its ciliary beat, it can have an unusually prolonged period of contact with the surface; Kotin has postulated that this is the first step in cell damage and, in the case of carcinogens, it produces metaplasia of cells.

The Secretion of Mucus

Much has been written of the secretions of the tracheobronchial tree — rate of formation, regulation, functions, physical characteristics and procedures for manipulating them. Unfortunately, most of this refers to *sputum*, which is a varying mixture of secretions of the tracheobronchial, salivary, nasal and lacrimal glands, plus entrapped foreign materials, dead tissue cells, phagocytes, leukocytes, erythrocytes, alveolar lining layer or pulmonary transudate or the products of bacterial or fungal infection. Sputum is relatively easy to collect, measure and analyze; pure tracheobronchial secretions are not.

Histologic examination shows that the surface of the trachea, bronchi and bronchioles is lined with about equal numbers of ciliated epithelial cells and mucus-containing goblet cells (see Fig. 17-1); these are derived from an underlying layer of "reserve" cells, which can differentiate into either ciliated or goblet cells. Between this surface epithelial layer and the cartilaginous rings or plates lie the gland cells. These are approximately 40 times as numerous as the goblet cells. Normally their secretions coat the epithelial lining of the tracheobronchial tree and protect it from mechanical or chemical injury or drying. Since it is these secretions that are carried up the tree by ciliary motion, they must be replenished at a regular rate.

Nerve impulses are unnecessary for the goblet cells to discharge their contents; they do this even when nerves to the airways have been cut and other gland cells responsive to parasympathetic nerve impulses have been blocked by large doses of atropine. Local mechanical or chemical irritation is an adequate stimulus to discharge them. The deeper gland cells are at least partly regulated by vagal nerve impulses, and their secretion is decreased by atropine.

In response to chronic irritation, both the gland cells and the goblet cells increase in number; the gland cells occupy more and more of the space between the epithelium and the cartilages, and the goblet cells crowd the ciliated epithelial cells out of the surface layer (the "reserve" cells seem to differentiate into more and more goblet cells and fewer ciliated cells). The result, in chronic bronchitis for example, is more mucus (possibly more viscid) and fewer cilia to propel it upwards.

Clinicians have observed that *sputum* is sometimes scant or sometimes unusually copious, sometimes thin and clear and sometimes thick, viscid, tenacious, stringy; they would like to reduce excessive secretion to normal, liquefy mucus globs or plugs and in general prevent airway plugging, promote the physiologic activity of the cilia-mucus conveyor belt and hasten the elimination of excess fluids. This requires more knowledge than we now have of the mechanisms regulating tracheobronchial secretion and of the chemical composition and physical characteristics of these secretions in pulmonary diseases such as bronchitis, bronchiectasis, emphysema and mucoviscidosis (also commonly called cystic fibrosis). We know that the most important chemical component of normal mucus is a mucopolysaccharide (complexed with sialic acid), which is closely linked with, and probably physically separable from, mucoproteins. Yet physicians have used, in an attempt to liquefy mucus, aerosols of: (1) crystalline trypsin, a proteolytic enzyme especially effective in lysing fibrin; (2) deoxyribonuclease (streptodornase, pancreatic dornase), which splits deoxyribonucleoproteins in cell debris, though not in living cells protected by intact cytoplasm; (3) streptokinase, an exotoxin from beta hemolytic streptococci, which acts specifically as a fibrinolysin; (4) hyaluronidase, which acts on hyaluronic acid (a constituent of intercellular cement) but not on mucus or fibrin, (5) lysozyme, which specifically dissolves mucus but does so rather slowly, and (6) acetylcysteine, which may open disulfide bonds in native proteins.

Rational therapy with enzymes should

require knowledge of the substrate, the optimal enzyme concentration, proper chemical environment and time necessary for effective splitting of the substrate. Enzymes that split mucus do not split protein, enzymes that split protein components of cell nuclei have no effect on mucus and inactive enzymes have no effect at all.

Defense Mechanisms of the Terminal Respiratory Units

Man normally inspires 10,000 to 12,000 L of air a day, and each L of urban air may have several million particles suspended in it. So, despite physiologic mechanisms to prevent it, some inhaled particles, particularly those suspended in fluid droplets, do reach the terminal air units—the respiratory bronchioles, alveolar ducts and alveoli. How do these structures, which have no cilia or mucus glands, defend themselves?

ALVEOLAR MACROPHAGES. These are large, mononuclear, ameboid cells that scavenge the surface of the alveoli (Fig. 17-2). Like other macrophages, they contain lysosomes capable of killing bacteria that they engulf; killing occurs more quickly than actual clearance from the alveoli. Macrophages also surround inhaled particles (hence their original name, "dust cells") and prevent contact between potentially harmful materials and alveolar tissues; most macrophages, with their contained load, migrate to the blanket of mucus on the walls of terminal bronchioles and ride this to larger airways where they can be coughed up in sputum.

Formerly studied only in fixed microscopic sections of lung tissue, macrophages can now be examined in a live, dynamic state by a new technic that has been used in both animals and man. A cuffed catheter is placed in a bronchus to one lobe and the cuff inflated. Then about 50 ml saline is injected into the airway and withdrawn; this is repeated 4 or 5 times with fresh saline. The lung washings obtained by this technic of irrigation or lavage are centrifuged; the cells so obtained are almost all alveolar macro-

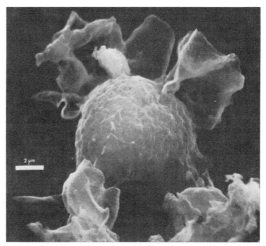

Fig. 17-2.—Alveolar macrophage from rabbit lung. Note the characteristic delicate, almost transparent, undulating membranes attached to the cell body; these may serve to entrap foreign particles. Fixed in glutaraldehyde and freeze-dried. (Courtesy of Drs. Alvin Warfel and Sanford Elberg.)

phages. They can be counted, and their properties of ameboid motion, phagocytosis and bacteria killing can be studied. From such studies, we now know that irritant materials (such as cigarette smoke) provoke an outpouring of alveolar macrophages so that there may be four times the normal number (their origin is not yet certain: from hematopoietic tissues? from circulating monocytes? from type II alveolar cells?). However, inhaled substances may also make these macrophages less effective in gobbling up particles and killing bacteria. Unlike peritoneal macrophages that function with a Po_2 of 10 torr, alveolar macrophages live in alveoli with a Po_2 of 100 torr. Presumably they function less well in hypoventilated alveoli with a very low Po_2. Much will be learned in the next few years about their metabolic processes and ways to promote their function by avoiding certain measures and instituting others.

OTHER MECHANISMS FOR CLEANSING ALVEOLAR SURFACES. When the number of particles reaching alveolar surfaces is small, alveolar macrophages can take care of them. When it is huge and exceeds the maximum that phagocytes can eat (even though "mac-

rophage" means "large eater"), the particles that remain on the alveolar surfaces
must be removed by other means. One of
these is movement of particles on a surface
film moving upward; this moves about half
the particles up to the mucus blanket in
about 24 hours. Another mechanism is cou-
pling of the sheet of respiratory tract fluid
with the mucus blanket, with upward movement of the two brought about by the pro-
pelling beat of bronchiolar cilia. A third is
flow of particles upward due to gradients of
surface tension from alveoli to bronchioles.
A fourth is penetration by particles of epithelial barriers and lodging in the interstitial
spaces for further phagocytosis by tissue his-
tiocytes for transport into lymph channels.
Or the particles may be broken up by surface
enzymes or managed by immunologic reactions. Water and small molecules can readily
leave the alveolar spaces and enter pulmonary capillary blood. Plasma and protein molecules are removed normally in the pulmonary lymph.

Obviously, some particles remain in the

Fig. 17-3.—Retention of dust particles in alveoli.
Following a bronchogram using tantalum dust, the
airways were cleared promptly. However, particles
(outlined by arrows) that settled in poorly ventilated
alveoli remained for weeks or months. (From Gamsu,
G., Weintraub, R. M., and Nadel, J. A.: Am. Rev.
Respir. Dis. 107:214, 1973.)

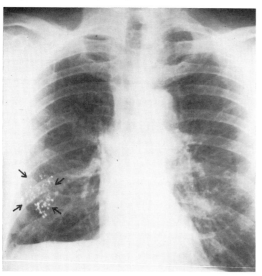

peripheral lung tissue (as in the patchy black
lungs of coal miners). Figure 17-3 shows
inert tantalum dust, inhaled several months
previously, sitting in terminal air units or in
interstitial tissue. Some particles, like tantalum, simply stay in lung tissue as squatters;
others, such as silica, generate a response of
fibroblasts, which in turn leads to serious
pulmonary restrictive disease; others, such
as pneumococci, tubercle bacilli or viruses,
cause specific lung infections; blue asbestos
fibers (crocidolite) appear to be a factor in
causing a specific tumor (mesothelioma) of
the pleura. There is also a definite association between the incidence of heavy cigarette
smoking in men and women and the incidence of bronchogenic carcinoma of the
lung.

REFLEXES FROM THE UPPER AND LOWER RESPIRATORY TRACTS

Chemical or mechanical irritation of the
nose of some animals causes reflex apnea,
closure of the larynx, bradycardia and sometimes bronchoconstriction; the afferent impulses travel in the olfactory and trigeminal
nerves. In the rabbit, prolonged and even
fatal reflex apnea may follow the passage of
ether or chloroform vapor through the nose,
pharynx and larynx; it is reasonable to consider this as a defense mechanism to prevent
potentially harmful gases from reaching the
alveoli and the pulmonary circulation. However, toxic gases that are nonirritant (such as
carbon monoxide) do not initiate these defense mechanisms. Mechanical stimulation
of the larynx causes laryngospasm, bradycardia, or even cardiac arrest and bronchoconstriction. Electrical stimulation of the
central end of the superior laryngeal nerve
often causes apnea and coordinated cough
movements.

In air-breathing diving animals, such as the
seal, immersion of only the nose in water
causes reflex apnea, marked bradycardia and
intense vasoconstriction of all arterioles
leading to skeletal muscles and abdominal
organs. This appears to be a beautifully coor-

dinated plan to prevent the animal from breathing during a dive, to decrease the work of the heart and to direct its left ventricular output wholly to vital organs such as the heart and brain that do not function anaerobically—and away from other tissues or organs that either can work anaerobically or can survive temporary ischemia.

Introduction of water (but not of amniotic or tracheal fluid) into the pharynx of newborn lambs causes apnea. Mature fetal lambs were delivered by Cesarean section and immersed in a warm, saline bath with only a tracheal cannula exposed to air. Each lamb began to breathe rhythmically when its umbilical cord was ligated; each stopped when water was introduced into its upper airway and did not breathe until the water was removed or the superior laryngeal nerves were cut. The receptors for the reflex were located at the entrance to the larynx. Since normal tracheal fluid did not cause apnea, it is unlikely that the reflex inhibits breathing in utero. Its role in sudden death in infancy or death in drowning remains to be explored.

In many species, swallowing results in reflex closure of the glottis and inhibition of respiration. The pharynx is a common passageway for air and for food and water, and this reflex effectively closes off the respiratory passages and stops respiration when food or water is passing from the mouth to the esophagus. This reflex is lost in unconscious patients; for this reason, the custom of forcing whiskey down the mouth of an unconscious patient can be a dangerous one. The reflex is also lost in anesthetized patients; to prevent gastric contents from entering the lungs, anesthetists usually place a soft tube, fitted with an inflatable balloon near the tip, in the patient's trachea. It is well to keep the stomach empty in unconscious patients to prevent aspiration of regurgitated contents. If a tube is placed in the stomach to empty it, the upper end must be pinched off when the tube is withdrawn so that the gastric fluid in it does not run into the trachea. This swallowing reflex is dulled during deep sleep, and occasionally, if the cardiac sphincter relaxes and gastric contents enter the esophagus, some may be aspirated.

When specific chemical irritants pass below the larynx, the pulmonary chemoreflex (see p. 86), consisting of reflex apnea, bradycardia and hypotension, may occur. Usually, however, the response is a cough (or a forced expiration, which is its equivalent in an anesthetized animal) and bronchoconstriction. Most of our recent knowledge of tracheobronchial reflexes comes from the work of Widdicombe. The respiratory tract is abundantly supplied with nerve endings, often called "irritant receptors," which have terminations that ramify between the mucosal cells, and these seem to be admirably situated to respond to mechanical and chemical irritants in the airways.

The reflex responses to irritation of the airways vary according to the site stimulated. Mechanical stimuli—foreign bodies or dusts—act mainly on receptors in the trachea and larger airways, concentrated at the carina; the receptors are rapidly adapting, and their primary effect is an expiratory effort (see Chapter 8). Deeper in the lungs lie receptors for chemical irritants (SO_2 and NH_3 have been chiefly studied); the primary reflex response is an inspiratory effort followed by an explosive expiration. These endings accommodate rapidly to repeated stimuli. Both types of receptors are excited by large inflations and deflations of the lungs, and irritant stimuli sensitize this response. This may explain the all-or-none nature of coughing, for a weak stimulation of the receptors is potentiated by its own reflex response, and also the paroxysmal character of coughing, since once cough receptors are stimulated, each vigorous respiration will initiate the next. The cough reflex, like the swallowing reflex, is depressed or absent in anesthetized or unconscious patients. It also becomes less active in older men and women, and this explains why they are more apt to aspirate material into their lungs.

A second, less obvious response to irritation of the airways is bronchoconstriction. Inert dusts, smokes and low concentrations of gaseous irritants increase airway resistance in humans, even when the concentration is too low for detection or for eliciting the cough reflex. Experimental studies with cats and dogs show that similar stimuli (as well as mechanical irritation of the larynx and trachea) cause a vigorous discharge of impulses in the nerves traveling to the trachea and lungs; the result is reflex tracheal constriction and bronchospasm, even when the irritant stimuli are too weak to cause skeletal muscle movements of coughing.

Smoking of a cigarette induces an immediate 2- to 3-fold increase in airway resistance, which lasts about 10–30 minutes. It does not cause dyspnea, because airway resistance must be increased 4- to 5-fold to cause noticeable shortness of breath and 10- to 20-fold to cause severe dyspnea, as in asthma. Inhalation of cigarette smoke causes a similar effect in both smokers and nonsmokers, with or without bronchopulmonary disease. Because similar increase in airway resistance occurs when men or women smoke cigarettes with a normal (2%) or very low (0.5%) nicotine content, and no increase occurs when they inhale aerosols of nicotine (2 mg nicotine/ml 0.9% saline), the bronchoconstriction is not due to inhaled nicotine but rather to the settling of submicronic particles on sensory receptors in the airway. The effect is reflex. The receptors are tracheobronchial cough receptors. The sensory fibers run up the vagus nerves, and the motor fibers (parasympathetic) descend in the vagi to end on the bronchi and bronchioles. Filters remove some of the particles (solids or droplets), but smoke and particles are synonymous. No particles (complete removal by millipore plus glass wool filters) means no smoke; only true gases and completely volatile compounds would emerge from a perfect filter for particles, and these are not visible.

Other air pollutants—irritant gases, vapors, fumes, aerosols, particles, smokes— may produce similar bronchoconstriction. If such pollutants produce severe and repeated bronchoconstriction, excessive secretion of mucus, depression of the activity of cilia and of alveolar macrophages, obstruction of fine airways and cell damage, they may make it possible for bacteria to penetrate to the alveoli and remain there for a long enough period to cause infectious lung disease. They may also be factors in production or aggravation of tracheobronchial diseases such as chronic bronchitis, emphysema and bronchogenic carcinoma. There is a statistically significant association between heavy cigarette smoking and pulmonary emphysema; however, some patients with severe emphysema have never smoked, have not been exposed to unusual air pollution and do not recall having inhaled toxic fumes.

18

Special Acts Involving Breathing

WE USUALLY THINK of respiration only as a mechanism for providing alveolar ventilation and pulmonary blood gas exchange. In many circumstances, a change occurs in the normal pattern of inspiration-expiration that is unrelated to the need for alveolar ventilation.

VALSALVA'S MANEUVER is an experimental act in which the subject voluntarily closes his glottis (or nose and mouth) and then maximally contracts his abdominal and thoracic expiratory muscles. The result is a marked elevation of intrathoracic and intraabdominal pressures—to as much as 200 mm Hg. A similar maneuver is carried out while straining during difficult bowel movements and during certain types of muscular effort (usually accompanied by straining and grunting). The high intrapulmonic pressure places no stress on alveoli or air ducts because it is generated by the thoracic and abdominal muscles and so causes an almost equal increase in intrapleural and alveolar pressures; as a result, transpulmonary pressure changes but little. It does, however, produce striking effects on the circulation. The high intrathoracic pressure decreases or even stops venous return to the right heart. For a few beats (Fig. 23-1), the left ventricle maintains its output because it continues to receive blood from the reservoir in the pulmonary circulation; then its output decreases. Systemic arterial blood pressure rises immediately because the increased intrathoracic pressure is transmitted to the heart and

large arteries; systemic pressure falls when venous return and cardiac output decrease. When the Valsalva maneuver is stopped, systemic arterial pressure rises well above control values ("overshoot") and then returns to normal.

The intrathoracic and intra-abdominal arteries are not stressed *during* the maneuver because the increase in intra-arterial pressure is balanced by an increase in pressure on the outside of these arteries. The arteries of the arms, legs, head and superficial structures of the trunk *are* stressed because the intra-arterial pressure rises without any increase in external supporting pressure. Veins and venules in these regions are also stressed by the accumulation of blood in them and the transmitted back pressure. The intracranial vessels are supported, *during* the maneuver, by a concomitant rise in cerebrospinal fluid pressure because the rise in intrathoracic and intra-abdominal pressure is immediately transmitted through the intervertebral foramina; in the overshoot period, spinal fluid pressure is now normal and no longer provides the extravascular support.

The Valsalva maneuver is sometimes used as a cardiovascular function test. In patients with congestive heart failure and increased systemic venous pressure, cardiac output and arterial blood pressure do not fall during the effort. In patients with impaired function of the sympathetic nervous system, "overshoot," which is a response to sudden flooding of the great veins and heart with blood, does not occur at the end of the test. However, dangers are associated with the test, the most important being sudden overload of the ventricles when the effort stops.

The playing of wind instruments involves a deep inspiration, followed by a slow expiration through a narrowed orifice. For reasons mentioned earlier, it does not rupture alveoli. The prolonged breath holding and increased intrathoracic pressure may produce circulatory changes during and after each inspiration.

A COUGH is a complex, highly coordinated act that results in the rapid expulsion of alveolar gas at a very high velocity, presumably to sweep the airway free of irritant gases, dust, smoke, excess mucus, cell debris or pus. The first step is similar to the Valsalva maneuver—by a forced expiratory effort against a closed glottis, the patient develops high intrathoracic and intrapulmonic pressures. The glottis then opens abruptly so that there is a large pressure difference between alveolar pressure and upper tracheal pressure (now atmospheric). This results in a very rapid flow rate. Equally important is dynamic compression of intrathoracic airways, including the trachea, due to high intrathoracic pressure (+40 mm water). Figure 18-1 shows that this inverts the noncartilaginous part of the intrathoracic trachea. Air rushing through a greatly narrowed trachea (16% of its original area) has a high linear velocity (calculated to be 500 miles/hour, or 85% of the speed of sound), and this dislodges foreign materials or mucus and pushes them into the throat. Although the membranous portion of a relaxed trachea folds in during dynamic compression and obliterates most of the lumen, the *contracted* trachea, at least in some species, resists compression by pulling the two ends of the cartilaginous ring into an overlapping configuration, thus creating a solid ring.

Does coughing harm the lungs? Some have stated that it favors alveolar wall rupture because of the high pressures generated in the alveoli during coughing. It is true that

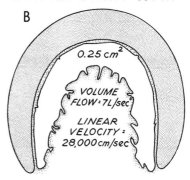

TRACHEA DURING NORMAL BREATHING

A

1.5 cm^2

←— 14 mm —→

VOLUME FLOW = 1 L/sec

LINEAR VELOCITY = 667 cm/sec

TRACHEA DURING COUGH

B

0.25 cm^2

VOLUME FLOW = 7 L/sec

LINEAR VELOCITY = 28,000 cm/sec

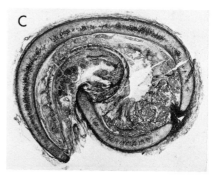

C

Fig. 18-1.—Changes in cross-sectional area of trachea. **A**, contours and dimensions of trachea during normal breathing. **B**, during a cough, the positive intrathoracic pressure inverts the noncartilaginous part of the intrathoracic trachea (see Fig. 10-21) and decreases its cross-sectional area to $\frac{1}{6}$ of normal. This, added to a 7-fold increase in flow rate, increases the *linear* velocity 42-fold. **C**, cross-section of relaxed human trachea that was compressed (post mortem) by 100 cm H$_2$O external pressure, rapidly frozen, fixed and sectioned. The membranous portion is inverted, and one free edge of the cartilage is curled inward. (From Olsen, C. R., *et al.*: J. Appl. Physiol. 23:35, 1967.)

alveolar pressure may rise to more than 100 torr during the violent expiratory effort. However, alveoli rupture when they are *stretched* beyond a certain volume, and this requires a high *transmural* pressure; because the high alveolar pressure during cough is generated by contraction of the respiratory muscles, which increases both intrapleural and alveolar pressure, transmural pressure does not increase *during* the expiratory act. The very high intrathoracic pressure does, however, cause compression of the intrathoracic venae cavae, marked decrease in venous return to the heart and a sudden increase in systemic venous pressure. At the same time, the sudden increase in intrathoracic and intra-abdominal pressure is transmitted through the intervertebral foramina to the cerebrospinal fluid; this in turn can produce temporary cerebral ischemia, especially if cardiac output is decreased simultaneously. The dangers of violent paroxysms of coughing are apt to be lightheadedness, syncope and hemorrhages from small venules in the face and neck rather than pulmonary damage.

MÜLLER'S MANEUVER. When a person sucks fluid at atmospheric pressure up a tube, the fluid moves because the intrapleural, intrapulmonic and mouth pressures are *sub*atmospheric. Healthy men can, by inspiring maximally against a closed airway, lower intrapulmonic pressure to as much as 60–100 torr below atmospheric. Because the force is generated by the respiratory muscles, and this lowers intrapleural and intrapulmonic pressures almost equally, no stress is placed on the alveoli or airways. As with Valsalva's maneuver, the important changes are circulatory. The low intrathoracic pressure permits greater filling of all intrathoracic vessels, and blood accumulates in them. If the lowering of intrathoracic pressure is cyclic, it can improve venous return under certain circumstances; thus, inspiring against a resistance prevents the fainting that may occur when man stands motionless on a tilt table.

BREATH HOLDING may be voluntary or a reflex action. Swallowing (see p. 227) is normally accompanied by breath holding. The act of swallowing initiates a reflex that appears to depress the respiratory center; voluntary breath holding can be prolonged by repeated swallowing, probably because of this reflex. In some animals, diving is accompanied by reflex breath holding (see p. 226). Crying infants may have alternating periods of deep breathing and breath holding.

Voluntary breath holding is terminated by many factors. Two important ones are the levels of arterial blood P_{O_2} and P_{CO_2}. Breath holding can be prolonged by preliminary hyperventilation (to decrease arterial P_{CO_2}); the breath can be held much longer if there is preliminary hyperventilation with O_2 (to decrease arterial P_{CO_2} and to provide a large reservoir of O_2 in the alveoli). Factors other than chemical stimuli are also involved; Fowler has shown that, at the breaking point of breath holding, a subject can hold his breath longer if allowed a few breaths, even of a gas mixture which *lowers* arterial P_{O_2} and *raises* arterial P_{CO_2}.

It is unlikely that serious harm can result from voluntary or reflex breath holding in man because an uncontrollable urge to breathe terminates it. However, we have observed a patient with medullary damage who could hold his breath well beyond ordinary limits of tolerance; his arterial O_2 saturation was 35% and the P_{CO_2} 77 torr when we asked him to resume breathing. Some animals, notably the rabbit, have such powerful inhibitory reflexes that chemical irritants drawn into the upper respiratory tract can produce prolonged apnea and even death.

PANTING is rapid, shallow breathing that moves fresh air into and out of the anatomic dead space far more frequently than does normal breathing. It is a mechanism to eliminate heat used by some species that sweat little or not at all. In these animals, local heating of specific hypothalamic centers governing heat elimination leads to panting. Man, faced with the problem of heat elimination (during fever, or in high ambient temperatures) responds by cutaneous vasodilation and sweating, not by panting. Indeed, increased body temperature in man is often associated with alveolar hyperventilation and a decrease in alveolar and arterial P_{CO_2}.

It is sometimes thought that small tidal volumes, equal to or smaller than the volume of the anatomic dead space, merely eliminate heat and produce no alveolar ventilation. Because air travels up and down the airway as a long cone and not as a square wave, some air moves in and out of alveoli even when tidal volume is only 60% of the dead space volume. Panting therefore does not prevent alveolar ventilation; it does prevent alveolar *hyper*ventilation while eliminating heat.

SNIFFING is one or more small, quick inspirations through the nose. It is a mechanism for bringing ambient air into contact with the olfactory receptors in the nose without carrying the air (which may contain irritant, toxic materials) deep into the lung. It also serves as the reverse of nose blowing and sweeps nasal mucus or foreign material into the nasopharynx, from which it can be expectorated or swallowed. Radiologists use a sniff test to detect unilateral paralysis of the diaphragm; the normal hemidiaphragm descends with the quick inspiration, but the paralyzed side rises in the chest.

SNEEZING is a deep inspiration followed by an explosive, almost uncontrollable expiration. It is initiated reflexly by irritation of sensory receptors in the nasal mucosa; impulses from them ascend in fibers of the trigeminal and olfactory nerves.

SPEAKING, SINGING AND WHISTLING are acts that require the passage of air and therefore modify the normal inspiratory-expiratory pattern. Although speaking requires frequent and often prolonged modification of respiration, we know little of its effect on alveolar ventilation and arterial blood gases. It is reported that loud, prolonged speaking may produce alveolar hyperventilation and a decrease in alveolar P_{CO_2}. Whether some political orators suffer from hypocapnia and cerebral vasoconstriction is not known; it might be in the public interest to find out.

SIGHING is a slow deep inspiration followed by a slow expiration. It occurs infrequently and irregularly in healthy man, frequently in some patients (with acute hypotension, neurocirculatory asthenia or anxiety) and at regular intervals in some animal species. In common with any deep inspiration, a sigh temporarily increases alveolar P_{O_2}, decreases alveolar P_{CO_2} and increases venous return to the heart. Because a single maximal inflation of the lungs opens collapsed alveoli and temporarily overcomes bronchial constriction, some believe that a sigh is a reflex initiated in scattered areas of atelectasis caused by regional hypoventilation. Some ventilators are constructed to permit delivery of an occasional deep breath to prevent or counteract atelectasis in patients not breathing spontaneously.

A YAWN is a long, deep inspiration with the mouth wide open, followed by a slow expiration; it is often accompanied by stretching and stiffening of the extremities and trunk. Yawning occurs in babies and in many species of animals. In adult man, it occurs especially under the following conditions: sleepiness, weariness, awaking from unrefreshing sleep and boredom. All of these have in common a state of decreased awareness of the environment. It has generally been observed that yawning is apt to spread from one to the other members of a group in a similar environment. Except for the observation that yawning, in common with a voluntary deep inspiration, causes increased venous return to the right heart, vasoconstriction in limb vessels and changes in alveolar gas tensions, little is known of the stimulus causing it, the pathways involved and its physiologic function. Yawning (and sighing) often occur in conscious hypotensive patients; the yawn may serve to increase venous return.

SWALLOWING inhibits breathing in the expiratory phase; this prevents inhalation of food or fluid during the swallowing act (see p. 227). In some animals, touching the larynx or injecting fluid into the pharynx inhibits breathing; reflex bradycardia and hypotension may accompany the apnea.

HICCUPING is an intermittent, spasmodic contraction of the diaphragm often accompanied by similar contraction of the accessory muscles of inspiration. It occurs in a wide variety of conditions, such as disorders of the esophagus or stomach, acute intra-abdominal inflammation, disease of the liver, kidney, mediastinum, heart, pericardium or brain and meninges. It also occurs in healthy persons for no apparent reason or after specific incidents such as prolonged laughter. There are many theories of its origin. It may be a reflex initiated by excitation of sensory receptors in the thorax or abdomen. It may be central in origin and due to unexplained excitation of the motor cortex or of a part of the inspiratory center. It may be due to peripheral excitation of a phrenic nerve or of the diaphragm itself. Experimentally, contractions of the diaphragm, synchronous with the heartbeat, may be produced by severing a phrenic nerve where it passes over the heart; the cardiac action potential spreads to and excites the peripheral end of the cut phrenic nerve. Direct excitation of intact phrenic nerves by cardiac injury currents may occur after occlusion of a coronary artery and consequent myocardial infarction.

Common treatments of hiccup include repeated swallowing (which inhibits the medullary respiratory center), breath holding, rebreathing or inhalation of 5% CO_2 from a paper bag (which stimulates it), sudden fright, phrenic nerve block or crush or drugs such as quinidine that prolong the refractory period and decrease the excitability of muscle. The paroxysms are occasionally so severe, frequent and prolonged as to prevent eating, drinking or sleeping and may even threaten life.

SNORING is noisy breathing caused by vibrations of the relaxed soft palate and the thin edge of the posterior pillars when sleeping man breathes through his mouth. It is not an abnormal type of breathing but normal breathing through an abnormal passageway.

VOMITING, like coughing and swallowing, is a complicated reflex act involving coordinated activities in many nuclei of the brain. The activities consist of salivation, swallowing, gastrointestinal reactions of a special nature, rhythmic, spasmodic respiratory movements and finally an upward squeezing action of the diaphragm and abdominal muscles. Wang and Borison have described a medullary emetic center with two anatomically close, but functionally separable, units; one is a chemoreceptive emetic trigger zone in the area postrema of the medulla and the other a vomiting center in the region of the tractus solitarius and the underlying lateral reticular formation. The trigger zone represents the site of the action of chemical substances such as apomorphine, morphine, digitalis and ergot. The vomiting center itself receives afferent messages from the gastrointestinal tract that are initiated by the action of irritants on the mucosa. It is of interest that veratridine, which excites the thoracic chemoreflex and causes apnea, bradycardia and hypotension, also causes reflex vomiting; it is possible that vomiting is an inseparable part of this reflex.

19

Respiratory Adjustments in Health

THE HYPERPNEA OF MUSCULAR EXERCISE

THE MAIN FUNCTION of the lungs is to provide proper exchange of O_2 and CO_2 between air and blood. It must do this nicely at all levels of metabolism, from basal conditions to maximal activity. Increased metabolism need not be due to greater activity of skeletal muscles; it may result from increased contraction of smooth or cardiac muscle, increased secretion of endocrine or exocrine glands, increased reabsorption or increased activity of nerve tissues. The respiratory response to muscular exercise is the easiest to study experimentally; practically every respiratory physiologist of the last 100 years has done so and has contributed either new methods, data, equations, theories or models. It is startling, therefore, to learn that we still do not know the cause or causes of the increased ventilation associated with muscular exercise and know very little about the effects on respiration of increased metabolic activity of tissues and organs other than skeletal muscle.

This means either that this seemingly simple, uncomplicated problem is an exceedingly difficult one or that respiratory physiologists have not been very perceptive or both. One of the difficulties is that most physiologists have been — and still are — searching for a single measurable stimulus and mechanism that will explain all the data. Another is that good respiratory physiologists are not

necessarily good neurophysiologists or good control-system engineers, and maybe they must be to solve the problem.

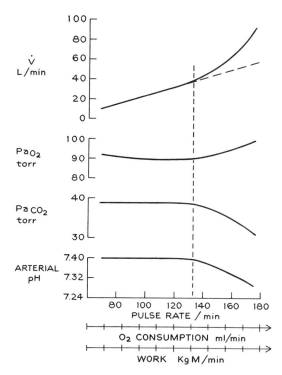

Fig. 19-1.—Ventilation during muscular exercise. $\dot{V}$ = total ventilation/minute; Pao_2 and $Paco_2$ = arterial O_2 and CO_2 tensions (corrected to existing body temperature during exercise). The 3 indices of the severity of muscular exercise (pulse rate, O_2 consumption and work) increase linearly from left to right; absolute values are given only for pulse rate. Ventilation increases in proportion to the severity of the exercise up to the point indicated by the dashed vertical line. (Redrawn from Holmgren, A., and McIlroy, M. B.:J. Appl. Physiol. 19:243, 1964.)

234

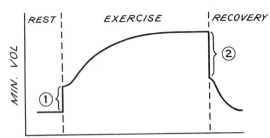

Fig. 19-2.—Schematic representation of changes in total ventilation/minute during exercise, showing (1) the abrupt increase at the onset and (2) the abrupt, larger decrease at the end of exercise. (Redrawn from Dejours, P., in Fenn, W. O., and Rahn, H. [eds.]: *Handbook of Physiology* [Washington, D.C.: American Physiological Society, 1964], sec. 3, vol. I.)

It is instructive to review some of the concepts and experimental approaches used over the past 100 years. But as we do, we must remember two observations which everyone agrees are true. The first is that in mild and moderate *steady* exercise, the ventilation increases directly as the metabolic rate increases (Fig. 19-1). The second is that there is an abrupt increase in ventilation at the onset of exercise—beginning within 1 second—and an equally abrupt decrease toward resting values at the end of exercise (Fig. 19-2).

CO₂ as the Stimulus

This is a straightforward, logical concept: active tissues produce more CO_2. The P_{CO_2} rises in the active tissue, in venous blood draining it, in mixed venous and pulmonary arterial blood. Unless there is an increase in alveolar ventilation at the precise moment that the venous blood, rich in CO_2, reaches the alveolar capillaries, the alveolar P_{CO_2} and arterial P_{CO_2} must rise. And after appropriate time lags, P_{CO_2} must rise in the arterial and medullary chemoreceptors.

The logical place to look for the stimulus is in the arterial blood. We know that inhalation of a gas rich in CO_2 increases arterial P_{CO_2} and increases ventilation in proportion. However, if we measure the ventilation and arterial P_{CO_2} of healthy men during increasing work loads (walking on a treadmill or pedaling a stationary bicycle), we find to our astonishment that their ventilation increases 5-, 10- or 15-fold without any change in arterial P_{CO_2} measured at body temperature (Fig. 19-1). Physiologists know that to produce similar increases in ventilation by inhalation of CO_2, 8–10% CO_2 must be inhaled and arterial P_{CO_2} must increase by 20–30 torr (see Fig. 5-1). The conclusion is obvious—if there is no appreciable change in arterial P_{CO_2} during exercise, CO_2 cannot be the stimulus which produces the hyperpnea of exercise. (Recently Bainton measured ventilation and alveolar P_{CO_2} in dogs exercising on a treadmill at 3 miles per hour. He changed only 1 factor—he increased the slope of the treadmill from zero (horizontal) to a 15% grade. Ventilation increased and so did alveolar P_{CO_2}, and the increase in ventilation was similar to that measured in these dogs when he increased their alveolar P_{CO_2} by giving them CO_2-rich gas to inhale. These experiments must be confirmed in man before physiologists can challenge the statements made above.)

Good physiologists are stubborn, however. Reasoning that CO_2 might stimulate receptors within or near the exercising muscles, they have perfused skeletal muscles with venous instead of arterial blood or with venous blood with added CO_2; this produces no hyperpnea. Further evidence against muscle chemoreceptors is Dejours' observation of an abrupt decrease in minute ventilation at the end of exercise even though tourniquets were applied to the limbs at that moment to prevent a decrease in chemical stimuli there. But there could be receptors in the veins or pulmonary arteries that respond to increased P_{CO_2}. So physiologists have devised ways to increase the blood P_{CO_2} only in the veins or only in the pulmonary circulation or only in the pulmonary arteries. But no matter how high the P_{CO_2}, how abrupt the change or how long it was maintained, no one has been able to stimulate respiration by changing blood P_{CO_2} in these regions alone, even in unanesthetized animals or man.

This does not mean that the proponents of

the CO_2 theory are wrong; they may be measuring the wrong quantity. For example:

1. Exercise may cause a tremendous increase in the number of sensory and motor messages that impinge on the respiratory centers, and this may make them far more sensitive than usual to CO_2. But CO_2 response curves measured before and during exercise are about the same and do not support the concept of increased sensitivity of the central respiratory mechanism to CO_2.

2. The CO_2 control mechanism may be so exquisitely sensitive that it can increase ventilation maximally with no measurable change in arterial P_{CO_2}. If the job of the control mechanism is to keep arterial P_{CO_2} at 40 torr and if it is sensitive to ± 1 torr P_{CO_2}, it could drive respiration to 50 L/minute or more without any measurable increase in arterial P_{CO_2}, *because its job is to control P_{CO_2} and keep it at a set level*. This is at first completely illogical, because every student who has inhaled a CO_2-rich gas thinks of ventilatory responses only in terms of response to *inhaled* CO_2. But it is logical to a control-systems engineer. An efficient air conditioner will keep a room at 70 F no matter what the heat load in the room *if the air conditioner is sensitive and has a proper capacity and an outlet for the heat. The efficiency of the air conditioner is judged by its ability to *prevent* any rise in room temperature with increasing heat loads; the air conditioner fails when it permits the temperature to rise. The same reasoning can be applied to the CO_2-producing and -eliminating systems. The lung is designed to eliminate CO_2 in a CO_2-free medium, air. When CO_2 is added to the inspired air, it clogs the mechanism for CO_2 elimination, and arterial CO_2 must rise. Yamamoto has shown that arterial P_{CO_2} does not rise when CO_2 is injected into the venous *blood* (to simulate an endogenous rise such as occurs during exercise), so that the CO_2-eliminating organ is not clogged with inspired CO_2; minute volume increases 5-fold as the CO_2 load increases in venous blood, but arterial P_{CO_2} does not rise measurably. No one

has yet infused CO_2-rich blood in unanesthetized animals or man to see whether "endogenous" CO_2 will produce large increases in ventilation without measurable increase in arterial P_{CO_2}. It is of interest that inhalation of a very low concentration of CO_2 (about 1%) increases ventilation with no measurable change in alveolar or arterial P_{CO_2}; dismissed in the past as an experimental error, this finding may be a key to the CO_2 control story.

3. The receptors sensitive to CO_2 may be sensitive to a *change* in P_{CO_2} rather than to a steady P_{CO_2}. Figure 2-3 (p. 12) shows that alveolar and arterial P_{CO_2} fluctuate during a normal respiratory cycle because expiration is essentially a period of breath holding during which P_{CO_2} rises, and inspiration a period of dilution of alveolar CO_2 during which P_{CO_2} decreases. Physiologists who draw samples of arterial blood over 30–60 seconds are impressed with the constancy of P_{CO_2}; if they drew samples of end-pulmonary capillary blood every second, they would be impressed by its fluctuations. When man exercises, mean alveolar and arterial P_{CO_2} remain constant, but the fluctuations increase because venous P_{CO_2} is higher. An increase in venous P_{CO_2} (endogenous CO_2) increases the fluctuations of arterial P_{CO_2} about the mean. An increase in CO_2 in inspired gas (exogenous CO_2) decreases the fluctuations because inspired P_{CO_2} is now very close to mixed venous P_{CO_2}. Neurophysiologists know that many receptors respond maximally to a *change* in their environment or to *rate of change*. The carotid sinus pressoreceptors are activated more by an increase in pulse pressure than by an increase in mean pressure; a progressive increase in pulse pressure, *mean* pressure remaining constant, progressively stimulates these receptors. If chemoreceptors behave similarly, they would be activated more by the fluctuations of P_{CO_2} above the mean than by the mean itself. It is possible, therefore, that *mean* arterial P_{CO_2} is not the proper value to measure in the search for an exercise stimulus. To settle the point, measure-

ments should be made in unanesthetized man or animals, because all general anesthetics depress the respiratory response to CO_2.

However, *medullary* CO_2 or H^+ receptors may not be exposed to these rapid fluctuations if these are smoothed out by the pool of extracellular, cerebrospinal fluid bathing them. (The carotid and aortic bodies are designed for rapid response.)

4. Instantaneous hyperpnea at the onset of exercise lowers arterial P_{CO_2} momentarily and may simultaneously reset the respiratory center to maintain an arterial P_{CO_2} of, say, 36 instead of 40 torr, without changing the slope of the CO_2 response curve.

Low O_2 as the Stimulus

If we rewrite the CO_2 story, substituting low O_2 for high CO_2, we will have another logical concept: active tissues consume more O_2; P_{O_2} must decrease in the active tissues, venous and pulmonary arterial blood. Unless ventilation increases, P_{O_2} might also decrease in arterial blood. However, there are no known O_2-sensitive receptors in muscle, veins or pulmonary arteries that regulate breathing, at least past fetal life. Careful measurements of mean arterial blood P_{O_2} during exercise show only small changes, and the carotid and aortic body O_2 receptors are not sensitive to these small changes. Since they represent the only known O_2-sensitive receptors, exercise hyperpnea cannot be due to a low O_2 stimulus.

The possibility exists that during exercise the blood flow to the chemoreceptors is specifically and sharply decreased by vasomotor reflexes and that the resulting decrease in chemoreceptor cell P_{O_2} stimulates breathing. This provides no way to increase ventilation in proportion to metabolic needs unless the signal for vasoconstriction increases with increasing exercise. However, Severinghaus found no change in the hyperpnea of exercise after the superior cervical sympathetic ganglia had been blocked in man. Further, Wasserman studied the ventilatory response to exercise in seven patients before and after

removal of both carotid bodies (see p. 53) and found no decrease in ventilation during exercise even though the ventilatory response to hypoxia was abolished; this finding seems to eliminate hypoxia or interaction of hypoxia and increased CO_2 acting on peripheral chemoreceptors as a factor of importance. Even so, before dismissing O_2 lack as a factor, any general theory of the hyperpnea of exercise must explain (1) the striking correlation between hyperpnea and O_2 consumption during mild and moderate exercise (Fig. 19-1) and (2) a $10-15\%$ decrease in ventilation that occurs during steady exercise when O_2 is inhaled instead of air.

(H^+) as the Stimulus

We could substitute (H^+) for P_{CO_2} in the CO_2 story, because muscle contraction also produces more H ions. But there is an additional factor. When arterial blood flow to exercising muscles increases sufficiently to meet the increasing needs for O_2, metabolism is aerobic. When blood flow can supply enough O_2 to meet only part of the needs, some metabolism is anaerobic, and lactic acid is not metabolized to CO_2 and H_2O. The result is an increase in local (H^+) and an increase in blood lactate or in blood (H^+). (When excess lactic acid spills into the venous blood, it can be measured by chemical determinations on blood or by breath-to-breath analysis of expired alveolar gas. The latter depends on the chemical release of CO_2 from blood bicarbonate by lactic acid; released CO_2, added to CO_2 formed in metabolism, increases alveolar P_{CO_2} relative to P_{O_2} so that R, or $\dfrac{CO_2}{O_2}$, rises from approximately 0.8 toward or above 1.0.)

Lactate is not a known respiratory stimulant; (H^+) is. Measurements of blood pH show a decrease in pH (rise in [H^+]) only during severe exercise (see Fig. 19-1); therefore, a decrease in arterial blood pH can only be a factor in explaining part of the hyperpnea of exhausting muscular exercise. Part of the decrease in ventilation when O_2 is inhaled during exercise may be due to suppression of carotid and aortic body O_2 receptors, and part may be due to suppression of anaerobic metabolism; an abrupt change is probably due to the former and slower changes to the latter.

Substance X as the Stimulus

Failure to explain the hyperpnea of exercise by detecting changes in mean arterial blood P_{CO_2}, P_{O_2} or pH led to search for unknown chemicals that may be formed and liberated during muscle metabolism and act locally or systemically. If there are such, they do not act on receptors in veins or in the pulmonary circulation. Dejours proved this by a simple experiment. During exercise of the legs, he occluded the veins by inflating cuffs around the thighs. Any chemical formed during exercise would accumulate in the trapped venous blood. Shortly after the end of the exercise, he released the cuffs and noted that tidal volume never increased until time had elapsed for the altered blood to reach the carotid arteries. More elaborate cross-perfusion experiments by Kao confirmed these findings.

Increased Temperature as the Stimulus

Increase in chemical reactions produces more heat and increases the temperature of active tissues. If heat production exceeds heat elimination, blood and body temperature rise. In moderate exercise, the heart of healthy man can pump enough blood to exercising muscles to meet their metabolic needs and enough to the cutaneous circulation (the radiators) to permit heat loss and maintain normal body temperature. During maximal exercise by healthy man or moderate exercise by patients with limited cardiac output, the heart cannot do both jobs. It tries to maintain muscle blood flow but gives up on cutaneous blood flow; as a result, body temperature rises.

Ventilation may increase either because the temperature of skeletal muscle increases or because blood and body temperature increase. Local temperature could increase quickly, body temperature only after a time lag. There are no known temperature-sensitive receptors in muscle that influence respiration; perfusion of limbs with heated blood or local heating of muscle does not increase respiration. Therefore, the immediate hyperpnea of exercise is not due to change in muscle temperature. Only part of the delayed response can be due to increase in body temperature, because exercise ventilation reaches its peak before blood and body temperature increase maximally. The immediate decrease in ventilation at the end of exercise is not due to a change in body temperature, because ventilation declines rapidly though body temperature is still high. However, the subsequent gradual decrease to normal ventilation has a time course similar to the decrease in body temperature to normal.

Impulses from the Motor Cortex

So far, we have discussed chemical concepts; some physiologists are convinced that the stimulus must be a chemical one, related directly to increased metabolism. Other physiologists are convinced that the answer will be in a nonchemical, or neural, concept. Krogh reasoned that muscles contract because they receive impulses from the motor cortex and the force of their contraction is related to the frequency of such impulses. A signal proportional to that going to the active muscles may be sent simultaneously to the respiratory (and vasomotor) center. Thus the brain tells the muscles what and how much work to do and informs the supporting cardiovascular and respiratory systems of their task. This is an attractive hypothesis, despite the lack of direct evidence. Some believe that the *rapid* decrease in ventilation at the end of exercise (see Fig. 19-2) might be due to withdrawal of the signals to the muscles but that the *slow* decrease following this must be due to *decline in the other stimuli*; this is based on the assumption that nerve signals to the respiratory center stop the instant that the muscle effort stops. Some do not accept Krogh's concept because stimulation of peripheral nerves to muscles causes hyperpnea even though the motor cortex is not directly stimulated; however, this does not rule out the possibility that the cortex *can* deliver an effective signal. The demonstration that *one* mechanism exists never rules out alternative mechanisms; the body often has several ways to do an important job. A critical experiment would be one in which stimuli are delivered to the motor cortex to produce a regular series of muscle contractions of the lower limbs that increase ventilation; one could then determine whether the same cortical stimulation increases ventilation after contraction of hind limb muscles is prevented by low spinal cord block or local (intra-arterial) injection of neuromuscular blocking agents to the hind limbs.

Mechanoreceptors in the Muscles or Joints

We mentioned earlier (p. 91) that respiratory stimulation occurs during passive movements of a limb.[1] It does not occur with cycles of stretch and recoil just of a muscle; there must be movement of the limbs about a joint. Impulses from joint mechanoreceptors or vibration receptors could explain the *immediate* increase in respiration that occurs with the first movement before any chemical stimuli could accumulate and be transported to sensitive regions, but they could not account for the close relationship between ventilation and metabolism; joint receptors can signal how much movement there is and how often it occurs but cannot indicate how much *force* was generated to produce the movement and how much energy was used. With isotonic contraction, the movement is great and the work little; with isometric con-

---

[1]Passive movements are not really passive. Movement of a limb must stretch muscles, which then send impulses to the spinal cord and initiate a contraction of the same muscles by a stretch reflex; for this reason, O_2 consumption increases during "passive" movements of a limb.

traction, the movement is minimal and the work great.

Other Peripheral Receptors

Electrical stimulation of limb muscles often causes marked hyperpnea. It is difficult to separate stimulation of motor fibers to muscle from stimulation of sensory fibers from the limb when mixed nerves or masses of muscle are stimulated electrically. Pain from limbs can stimulate breathing and may contribute to the hyperpnea of *static* exercise. This hyperpnea is easy to demonstrate: lie in bed, raise one leg and thigh to an angle of 45 degrees with the bed and hold it there by active contraction of the thigh muscles. This maneuver, besides contracting muscles, also causes pain, probably because the tonic contraction occludes fine blood vessels, makes the muscle ischemic and permits the local accumulation of chemical materials.

Kao believes, on the basis of elaborate cross-perfusion experiments, that the limbs contain "ergoreceptors" that drive respiration reflexly; the precise nature of these and their physiologic stimulus are not yet defined. Possibly these are deep mechanoreceptors that are excited by hyperosmolality that occurs in exercising muscle. Phillipson has shown in unanesthetized dogs that the vagi are not essential for the normal ventilatory responses to exercise.

Conditioned Reflexes

Many observers have noted an increase in ventilation just before exercise begins. Wasserman has reported that this does not occur in all of his subjects and believes that it is a learned response rather than an essential component of the hyperpnea of exercise.

Multiple-Factor Theory of Regulation of Ventilation

The inability to find a single mechanism to explain exercise ventilation led to the concept that *multiple factors* are involved and that it is the interplay, potentiation or algebraic sum of these that really determines the final ventilatory response. The first elegant mathematical approach to this interplay was made by Gray. On the basis of all available data on healthy man, he proposed the following equation to predict change in ventilation when certain chemical changes occurred in arterial blood in (H^+), Po_2 or Pco_2:

$$V_R(\text{chemical}) =$$
$$0.22(H^+) + [0.262\ Paco_2 - 18]$$
$$+ [2.118 \times 10^{-8}(104 - Pao_2)^{4.9}]$$

In this equation, $V_R(\text{chemical})$ is the ventilation during chemical stimulation of breathing, expressed as multiples of the control minute volume; (H^+) is expressed as moles/L $\times 10^{-9}$, and $Paco_2$ and Pao_2 are arterial gas tensions in torr.

Several problems are associated with this mathematical formulation of the ventilatory response to multiple factors. First, this equation deals only with *chemical* stimuli and only with three *known* chemical stimuli. Second, such an equation must be based on data, and these are usually the responses of healthy men to change in arterial blood (H^+), Pco_2 and Po_2. The assumptions must then be made that (1) the data for the small group used as subjects are typical of a large population; (2) the same data would be obtained in the small group if the measurements were repeated in them on another day; (3) changes in arterial blood (H^+), Pco_2, and Po_2 are the only stimuli involved in the chemical regulation of respiration; (4) one chemical stimulus simply adds to or subtracts from another and there is no potentiation; (5) no other factors alter this relationship. Men of the same age and size, and even identical twins, respond differently to the same chemical stimulus, and the same man may respond differently to the same stimulus presented at successive experiments during the same day. And, of course, the equation fails to predict ventilation in patients with severe obstructive or restrictive disease of the lungs or with neuromuscular or central depression or paralysis (due to disease, drugs or anesthesia); in these patients with

severe hypoventilation, low arterial blood Po_2 and high Pco_2 and (H^+), the equation would predict extraordinarily high values for minute ventilation (higher than the maximal voluntary ventilation), yet minute ventilation is below normal.

Even in healthy man, there are mechanisms that depress ventilation. Inflation of the lungs inhibits breathing; so do increased mean pressure and increased pulse pressure in the aortic arch and carotid sinuses and increased cerebral blood flow. Tidal volume increases markedly during exercise, and this stretches the lungs and should check the depth of inspiration. Arterial blood pressure and cerebral blood flow increase and should cause inhibition of breathing. Why do these not depress ventilation? The "answer" is that in some circumstances, some mechanisms are prepotent (take precedence over others) and in other circumstances, others have priority. The brain usually seems to accept good advice and to turn a deaf ear to bad advice; in short, it is a wondrous organ.

In muscular exercise (unless it is exhausting and arterial blood pH has decreased), there are no measurable changes from normal arterial blood, and the equation therefore says that no change in ventilation has occurred *as a result of chemical factors*. This of course is a main use of mathematical equations and models; if the observed ventilation is far in excess of that predicted, then other factors (in this case, nonchemical factors) must be involved or the equation was based on the wrong data (e.g., ventilatory response to inhaled CO_2 rather than to endogenous CO_2). As we acquire more facts, mathematical models will be modified to include more factors and information on interaction among these. At the moment, a fascinating field of inquiry is why the responses of men to standard stimuli differ and why responses of the *same* man differ at various times. We know, for example, that norepinephrine and certain afferent stimuli that excite the reticular activating system increase the respiratory response to chemical stimuli such as CO_2. What else does this? What is the importance of these factors?

Until we learn more, we must conclude that many factors are involved in the hyperpnea of muscular exercise. These include chemical stimuli (known and possibly unknown, acting on known and possibly unknown peripheral and central sites), temperature change and nervous influences (both reflex and central). Some are responsible for the rapid change at the beginning and end of exercise, some for the slower on-and-off responses and some for both. And, as Dejours has pointed out, the influence of each may vary with the type of exercise, its intensity and duration and with environmental factors.

RESPIRATION IN THE FETUS AND NEWBORN

Gas Exchange in the Fetus

In the adult, gas exchange occurs in the lungs, between air and blood separated by alveolocapillary membranes. In the fetus, completely surrounded by amniotic fluid, the lungs have no gas exchange function, and O_2 and CO_2 are transferred to and from maternal blood and fetal blood in near contact in the placenta. The mother's heart pumps arterial blood through her aorta and uterine arteries into the spiral arteries of the placenta; from these it spurts or surges into intervillous sinusoids. The fetal heart pumps blood through the umbilical arteries to cotyledonary arteries in the placenta; from these blood flows into the fetal placental capillary loops, which dip into the intervillous spaces and sinusoids fed with maternal blood. Here gas exchange occurs. Fetal blood richer in O_2 and poorer in CO_2 returns to the umbilical veins and then to the inferior vena cava (Figs. 19-3 and 19-4).

The precise anatomic relationships between the fetal and maternal vessels within the placenta vary from species to species. The possible arrangements are shown schematically in Figure 19-5; which one represents the human placenta is not known for sure, though many believe it is closer to D than to A, B or C. In any case, the fetal blood leaving the placenta contains less O_2/100 ml than maternal arterial blood entering it. Maternal blood to the placenta has a Po_2 of about 100 torr, and its hemoglobin is about 98% saturated with O_2. Fetal blood entering the placenta has a Po_2 of about 22 torr, and its hemoglobin is 45–55% saturated with O_2; that leaving the placenta has a Po_2

Fig. 19-3.—Schematic representation of human fetal circulation. Numbers refer to the Po_2 of blood (torr) in different parts of the circulation; note that the coronary and cerebral vessels receive the arterial blood that has the highest Po_2. (Based on data of A. M. Rudolph.)

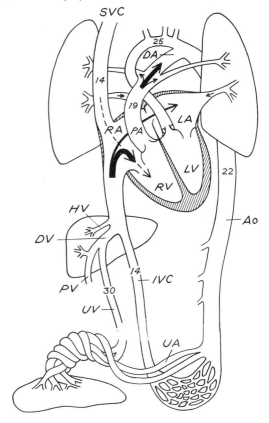

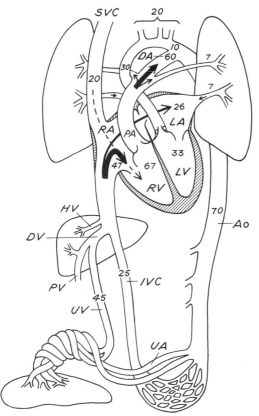

Fig. 19-4.—Schematic representation of human fetal circulation. Numbers refer to blood flow in milliliters per minute through the main vascular channels. (Based on data of A. M. Rudolph.)

lung is a nearly perfect system for gas transfer; the ideal placenta is a less effective system. Both systems are subject to impaired effectiveness for the same causes (see Chapters 12 and 13): "hypoventilation," shunts (in the placenta, between the umbilical artery and vein that bypass the gas exchange vessels), impaired diffusion and abnormal "ventilation"/perfusion ratios. "Ventilation" (uterine blood flow) can increase and decrease relative to "pulmonary" (umbilical) blood flow, and the change can affect either the whole gas exchange system or only certain regions. Umbilical vessels can at times be occluded by kinking or knotting of the cord. Uterine blood flow varies with maternal blood pressure, with the relative resistance to flow in its branches to the uterine muscle and those to the placenta and, during labor, with pressure exerted on vessels by the contracting uterine muscle. And just as the Po_2 of inspired air can change (e.g., at high altitude), so the Po_2 of maternal uterine blood can change under abnormal circumstances. In addition, fetal hemoglobin (F) has different characteristics from adult hemoglobin (A) (see p. 192).

of about 30 torr, and its hemoglobin is 65–75% saturated (depending on its pH).

In gas exchange, the placenta functions in many respects like the lung except that it brings arterial blood instead of air into intimate contact with blood that requires arterialization (Fig. 19-6). The maternal uterine arterial blood is equivalent to the lung's inspired gas, high in O_2 and low in CO_2. The maternal placental blood pool is equivalent to the lung's alveolar gas; the uterine venous blood is equivalent to the lung's expired gas. The fetal umbilical circulation is the counterpart of the lung's pulmonary circulation; in each circulation, arteries bring blood low in O_2 and high in CO_2 to a capillary bed for arterialization, and veins conduct blood high in O_2 and low in CO_2 back to the pump for distribution to organs and tissues. The ideal

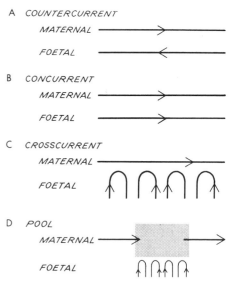

Fig. 19-5.—Diagrams of possible arrangements in maternal and fetal vascular channels in the area of gas exchange of a placenta. (From Dawes, G. S.: *Foetal and Neonatal Physiology* [Chicago: Year Book Medical Publishers, Inc., 1968.])

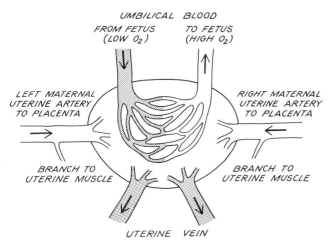

UMBILICAL BLOOD
FROM FETUS   TO FETUS
(LOW O₂)   (HIGH O₂)

LEFT MATERNAL   RIGHT MATERNAL
UTERINE ARTERY   UTERINE ARTERY
TO PLACENTA   TO PLACENTA

BRANCH TO   BRANCH TO
UTERINE MUSCLE   UTERINE MUSCLE

UTERINE VEIN

Fig. 19-6.—Schematic representation of fetal and maternal blood flow through the placenta.

The best-oxygenated blood in the fetus is that in the umbilical veins. Before it gets to the fetal systemic arterial circulation, its O_2 saturation is decreased by admixture with venous blood from the portal veins and inferior vena cava. Some of it—that which enters the right atrium—has a further reduction in O_2 saturation by mixing with superior vena caval blood. However, most of it flows directly through an opening between the inferior vena cava and the left atrium—the foramen ovale—into the left atrium and the left ventricle and is then pumped to the ascending aorta, and into arteries to the heart, brain, arms and upper trunk (see Fig. 19-3). Thus the best-oxygenated fetal blood is directed to the heart muscle and brain. The right atrial blood, with less O_2, enters the right ventricle and is pumped largely through a short, wide fetal artery (the ductus arteriosus) to the beginning of the descending aorta, and this supplies most of the other tissues and organs.

Little blood flows through the fetal pulmonary circulation—only about 10% of the combined output of the right and left ventricles. Because of the wide communication between the aorta and pulmonary artery, the pressures in the right and left ventricles are about the same. Since blood from the two ventricles can enter either the pulmonary circulation or the aorta, the former must have a relatively great vascular resistance. The fetal pulmonary vessels are very reactive; they can be actively constricted by low Po_2 and even more by concomitant hypoxia and acidosis. Why does *any* blood flow through the fetal pulmonary circulation, since it has no gas exchange function? Probably in part because flow is essential for the development of this huge vascular bed that is destined to carry the entire right ventricular output shortly after birth. It is also essential for cells that carry out the nonrespiratory functions of the pulmonary circulation (see p. 287) and for delivering materials to the alveolar walls and alveolar ducts; these tissues have a high metabolic rate and are very active in the synthesis of lipo-proteins, which become the alveolar surfactant (see p. 111).

During early fetal life, the lung is solid. Later it develops tubes that still later become airways and alveoli. But the alveoli are lined with cuboidal epithelium and are not coated with surfactant; the "airways" and alveoli are not collapsed but are filled with fluid. It was long believed that this was amniotic fluid that drifted into the lung or was drawn in during occasional gasps. Studies by a variety of technics (chemical analyses of lung and amniotic fluid; ligation of the fetal trachea; intubation and collection of tracheobronchial fluid in the fetus) have demonstrated clearly that most of the lung fluid originates in the lung and indeed contributes to the amniotic fluid. Some of the pulmonary fluid is secreted by alveolar cells and the tracheobronchial glands; some may be a filtrate from blood flowing through the pulmonary capillaries.

Respiration in the Newborn

Dawes has shown that the fetal lamb makes rapid shallow respiratory movements in utero during part of each day and occasionally produces a larger gasp. One can only speculate why; possibly it is a way of developing respiratory muscles that later must expand the thorax to produce the first breath when the fetus becomes a newborn. For this event, the lung must also mature: cuboidal cells lining alveoli must become thin to permit lung expansion, and surfactant must form and coat the alveolar surfaces.

The cardiovascular-pulmonary events that occur at the birth of a baby are by far the most dramatic of its lifetime. These are remarkable in their magnitude, diversity and timing. At birth, the umbilical cord is clamped, tied and cut. The newborn infant can no longer depend on the maternal circulation; it must breathe soon or die. What events make it breathe? Some of these are the multiple, strange and varied sensory stimuli which, for the first time, bombard the respiratory and associated centers of the previously insulated newborn: sounds beat against its ears; bright lights shine into its eyes; the tissues experience the effects of gravity; the limbs move and stretch receptors are excited; the skin experiences cold and touch and pain, and odors assail the nose. The immersion reflex, which could inhibit breathing in utero, is no longer excited. And at the same time, the tissues are using blood O_2 without replenishing it and are adding CO_2 and H ions without eliminating them; blood Po_2 and pH fall, Pco_2 rises, and peripheral and central chemoreceptors are soon maximally stimulated.

Are all of these sensory receptors properly connected at birth by nervous paths to the center, and are the centers in turn connected by motor paths to the respiratory muscles? In a baby born at full term—yes; in an in-

fant born quite prematurely—probably no. Healthy newborn babies at term increase their ventilation when they inhale CO_2-rich gas; their breathing is depressed by inhalation of O_2 and stimulated by inhalation of O_2-deficient atmosphere. The inflation and the Head paradoxical reflexes are active at birth (though their effectiveness decreases in the next few days). A combination of events makes the infant take its first breath; probably the chemical stimuli are the most urgent of all.

The first breath requires unusual effort by the respiratory muscles. The fetal lungs contain fluid. When the head emerges first from the birth canal, the nose and mouth are at atmospheric pressure while the thorax is still subject to increased intrauterine pressure. A uterine contraction may squeeze the thorax and empty it of much fluid, but some remains. The first inspiration must pull fluid that is 36 times more viscous and 1,000 times denser than air through the fine air ducts. Figure 10-9 (p. 106) shows that less pressure is needed to distend a fluid-filled lung than an air-containing lung. However, this is a graph of compliance, with volume and pressure measured under *static* conditions, and frictional, viscous resistance does not play a role. Further, Figure 10-9 shows a fluid-fluid interface—not fluid-air—and no surface forces are involved. The first breath must also overcome the forces of surface tension at each of the fluid-air interspaces, in addition to the usual work of overcoming elastic recoil and tissue resistance. As the air enters smaller and smaller tubes and the radii of curvature of the air-fluid interface become smaller, the pressure required to overcome surface tension increases, as expected from Laplace's law. A transpulmonary pressure of as much as 80 cm H_2O may be needed to overcome all resisting factors.

The first expiration is equally important. If all the air that entered the lung during the first inspiration and was not absorbed left it during the first expiration, atelectasis would occur, with cohesion of the walls of alveoli, ducts and bronchioles. The second inspiration would require another tremendous effort and, if this were repeated over and over again, breathing would soon exhaust the infant. This does happen in infants with the respiratory distress syndrome, but in normal infants a reserve volume of air (the functional residual capacity) is built up in the lung beginning with the first breath. The newborn lung expands fully within a few minutes, and its FRC is then reasonably stable. Why does breathing continue after the first breath removes the low Po_2 and high Pco_2 stimuli? Removal of inhibitory influences, the existence of alerting and arousing stimuli and excitatory impulses to the spinal cord from the once-stretched respiratory muscle spindles may all be important. The Head paradoxical reflex, a positive feedback mechanism that can increase a modest inspiration into a maximal one, may also be a factor early in life.

Although the mechanical events during delivery eliminate much of the lung fluid, some must be removed by other means; these include absorption into blood now rushing through the pulmonary circulation (see p. 287), entry into lymphatic channels and possibly evaporation. Most of the fluid is removed within minutes of birth.

Circulatory Changes in the Newborn

Inflation of the lungs is only one event in the changeover from fetal to newborn life. Ventilation accomplishes little until the pulmonary circulation becomes a low-resistance, high-flow system. This it does with the first breath. Part of this change may be due to mechanical forces associated with pulmonary expansion because it occurs even when the gas inhaled is N_2. Most of it, however, is due to the increase in alveolar and arterial Po_2. (In some newborn animals, inhalation of low O_2 mixtures produces a prompt and almost complete reversion of the pulmonary circulation to a high-resistance–high-pressure system.)

The changes in the lungs and pulmonary

circulation are followed by closure of the special openings that are useful to the fetal circulation but not to that of the newborn. The foramen ovale closes functionally within a minute of the first breath. When the pulmonary vascular resistance decreases and pulmonary blood flow increases, the left atrial pressure increases above that in the right atrium and inferior vena cava and the reversal of the pressure gradient holds the flaplike valve closed. At about the same time, closure of the umbilical vessels and elimination of this large, low-resistance vascular bed decreases venous flow through the inferior vena cava and more firmly establishes the difference in pressure between the left and right atria (Fig. 11-1). Anatomic closure of this foramen occurs in 2 to 3 weeks, except in about 10% of persons in whom it never closes anatomically.

The ductus arteriosus narrows in about 10–30 minutes after the onset of ventilation. This is probably due to a direct action of O_2 on its smooth muscle, resulting in active constriction, because it occurs *in vitro* as well. In the fetus, the direction of flow through the ductus arteriosus is right to left; within an hour after birth, it becomes left to right. This is because elimination of the low-resistance placental circulation increases systemic vascular resistance, and simultaneously pulmonary vascular resistance decreases. Later—near the end of the first day—there is complete closure of the ductus as a shunt; until then, the left ventricular output exceeds the right. The right ventricular and pulmonary arterial pressures decrease to adult values in 1½–2 weeks. In 2–3 weeks, the wall of the left ventricle becomes thicker than that of the right. Within 3–4 weeks the pulmonary arterioles lose most of their thick ring of smooth muscle. The number of pulmonary alveoli increases about 10-fold from birth to adult life; most of this increase occurs in the first 8 years. Between 8 and 25 years, the lung volume doubles, but this is due largely to increase in the linear dimensions of existing units.

Because the Po_2 of the best-oxygenated

fetal blood is only 30 torr, the fetus must develop mechanisms for insuring adequate O_2 transport. One of these is an increase in red blood cells to about 6,000,000/mm³ and an increase in hemoglobin to about 20 gm/100 ml of blood. Another is that fetal hemoglobin (F) differs in several respects from adult (A) hemoglobin. Pure hemoglobin F has a slightly lower affinity for O_2 than hemoglobin A, but *red cells* containing mainly hemoglobin F have a high affinity for O_2 (Fig. 14-2), presumably because 2-3 diphosphoglycerate (DPG) does not bind to fetal hemoglobin (see p. 192); this favors greater uptake of O_2 by Hb. The newborn baby, now functioning at the arterial blood Po_2 of an adult, sheds its fetal mechanisms for insuring O_2 transport; hemoglobin and red cell levels fall to adult levels (or below) by 4 weeks and hemoglobin F is replaced by hemoglobin A.

Respiratory Problems of the Newborn

The first few days of life are the most hazardous of all, and many of the newborn's problems are respiratory. The respiratory distress syndrome has been discussed earlier (p. 112). In addition, a premature infant suffers from incompletely developed and weak respiratory muscles at a time when these must make maximal efforts because of low pulmonary compliance and a deficiency of surfactant lining the alveoli. The medullary respiratory centers of any newborn infant may be depressed because of overdose of drugs given to the mother for analgesia or anesthesia or because of trauma to its head during birth. Aspiration of fluids into the lungs is another hazard, and long-continued hypoxemia—due to failure of fetal circulatory shunts to close or atelectatic areas of the lungs to open—is another. Occasionally, pneumothorax results from alveolar rupture due to the development of very large transpulmonary pressures during the first few breaths.

The ductus arteriosus often fails to close in prematurely born infants, possibly because

an important mechanism of closure—responsiveness to high blood Po_2—has not fully developed. As a result, there is a large left-to-right shunt that can produce heart failure and pulmonary edema; the latter creates a special problem in pulmonary ventilation, since the respiratory muscles of prematurely born infants are weak.

Newborn babies breathe through the nose and seem not to learn how to breathe through the mouth for 3–4 months; Shaw noted that about 30% of babies have difficulty in adopting oral respiration up to 5–6 months of age. Even if the nares of newborn are gently occluded, only a few respond promptly by mouth breathing. Obviously it is inappropriate to determine whether occlusion of the nares for longer times will initiate mouth breathing, but the observation suggests that it may be important to insure open nares in young infants.

The newborn of all species tested can survive total anoxia (e.g., life in an atmosphere of N_2) longer than can adults of the same species. A newborn rat can survive for 25–30 minutes without O_2, while an adult rat dies in 3–4 minutes; the difference is less marked in species in which the newborn is more mature at birth. The prolonged survival probably depends on the utilization of glycogen and therefore on the amount of glycogen stored in the heart, for example. The fetal and newborn lamb reacts to hypoxia with a fall in O_2 consumption; the same is true of newborn babies. This may be part of a pattern for survival, in which blood flow is reduced to some tissues that can exist anaerobically to insure survival of vital organs that cannot. Another factor in anoxic survival may be differences in enzyme systems and substrate utilization in the premature infant.

The newborn possesses one additional advantage over the adult. Its pulmonary arterial pressure is high at birth, and by 3–4 weeks after birth has fallen to adult levels but not below. The infant, and indeed the child, because of its small size, coupled with the adult level of pulmonary artery pressure, has no problem in perfusing the top of its lungs with an unbroken supply of blood.

RESPIRATION DURING GENERAL AND SPINAL ANESTHESIA

General Anesthesia

AIRWAY OBSTRUCTION. Both preanesthetic drugs and procedures and the unconscious state favor the development of airway obstruction. Atropine, a parasympathetic blocking agent usually administered to decrease the volume of tracheobronchial secretions, may result in thicker mucus. Morphine and barbiturates given to decrease apprehension also depress respiration and the cough reflex. Volatile anesthetic agents may cause bronchiolar constriction, diminish the activity of cilia and increase the secretion of mucus despite prior use of atropine. Some anesthetic agents cause laryngospasm, as does the introduction of an endotracheal tube. All general anesthetic agents diminish or abolish reflexes that protect the airway. The unconscious state (often aided by drugs that block neuromuscular junctions and cause paralysis of skeletal muscles) also causes the tongue to fall back against the posterior pharyngeal wall, the palate to relax and the head and neck to fall into a position that obstructs the airway. Fortunately, anesthetists are prepared for all of these events, but they may well become problems in the *post*operative hours before all of the patient's functions return to normal.

EFFECTS ON RESPIRATION. One action of all general anesthetic agents is to decrease the respiratory response to inhaled CO_2. This does not mean that all general anesthetic agents decrease minute ventilation to less than normal values; some do, some don't, and some actually increase ventilation. A second effect has been mentioned earlier: decreasing the Pco_2 of arterial blood to subnormal values (by hyperventilation) is followed by apnea. A third phenomenon may be seen with *deep* general anesthesia—apnea follows the administration of O_2. These observations put together probably mean: (1)

General anesthetics tend, by a central action, to depress breathing, but some, by other actions, tend to stimulate it. Ether, vinethene, chloroform, ethyl chloride and halothane act on sensory receptors in the lungs and increase respiration by vagal reflexes; the last of these is known to sensitize the receptors for the inflation reflex and increase respiratory rate. Ether may also stimulate receptors in the limbs or certain cells of the central nervous system. Nitrous oxide, if given in greater than 80–85% concentration, causes hypoxemia and may increase respiration by carotid and aortic body reflexes. (2) The medullary chemoreceptors that respond to changes in Pco_2 are sensitive to respiratory depressant drugs, either because these drugs directly depress them or block other areas essential for the full CO_2 response. (3) The reticular activating system, which responds in awake man to a wide variety of sensory or alerting stimuli, is depressed by light anesthesia; this explains why breathing may continue in an awake man whose Pco_2 is less than 20 torr (because his reticular activating system is still functioning) but not in an anesthetized man in whom both the reticular activating system and medullary chemoreceptors are depressed. (4) Even when the medullary chemoreceptors and the reticular activating system are much less active owing to general anesthesia, the peripheral chemoreceptors are still functioning and maintain breathing reasonably well as long as the patient is hypoxemic. Inhalation of O_2 by a deeply anesthetized patient in whom there is no respiratory drive other than hypoxemia will lead to physiological denervation of the peripheral chemoreceptors and to apnea. As anesthesia deepens, there is thus a shift in the control of respiration from the medullary chemoreceptors to the peripheral chemoreceptors; sensitivity to change in CO_2 decreases markedly, but reactivity to low O_2 persists. If the anesthetist is not aware of this shift, he may note only that breathing seems to be approximately normal and may not appreciate that this is due only to a peripheral chemoreceptor drive. Failing to realize the significance or even the presence of hypoxemia, he may be unprepared for cessation of respiration or sharp decline in arterial blood pressure following inhalation of O_2 or the addition of subsequent doses of the anesthetic agent.

When 100% O_2 is administered along with respiratory depressants such as pentothal, cyclopropane or halothane, the full depressant action of the anesthetic agent becomes evident. The anesthetist prefers to prevent the hypoxemia by providing high concentrations of O_2 in the inspired gas mixture; this of course removes the reflex drive and may even lead to apnea. He then assists ventilation by some mechanical device to keep arterial P_{CO_2} from rising during the operation. The pink color of the skin of a patient inhaling O_2 does not mean that ventilation is adequate; *oxygenation* may be excellent under these conditions, but arterial and tissue P_{CO_2} will rise unless the *volume* of alveolar ventilation/minute is adequate.

Spinal Anesthesia

Ideally, local anesthetics injected in low concentration into the fluid around the spinal cord or spinal roots block sensory and not motor nerves. In fact, sensory fibers carrying impulses from pain receptors are more readily blocked than motor fibers, but the amount and concentration of the local anesthetic used may block both. If the anesthetic is confined to the body below the diaphragm, the intercostal and phrenic nerves are not blocked; if it reaches the thoracic level, the intercostal nerves may be blocked but the phrenic nerves are still unaffected; if it reaches the cervical region, the phrenic nerves to the diaphragm are also blocked, and artificial ventilation is necessary.

Sensory nerve block may produce respiratory depression even though motor paths still conduct. Block of the thoracic posterior roots may depress the neurons that drive the main intercostal muscle fibers by eliminating sensory input from muscle spindles (p. 83). Block of the surface chemosensitive zones of the medulla may diminish breathing markedly; upward diffusion of the local anesthetic agent may produce a concentration surrounding the medulla sufficient to depress these zones even though it is not enough to paralyze cranial motor nerves.

After Anesthesia

The main risk in patients subjected to anesthesia is in the *post*operative period if the anesthesiologist is not present to control or assist ventilation and to maintain an open airway. This is because a number of factors can reduce ventilation postoperatively: The preanesthetic medication has probably been reinforced by postoperative injections of morphine for the relief of pain. The neuromuscular blocking agent or the anesthetic agent itself may have an unaccountably prolonged effect. A patient with poorly ventilated areas of the lungs eliminates gaseous anesthetics slowly. Postoperative incisional pain discourages the patient from coughing up secretions even though he may be awake. The effect of preoperative atropine on secretions has worn off, but the airways cannot be cleared of mucus because ciliary activity is weak and coughing is suppressed; secretions accumulate, block the airway and lead to atelectasis and pulmonary infection. Vomitus may be inhaled into the respiratory tract. Sometimes the patient leaves the operating room with a high concentration of O_2 in his alveoli. If some of the airways to these alveoli become blocked or poorly ventilated, the O_2 may be removed by capillary blood flow, and atelectasis may result. The effect of anesthetic agents, particularly the volatile ones, on the phospholipid surfactant lining alveoli is unknown, but interference with its activity could also contribute to atelectasis.

There is an additional postoperative hazard in patients whose lungs have been mechanically *hyper*ventilated throughout long operations. In such patients, body stores of CO_2 are depleted and must be restored before ventilation responds adequately to rising blood P_{CO_2}. They are restored physiologically by CO_2 production in excess of CO_2 elimination; this requires hypoventilation, despite the hypoxemia produced by it. Inhalation of air enriched with O_2 may be needed to correct the hypoxemia.

Hypoxemia may also occur after N_2O anesthesia is stopped. Just as the presence of CO_2 (40 torr) and water vapor (47 torr) in alveolar gas lower the sum of P_{O_2} and P_{N_2} from 760 to 673 torr, so N_2O molecules leaving tissues and blood and entering alveolar gas temporarily lower the $P_{O_2} + P_{N_2}$ even more — depending on the quantities of N_2O being excreted.

RESPIRATION AT HIGH AND LOW PRESSURES

Changing Pressure

CHANGE IN VOLUME OF GASES. Boyle's law states that $PV = P'V'$. If P and V are 1 atmosphere of pressure and 1 L of gas respectively, then the new volume, V', must be ½ L if the new pressure, P', is 2 atmospheres, or the new volume must be 2 L if the new pressure is ½ atmosphere. Therefore, gas within the body is compressed when man is under water (every 33 feet below the surface of sea water = 1 atmosphere of pressure) and decompressed when man goes to a high altitude (the pressure at 18,000 feet above sea level is about ½ atmosphere and at 33,000 feet about ¼ atmosphere).

Decompression and compression and the accompanying expansion and contraction of gases matter little if they have free access to the outside air. When ambient pressure decreases, gas in the gastrointestinal tract, lungs, middle ear and sinuses expands and the extra volume escapes to the outside air. However, if the exit for gas is blocked, the consequences can be painful or serious. There can be intestinal distention and cramps (if there is intestinal obstruction), severe sinus pain (if the ostia are closed), rupture of the eardrum (if the eustachian tube is blocked) or alveolar rupture (if large or small airways are blocked). Alveolar rupture can cause pneumothorax (air between the lung and chest wall) and air bubbles can enter torn pulmonary vessels and cause air embolism in the coronary, cerebral or other systemic circulations. These events can occur either during too rapid ascent from deep water to sea level or from sea level to high altitude; divers must not hold their breath with the glottis closed during ascent because of the sudden large increase in lung volume.

Middle ear problems are more common during compression than during decompression. The air-containing middle ear communicates with the pharynx through the eustachian tube; this is normally closed by flaplike valves that can be opened by specific muscles which contract as part of the act of swallowing. During decompression, the gas volume increases in the middle ear; this tends to bulge or even rupture the drum but, unless the eustachian tube is completely occluded (e.g., by congestion), the gas simply forces the valve open, and pressure in the middle ear and pharynx and outer ear becomes equal, even though there is no active act, such as swallowing. If a person has been at a high altitude and descends rapidly, the gas in the middle ear shrinks to a smaller volume, and air from the pharynx must enter the tube to equalize pressures. But during recompression, the air pressure in the pharynx is rising and can mechanically hold the eustachian flaps shut; active muscular effort is needed to open the orifice and let air into the middle ear. The act of swallowing usually does this. Until this is accomplished, the gas in the middle ear is at lower pressure than air pressure in the external ear. The drum is pulled sharply inward, and hemorrhage may occur in the membrane.

FORMATION OF GAS BUBBLES IN TISSUE AND BLOOD. Table 22-2 (p. 276) shows gas tensions in air and blood of a man breathing air at sea level. There is a high partial pressure of N_2 in blood and in tissues because man breathes 79% N_2 and is surrounded by 79% N_2. Since N_2 is not used in metabolic processes, it acts as an inert gas and simply dissolves in blood and body tissues.

Henry's law states that such gases dissolve in liquids in direct proportion to their partial pressure. If man ascends to a high altitude, the P_{N_2} decreases in inspired air and alveolar gas but is still high in tissues and blood. Dissolved N_2 must then diffuse from tissues to blood and from blood to alveolar gas until tissue and blood and air tensions of N_2 are again equal. If the ascent and resulting decrease in ambient P_{N_2} occur slowly, nitrogen gradually leaves the tissues and blood by diffusion and no symptoms occur. If however, the ascent is abrupt, the dissolved N_2 in tissues and blood comes out of solution too rapidly to be carried away by diffusion, and gas bubbles form (just as when water that has been equilibrated with air is exposed to a vacuum). If O_2 bubbles form, these can be used locally in tissue metabolism; CO_2 is not involved, since there is very little CO_2 in ambient air. Thus the problem is largely one of N_2 bubbles, which can be removed only by diffusion. These bubbles produce a syndrome called decompression sickness or caisson disease. It consists of pains in the muscles and joints ("bends"), sensory disturbances, weakness or paralysis, shortness of breath ("chokes"), dizziness, deafness and convulsions; the symptoms are believed to be due to bubble formation in muscles, joint cavities, peripheral nerves and central nervous system and, in very severe cases, to actual bubble formation in venous blood and plugging of the pulmonary microcirculation by these. In mild cases, there may

be only muscle and joint pains; in severe cases, death may occur unless the person is *recompressed* promptly and then *gradually* *de*compressed over a much longer period.

It is easy to understand how N_2 bubbles form when man suddenly ascends to a high altitude; it is harder to see why they form when man ascends to the surface after swimming freely or working in a caisson (compression chamber) under water. The answer is they would *not* form if man was exposed briefly to high pressures and there was no time for additional N_2 to dissolve in his tissues at pressures of 2, 3 or 4 atmospheres. N_2 is relatively insoluble in water and blood. When man breathes air at 3 atmospheres, his alveolar P_{N_2} rises about 3-fold. This causes 3 times as much N_2 to dissolve in pulmonary capillary blood, and the blood distributes this to body tissues. But the blood volume is only 8% of the body volume, and considerable time is needed for blood to carry enough N_2 to tissues to saturate them at the new P_{N_2}. Some tissues that have a rapid blood flow and dissolve little N_2 comes to the new P_{N_2} quickly. Other tissues, such as fat cells full of fat droplets, have less blood flow per gram of tissue but dissolve 5 times as much N_2 per gram; these come to the new P_{N_2} much more slowly. If man goes to 3-atmosphere pressure for brief periods, he adds little N_2 to his tissues and will not suffer if he ascends rapidly. If he stays long enough for his tissues to load up more N_2, he must come up (decompress) slowly. There are tables of safe times that man may stay at each pressure without needing slow decompression.

A diver or caisson worker can escape the bends and chokes by breathing O_2 for several hours before diving; this eliminates dissolved N_2 from the tissues. If he then dives breathing O_2, he avoids the problem of N_2 bubbles but substitutes that of O_2 toxicity (p. 282). If after N_2 elimination, he dives, breathing air at high pressures, he will accumulate N_2, but the total body N_2 will be much less because his tissues started near zero level of N_2. Alternately, he could, after denitrogenation, dive while breathing 80% He and 20% O_2. Helium has the advantage over N_2 that it is only half as soluble in water, and twice the time is needed for a comparable volume of dissolved He to accumulate in tissues; breathing He-O_2 does not prevent decompression sickness but increases the safe period at high pressures.

High Altitude

Above sea level, the total barometric pressure is less than 1 atmosphere, or 760 torr (Table 19-1); since the percent of O_2 remains the same (20.93) as far out as our atmosphere has been sampled, there are fewer molecules of O_2 per unit volume and the P_{O_2} of inspired air must decrease as one goes to higher altitudes. Some arterial hypoxemia must occur, therefore, unless one is in a pressurized plane or space capsule or inhales O_2. Although some birds soar over the Himalayas (without O_2 masks!), man cannot climb to the top of Mount Everest (inspired $P_{O_2} = 49$ torr) without raising the P_{O_2} of inspired air by adding O_2. Above 40,000 feet, he would be hypoxemic even if pure O_2 were inhaled because the total alveolar pressure there is 141 torr, and 87 torr of this must be CO_2 and water vapor, leaving only 54 torr for alveolar P_{O_2}.

The effects of hypoxia vary with individuals and with acclimatization of any one individual. A healthy man going to high altitude at once feels breathlessness (extreme on exertion), has palpitation (consciousness of vigorous cardiac contractions), headache, fatigue, dizziness, weakness, nausea (even vomiting), impairment of judgment and other mental processes, dimness of vision and often insomnia; this group of symptoms is called "acute mountain sickness." After a few days at the same altitude, his symptoms diminish, and some even disappear. In a few weeks they become less annoying, and a reasonable amount of exertion is possible without real distress.

Some people live permanently at high altitudes; more than 10,000,000 persons live at altitudes above 10,000 feet. The highest village is at 18,000 feet (380 torr total barometric pressure), and some Peruvians daily go to work in a mine 19,000 ft above sea level. Obviously, there are short- and long-term physiologic and biochemical adjustments that permit long life at high altitudes. The body makes certain immediate adjustments to hypoxemia. We have already discussed the respiratory changes (p. 62). These consist of an increase in tidal volume and, with more severe hypoxemia, in frequency of breathing; if man behaves like laboratory animals, hypoxemia also causes some tracheobronchial narrowing and a decrease in anatomic dead space. The increase in tidal volume and decrease in dead space increase alveolar ventilation and bring the alveolar P_{O_2} closer to the inspired P_{O_2}; the increase in frequency also increases alveolar ventilation per minute. Another immediate adjustment is an increase in heart rate and cardiac output; this results in an increased blood flow to tissues per minute and partially compensates for the decreased O_2 content of each unit of blood.

Over a longer period, hypoxemia results in polycythemia (increased number of red blood cells/mm^3 of blood); this is due to the formation of additional erythropoietin, a hormone secreted by kidneys (and possibly by other tissues, including, according to Tramezzani, the carotid bodies), which acts on bone marrow to increase the rate of production of erythrocytes. This provides more hemoglobin/mm^3 of blood and helps to compensate for the decreased P_{O_2} and HbO_2 saturation. If hypoxia also results in an increased concentration of diphosphoglycerate

TABLE 19-1.—ALTITUDE, BAROMETRIC PRESSURE AND P_{O_2}

ALTITUDE		BAROMETRIC PRESSURE	O_2	INSPIRED P_{O_2}
Feet	Meters	Torr	%	Torr
0	0	760.0	20.93	159.1
5,000	1,524	632.3	20.93	132.3
10,000	3,048	522.6	20.93	109.4
15,000	4,572	428.8	20.93	89.7
17,962	5,475	380.0	20.93	79.5
20,000	6,098	349.2	20.93	73.1
25,000	7,620	281.9	20.93	59.0
30,000	9,144	225.6	20.93	47.2
35,000	10,668	178.7	20.93	37.4
40,000	12,192	140.7	20.93	29.4

within red cells, this would facilitate release of O_2 from HbO_2. These compensatory mechanisms operate to maintain the supply of O_2 to tissues and a near-normal tissue Po_2. Sometimes polycythemia progresses too far, and the person then has 9–10 million instead of 5 million erythrocytes/mm³; this increases blood viscosity, increases the work of the heart and favors mechanical block of fine blood vessels with erythrocyte masses or actual clots. This extreme response is seen at sea level in patients with congenital heart defects or artery-to-vein shunts across the lungs (pulmonary hemangioma), in whom hypoxemia is severe. The physician must decide whether (1) to reduce the red cell count by bleeding in order to lessen the risk of cardiovascular complications, or (2) to maintain maximal O_2-carrying capacity of the blood. He usually decides to decrease the polycythemia because marked increase in viscosity usually decreases blood flow through capillaries and so decreases the O_2 supply of tissues.

Prolonged residence at high altitudes also leads to hypoxic pulmonary arteriolar constriction and pulmonary hypertension (see Table 11-2, p. 156); as a rule pulmonary artery pressure returns to near normal after two weeks' residence at sea level.

Another delayed compensation is maximal opening of the capillary bed or growth of new capillaries; the mechanism of this is not known, though its effect is obvious—i.e., to decrease the distance that O_2 must diffuse between capillary and tissue cell.

When hypoxemia leads to hyperventilation, arterial and tissue Pco_2 falls. Unless there is an associated decrease in plasma (HCO_3^-), arterial blood pH rises (respiratory alkalosis). Renal mechanisms eliminate blood HCO_3^- to lessen the change in blood pH and some mechanism lowers CSF (HCO_3^-) to restore its pH toward its normal value of 7.32. The immediate and delayed changes in blood and CSF during hypoxia and its correction are illustrated in Figure 5-5 (p. 62).

Two other aspects of life at high altitude or of chronic hypoxemia at sea level deserve mention. (1) Arterial hypoxemia at either high altitude or sea level may cause a metabolic acidosis due to partial anaerobic metabolism of some tissues. (2) Hypoxemia in normal man living at high altitudes is always associated with hyperventilation and decreased arterial blood Pco_2 (respiratory alkalosis). Hypoxemia in some patients at sea level (artery-to-vein shunts; alveolar capillary block) may be associated with alveolar hyperventilation and respiratory alkalosis. Hypoxemia in others (restrictive or obstructive pulmonary disease) may be associated with alveolar hypoventilation and respiratory acidosis.

BLUNTED CHEMORECEPTOR FUNCTION IN CHRONIC HYPOXIA. In 1957 Chiodi observed that, although inhalation of O_2 led to decrease in ventilation in hypoxic man at sea level and in newcomers to high altitudes (by abrupt removal of carotid and aortic body drives), it did not depress respiration of natives at high altitudes who were born there and had lived there for years. This suggested to him that they no longer had effective peripheral chemoreceptors. A decade later, several groups confirmed this and found that the chemoreceptor response was blunted even after natives, long residents at high altitudes, had come back to live at sea level for as long as 10 months. A blunted response to hypoxia was also found in children who had congenital cyanotic heart disease.

This could be an inherited trait, because some healthy adults have little or no response even to extreme hypoxia. However, Grover found that men born at sea level who later went to live and work at high altitude also had severely depressed response to hypoxia. Why do carotid bodies, presumably once normal, lose their effectiveness after years of hypoxic stimulation? Many explanations have been offered: (1) the polycythemia caused by chronic hypoxemia could produce emboli or thrombi in blood channels essential for chemoreceptor function; (2) polycythemic blood contains more O_2/ml and, if the blood channels in the carotid body have become larger or more numerous, blood flow delivers more O_2/minute and so raises Po_2 in the carotid body; (3) DPG, increased in hypoxia, could release more O_2 from HbO_2 and raise the Po_2 of the carotid body; (4) carotid bodies are large in natives who have lived for years at high altitudes and increase about 2 to 3 times in size in experimental animals made hypoxic; if the increase in mass is due to increase in non-chemoreceptor cells, these could crowd out the chemosensory tissues; (5) long-continued hypoxic stimulation of chemoreceptor cells could eventually lead to adaptation of receptors (fewer impulses generated in response to the same stimulus); (6) chronic hypoxia could cause depression of the medullary centers that receive chemoreceptor impulses, even though medullary chemoreceptors still respond normally to increased Pco_2; (7) the peripheral chemoreceptors and medullary centers might be normal, but other centers in the brain may process incoming information to favor inhibitory influences and suppress excitatory influences.

We do not yet know whether patients with chronic *pulmonary* disease and hypoxemia have lost much of their hypoxic drive to ventilation; it is more difficult to measure ventilatory responses in a patient whose diseased thorax or lungs have imposed mechanical limitations to increased ventilation. However, some patients with chronic emphysema hyperventilate and keep their arterial blood Pco_2 near normal, while others with similar disease do neither; it is possible that the first group has maintained normal chemoreceptor function and the second group has depressed function.

Persons with a blunted response to hypoxia may still hyperventilate relative to healthy persons with a normal arterial Po_2; presumably such hyperventilation is due to anaerobic metabolism (including anaerobic cerebral metabolism) with glycolytic formation of lactic acid and stimulation of medullary chemoreceptors.

Manned Space Ships

When a capsule or other craft passes beyond the earth's atmosphere, the man inside is completely dependent on an artificial gaseous environment. The gas could be 20.9% O_2 and 79.1% N_2 and the total pressure could be atmospheric — just as on earth at sea level; presumably this was the gaseous environment of the Russian astronaut who made the first 5-day orbital flight. Another environment could be pure O_2 at a low total pressure of about $\frac{1}{4}$ of an atmosphere (O_2 at 760 torr is toxic; see p. 282). A third might be 50% O_2 and 50% N_2 at a total pressure of 380 torr. The selection in part depends on engineering considerations (weight and space required for the gas or gas mixtures; fire hazards; heat conduction; etc.) and partly on physiologic considerations. The latter include the problems of the toxicity of O_2 for cells, absorption of O_2 from closed spaces (see p. 276) and decompression sickness during rapid change in pressure.

Man in space also faces the problem of rapid acceleration during the launching, rapid deceleration during re-entry into the earth's atmosphere and the effect of prolonged weightlessness on body function. In manned space flight, the vehicle and crew starting from rest must attain a velocity of 11,600 meters/second to escape from the earth's gravitational field. The acceleration required for this increases the weight of body tissues and leads to displacement of those that are free or relatively free to move. The effects on columns of blood in systemic arteries and veins are well known; similar effects occur in the pulmonary circulation and to a lesser extent on lung tissues, chest wall and abdominal viscera. The chest wall decreases in size, and therefore lung volume decreases. Blood leaves the top of the lung and goes to the bottom. ("Top" means apices and "bottom" means bases when acceleration occurs along the long axis of the body; if the astronaut is supine, "superior" or "ventral" and "inferior," "dependent" or "dorsal" regions are equivalent to "top" and "bottom.") This leads to ischemia of upper lung regions and to increased pressure, congestion and edema in the lower lung regions. The normal difference of 7.5 cm H_2O between intrapleural pressure at the top and bottom of the lung of erect man at 1G* becomes much greater (as much as −40 cm H_2O at the top and +40 cm at the bottom). This produces a marked exaggeration of the usual high $\dot{V}A/\dot{Q}c$ ratio at the top of the lung and of the usual low $\dot{V}A/\dot{Q}c$ ratio at the bottom. Alveolar ventilation at the top of the lung approaches dead space ventilation; blood flow at the bottom approaches venous-arterial shunting as congestion and edema cause airway collapse and trapped gas (measured by tests of "closing volume"). It also decreases diffusing capacity by about one third.

Up to 4–6 G the respiratory muscles have enough strength to lift the increased weight of the chest cage and to move the diaphragm and attached abdominal viscera. However, during acceleration, respiratory rate increases and tidal volume decreases. These changes are probably reflex in nature and of multiple origins, e.g., upper lungs are overdistended, lower lungs are collapsed, carotid sinus pressure is very low, the brain and carotid bodies are ischemic.

Once the space vehicle has attained a steady speed, there are no effects of acceleration; when it is no longer subject to the earth's gravitational field, there is no longer any effect of gravity on blood and tissues. This state of weightlessness should improve

matching of gas and blood in the lungs and bring it toward an "ideal" lung. However, the effects of prolonged weightlessness on reflex control and intrinsic autoregulation of smooth muscle in the systemic and pulmonary circulations and airway are not known, nor are the adjustments that may be required on return to earth.

Underwater Exploration

If a man walks into deeper and deeper water breathing air through a tube leading to the surface, he has more and more difficulty inspiring and, when his thorax is 4–5 feet below the surface, he can no longer draw air into his lungs. This is because his inspiratory muscles, by their maximal effort, can lower pressure by not more than 100 torr. His alveolar gas pressure is still atmospheric, but 4.5 feet of water is pushing on his thorax, opposing the action of his inspiratory muscles (4.5 feet of water is equal to à column of Hg 100 mm long). This example illustrates that except for very short periods and for very small pressure differences, air pressure in alveoli should be the same as the air or water pressure about the thorax. This must be true for a worker in a caisson (in which the air pressure must be raised to equal the surrounding water pressure to keep the water out), a diver in a suit or a diver using SCUBA (self-contained underwater breathing apparatus).

The problems encountered with high pressures and in changing from high to low pressures or vice versa have been discussed earlier in this chapter. Divers and underwater swimmers should read Lanphier's excellent review "Diving Medicine."

---

*G is the symbol for accelerative forces, a dimensionless expression for the ratio of gravitational or accelerative forces divided by the force of earth's gravity, symbolized by g.

Manifestations of Pulmonary Disease

THE PHYSICIAN has many ways to detect the presence of pulmonary disease, identify it and determine its extent and severity: by a skillful history, by a careful physical examination, by fluoroscopic, radiologic and angiographic studies, by physiologic tests and by bacteriologic, immunologic, histologic and biochemical studies. I shall discuss briefly here some of the manifestations of pulmonary disease that are due to altered function; in Chapter 21 is a discussion of the usefulness of pulmonary functions tests in identifying and evaluating cardiopulmonary-respiratory disorders.

HYPOXEMIA AND CARBON DIOXIDE RETENTION

Pulmonary insufficiency is usually defined as an inability of the lungs to maintain arterial blood gases at normal levels when the patient breathes air at sea level. On the basis of arterial blood gas studies, pulmonary insufficiency is sometimes subdivided into (1) insufficiency for oxygenation of mixed venous blood, (2) insufficiency for CO_2 removal and (3) insufficiency for both. Pulmonary insufficiency only for oxygenation always occurs in patients with pure impairment of diffusion (rarely a pure disorder) and may occur in patients with uneven matching of gas and blood and in patients with right-to-left pulmonary shunting of blood if they can still ventilate enough to eliminate CO_2. Pulmonary insufficiency for both occurs when there is hypo-

ventilation or when there is uneven matching of blood and gas in patients unable to increase their ventilation. Pulmonary insufficiency only for CO_2 removal occurs when the patient is hypoventilating but the hypoxemia is corrected by adding extra O_2 to the inspired air. Sometimes the clinical manifestations of hypoxemia, of CO_2 retention or of hypoxemia plus CO_2 retention provide important clues to diagnosis.

Hypoxemia

Acute hypoxemia increases respiratory frequency, tidal volume and minute volume in almost all subjects (Fig. 4-1); for the same hypoxemic stimulus chronic hypoxemia increases these even more (Fig. 5-5). When this increase in respiration is present and is promptly abolished by inhalation of O_2, it is of some diagnostic value, but the respiratory response to mild or moderate hypoxemia may be barely measurable or there may be none at all (Fig. 4-1).

The increase in heart rate associated with hypoxemia (Fig. 4-1) is a better index of the presence of hypoxemia. But so many other factors increase the pulse rate of patients (fever, low blood pressure, pain, apprehension, drugs) that it is difficult to assess the rather small changes in heart rate resulting from the moderate degree of hypoxemia encountered clinically. An O_2 test is again helpful; hypoxemia was probably present if the patient's pulse rate decreases by 10 or more beats per minute within a minute or two after beginning inhalation of O_2.

There are only a few observations of the effects of moderate hypoxemia on blood pressure in man; there is a tendency for systolic blood pressure to rise. However, the wide variations in response make measurements of arterial blood pressure of little value in the diagnosis of hypoxemia.

Many physicians regard cyanosis as the most characteristic clinical manifestation of hypoxemia. Cyanosis is a blueness of blood or tissues due to an increase in the amount of deoxyhemoglobin. Cyanosis is best recognized as the blueness of capillary blood seen through mucous membranes or skin, where capillaries are numerous and close together and the tissues over them are thin and transparent, as in the lips and nail beds.

There are numerous pitfalls in diagnosing arterial hypoxemia by blueness of the fingers or lips. In patients with severe anemia, because of insufficient coloring material (hemoglobin), it is difficult to detect blueness; the same is true of patients in shock because their surface vessels are constricted and contain little blood. In both anemia and shock, there is pallor rather than either a pink or blue color, and so severe or fatal tissue hypoxia may occur without the warning sign of cyanosis. Again, in two other types of grave tissue hypoxia, the skin and arterial blood may be of normal color or even be bright red; in cyanide poisoning, tissues are unable to utilize blood O_2 even though it is abundant, and in carbon monoxide poisoning, blood contains a bright red pigment, HbCO, which does not permit proper combination of O_2.

On the other hand, blueness of the skin may occur without arterial hypoxemia — especially when cutaneous arterioles are narrowed because of cold or certain nervous influences. In such cases, capillary blood flow continues but is so slow that much more O_2 is extracted from each unit of blood.

In those persons in whom cyanosis is present solely because of arterial hypoxemia, can one correlate the degree of cyanosis with the degree of hypoxemia? Lundsgaard and

Van Slyke concluded in 1923 that cyanosis is present when there is 5 gm or more of deoxyhemoglobin in 100 ml of capillary blood. Assuming that capillary blood is equivalent to an average of arteriolar and venular blood, this means under ordinary circumstances that cyanosis is discernible when the *arterial* blood is 80% saturated. This represents moderately severe hypoxemia; most patients with pulmonary disease have saturations in the range of 85–95%. But recognition of cyanosis also involves a subjective component of color perception, and this is neither so precise nor so consistent as spectrophotometric analysis of color. A nice demonstration of the variability in such perception can be done by giving subjects high, normal and low O_2 mixtures to breathe and checking observers' statements of "pink," "slight cyanosis" or "definite cyanosis" against continuously recorded arterial O_2 saturation (ear oximeter). In one such study, when the subjects' arterial O_2 saturations were in the range of 81–85%, 14% of the observations were "pink," 37% were "slight cyanosis" and 49% were "definite cyanosis"; there is also apt to be inconsistency on the part of a single observer watching the same subject pass through several cycles of severe, mild or no hypoxemia.

Other clinical manifestations of hypoxemia (see p. 46) also occur in other disorders so that, although they serve as clues, they are not really diagnostic of hypoxemia.

An event that occurs to compensate for hypoxemia may be useful in diagnosis. Most patients who are hypoxemic are polycythemic if they have not bled recently from any cause. In some patients with chronic pulmonary disease, the polycythemia is less severe than in dwellers at high altitudes; this may be due to the presence of chronic pulmonary infection, which depresses red blood cell formation. In any case, an increase to above normal in the red blood cell count or packed cell volume points to tissue hypoxia, which may be of cardiopulmonary origin, and this must be ruled out before a diagnosis is made of primary polycythemia or of polycythemia due to inadequate release of O_2 from HbO_2.

Carbon Dioxide Retention
(Hypercapnia; Hypercarbia)

This may occur because alveolar ventilation does not keep pace with body metabolism and CO_2 production because of uneven matching of gas and blood (without compensatory hyperventilation) or because the inspired air contains added CO_2. Our knowledge of the manifestations of hypercapnia (increased CO_2 concentration in arterial blood) comes largely from observing the acute effects during and immediately after inhalation of CO_2 by healthy men. When 42 young men breathed 7.6% CO_2 in air for 3 – 8 minutes, their respiratory rate increased to 28/minute, tidal volume to 2,100 ml, pulse rate by 17 beats/minute and blood pressure by 31/22 mm Hg; these are average values — individual variations were great. Of the 42, 13 experienced dyspnea; 9, dizziness; 8, sweating; 3, fullness in the head; 1, headache, and 1 became unconscious. Other symptoms noted were palpitation; mental clouding; dimness of vision; muscle tremor or twitching; "generally uncomfortable"; tingling, cold extremities; exhaustion, and mental depression. An additional 12 had headache immediately *after* the inhalation of 7.6% CO_2 was stopped (and only then), another 5 experienced dizziness then and some had an abrupt fall in diastolic blood pressure. When very high concentrations (25 – 30%) of CO_2 are inhaled, a curious mixture of unconsciousness, anesthesia and convulsions occurs.

This does not mean that these symptoms will occur when a patient with pulmonary insufficiency gradually retains CO_2 over a period of days or months; in his case (1) the blood and tissue CO_2 rises slowly and compensatory changes that counter severe acidosis have time to occur, (2) blood O_2 is low unless he is breathing O_2-enriched gas, (3) the mean P_{CO_2} in the airway is much lower and does not initiate irritant reflexes from the nose, mouth and air tubes and (4) there may be mechanical limitation to thoracic movement that prevents the hyperpnea. For example, an emphysematous patient, kept alive for more than a year by O_2 therapy, was mentally alert even when his arterial P_{CO_2} was 140 torr; such a level would surely produce unconsciousness if attained in a few minutes.

The respiratory effects of hypercapnia have already been discussed (p. 55). The circulatory effects of excess CO_2 are complex: (1) by a direct stimulant action on the vasomotor center (augmented by reflex stimulation from the carotid and aortic bodies), it increases cardiac rate and force of contraction and narrows vessels with a sympathetic vasoconstrictor innervation; (2) by a direct action on systemic arterioles, it dilates them. In conscious man, the first action predominates, and blood pressure and heart rate increase; when the vasomotor center is unable to respond (because of deep anesthesia, brain damage, severe ischemia or hypoxia) or is disconnected from the peripheral parts of the sympathetic nervous system (because of spinal anesthesia, spinal cord damage or blocking drugs), direct vasodilation is the only or dominant effect and blood pressure falls. Hypercapnia has additional effects on the heart. The heart may appear to be normal when the blood P_{CO_2} is high because it maintains a normal cardiac output and blood pressure. However, *sudden* reduction of blood CO_2 from very high levels leads to ventricular arrhythmias or even fatal ventricular fibrillation; presumably this indicates that there were changes in the ionic composition of heart muscle due to alterations in the mechanisms regulating ion transport.

Carbon dioxide excess dilates cerebral blood vessels and increases cerebral blood flow. Some patients with severe CO_2 retention have an increase in cerebrospinal fluid pressure and papilledema (edema of the retina surrounding the region of exit of the optic nerve), presumably due to the increased volume of blood within the near-rigid cranial cavity.

The effects of hypercapnia on the central nervous system represent a curious mixture of stimulation and depression—muscular twitching and convulsions occur along with unconsciousness and anesthesia.

Excess CO_2 of course tends to cause respiratory acidosis and decrease in pH of blood and tissues; pH need not change much if (HCO_3^-) and buffer base increase at the same time (p. 213).

In many patients with pulmonary insufficiency, hypoxia and hypercapnia occur together. Some patients with this combination complain of headache, somnolence, mental confusion, weakness, lassitude and irritability. As the condition becomes more severe, they may become unconscious, have depressed reflexes or even flaccid paralysis, tremors and convulsions. Occasionally, a patient with pulmonary insufficiency, hypoxemia and CO_2 retention will become comatose when treated with O_2. Because the inhalation of O_2 relieves the hypoxemia, removes the hypoxemic drive to breathing, depresses ventilation and permits further accumulation of CO_2 (see Table 4-3 p. 51), the coma is often called "CO_2 narcosis." Certainly it permits the dominant pattern of cortical depression to become evident, although it has not yet been proved that the concomitant rise in arterial P_{CO_2} (as opposed to the abrupt relief of hypoxemia and removal of hypoxemic reflex drive to the brain) is the immediate and sole cause of the coma (see p. 281).

We mentioned previously that the pH of CSF is maintained within narrow limits, either by changes in its P_{CO_2} (effected by changes in alveolar ventilation) or in its (HCO_3^-) (effected by active transport mechanisms). Marked decrease in the pH of CSF is often associated with coma, and such a change may be the cause of stupor and unconsciousness seen in patients with severe pulmonary insufficiency. Since such patients cannot increase their ventilation and since intravenous injection of bicarbonate changes pH of CSF only slowly, it is important to increase their ventilation mechanically to decrease promptly the P_{CO_2} in blood and CSF and increase the pH of CSF.

HYPERVENTILATION (HYPOCAPNIA; HYPOCARBIA)

Hyperventilation is defined as alveolar ventilation in excess of that needed to eliminate metabolically formed CO_2. Patients may *hyper*ventilate because of anxiety, certain types of injury or infection of the brain (p. 30), neurocirculatory asthenia (effort syndrome), fever, hypoxia, metabolic acidosis, pulmonary disease, improper use of a mechanical respirator or administration of certain drugs (epinephrine, progesterone, salicylates). Alveolar hyperventilation leads to "washing out" of CO_2 by causing a decrease in P_{CO_2} of alveolar gas, and then in arterial blood, tissues and venous blood. Unless (HCO_3^-) decreases simultaneously and sufficiently to maintain a normal HCO_3^- to CO_2 ratio, blood pH must rise and respiratory alkalosis occurs. Associated with moderate to severe alkalosis are a wide variety of symptoms. Some are nonspecific, such as fatigue, headache, irritability, inability to concentrate and lightheadedness. Others are highly characteristic of increased excitability of nerve and muscle; these include numbness and tingling of the hands, feet, mouth and tongue, stiffness, aches and cramps of muscles, actual spasms of hands and feet (carpopedal spasm) and twitching and convulsions. Two simple tests are used to demonstrate this hyperirritability: (1) when the facial nerve is tapped in front of the ear, the facial muscles about the mouth contract (Chvostek's sign) and (2) when the brachial artery is compressed for 1–5 minutes, muscles of the hand and wrist go into spasm (Trousseau's sign). All of these rather alarming changes can be reversed by stopping the hyperventilation or supplying 5% CO_2 in air to restore the blood and tissue P_{CO_2} to normal.

The increased excitability of nerve-muscle has been attributed to (1) a decrease in total plasma calcium due to the alkalosis, but this does not occur, (2) a decrease in ionized Ca^{2+}, due to increased capacity of plasma proteins to bind Ca^{2+}, but this is difficult to demonstrate, or (3) an alteration in the polarization of nerve and muscle cell membranes due to loss of intracellular potassium during alkalosis. When normal men hyperventilated for an hour (blood Pco_2 22 torr and pH 7.56), serum calcium, potassium, sodium and magnesium and blood sugar remained normal, but serum inorganic phosphate decreased to half of the control values.

Hyperventilation is also known to decrease cerebral blood flow because of the reduction in arterial Pco_2; the lightheadedness, convulsions and unconsciousness may be due in part to cerebral ischemia. Prolonged experimental hyperventilation may also be followed by irregular respiration, possibly because of cerebral ischemia.

DYSPNEA

Patients with cardiopulmonary disease often complain of "shortness of breath," "breathlessness," or of being "unable to get their breath"; the physician calls these complaints *dyspnea* (difficult breathing). Pulmonary disability (inability to work because of pulmonary disease) is usually due to dyspnea. Dyspnea cannot be measured objectively as can vital capacity or arterial Pco_2; like pain, it is subjective and can be identified and graded only by the patient.

It might be profitable to compare the symptom *dyspnea* with the symptom *pain.* Pain can be characterized by an instructive variety of terms, such as stabbing, throbbing, aching, burning, oppressive or bursting. However, the patient's description of respiratory distress is channeled by most physicians into the term "dyspnea." More precise recording of the patient's own characterization of his difficulties in breathing might lead to better correlation of these with mechanisms responsible for dyspnea. Is the respiratory discomfort experienced in acute respiratory obstruction, chronic emphysema, congestive heart failure, pulmonary embo-

lism, acute neuromuscular paralysis, anemia, acidosis, neurocirculatory asthenia or pulmonary fibrosis really identical in each? How much of the distress is pain, how much is fatigue or exhaustion, how much muscular aching and how much is apprehension or fear?

Experimentally, one can induce respiratory distress by (1) requiring subjects to breathe against added inspiratory or expiratory resistance, (2) requiring subjects to breathe in and out of closed rigid containers, without added resistance to air flow, (3) strapping the thorax so that the subjects must breathe from near-residual volume, (4) adding CO_2 to inspired gas to produce increased ventilation, (5) asking subjects to hold their breath to the limit of tolerance or (6) requiring subjects to exercise to near their limit of tolerance. The symptoms experienced may be different in these different situations (ranging from simple awareness of increased breathing or a satisfying sensation of deep breathing, to a sense of suffocation). And the sensations induced in acute experiments may not be those experienced by patients with different acute and chronic disorders.

If we agree that dyspnea is a symptom just as pain is a symptom, there must be a neuroanatomic basis for it. As with pain, there may be only a central basis or there may be both peripheral and central components. Therefore, we must look for the sensory receptors, sensory pathways and thalamic or cortical centers that are responsible for the perception of respiratory discomfort and for the reaction to these unpleasant stimuli. Again, just as some patients have little pain (minimal sensory stimulation) but suffer greatly (maximal central response), or have much pain and suffer little, similarly some patients might have little respiratory difficulty and much dyspnea, or much respiratory difficulty and little dyspnea.

What and where are the sensory *receptors* that initiate afferent impulses leading to dyspnea? Are they the same mechanoreceptors or chemoreceptors involved in the normal processes of breathing—those that regulate the rate and depth of respiration? Is dyspnea caused by a barrage of impulses from these directed to the medullary respiratory center which, when in excess, spill over into the areas of consciousness? Is it caused by the activation of special receptors, not normally tonically active, which send impulses directly to the centers of consciousness and not primarily to the respiratory center? Or is it caused by a change in the pattern of impulses—too few of some, too many of others or an asynchrony of several (cf. dysesthesia)? Are these receptors located in the tissues surrounding the airway, the alveoli, the pulmonary circulation, the pulmonary parenchyma, the pleura, the bones, joints or ligaments of the thoracic cage or the muscles of respiration? Are they receptors for touch, change in temperature, in pressure or tension, in stretch, distention, volume or position or in chemical composition? Do their afferent fibers run centrally in the vagi, in the sympathetic nerves or in the somatic nerves?

One theory proposes that dyspnea, like the limb pain of patients with partially occluded arteries during walking or the substernal pain of patients with obstructed coronary arteries, occurs when the work of the exercising muscle is great relative to the flow of oxygenated blood through capillary beds; as a result, chemical products of metabolism accumulate to a level that excites sensory nerve endings in muscle, thus producing dyspnea.

Another is that of George Wright, who proposed that breathlessness may be caused by undue intensity and prolongation of the discharge of the medullary inspiratory neurons. The intensity could result from unusually strong, continuous stimuli bombarding the center and the prolongation from abnormally weak inhibitory impulses from stretch receptors in the lungs that normally interrupt the inspiratory neurons rhythmically. Breath holding in full inspiration or expiration does not lead to immediate dyspnea, so dyspnea is not caused simply by an extreme inflation or deflation of the thorax or lungs. However, breath holding extended to

the breaking point causes unpleasant respiratory distress that is relieved promptly by a deep inspiration even when the gas inhaled is N_2 or 7.4% CO_2 in air. The same is true of exercising patients with mechanical limitation to full inspiration induced by strapping of the thorax; their dyspnea is also relieved by full inspiration. This concept implies that continuous excitation of the inspiratory center ultimately showers the centers of consciousness with impulses that cause dyspnea.

Campbell and Howell developed an intriguing concept of the neural basis of dyspnea. They believe that an unpleasant sensation of breathlessness arises when there is a state of inappropriateness in the neural pathways subserving the respiratory act. Initially, they expressed this as "length:tension inappropriateness" because in studies of the sensation induced by mechanically hindering the breathing they found an unpleasant sensation was induced when the pressure (tension) required to cause a given tidal volume (change in length) was increased. It is obvious from what has been said before that the alpha and gamma systems may be involved in such a sensation, but it is unlikely that the sensation as such arises simply in the muscle spindles whose afferent discharge has often been shown not to relay directly to consciousness. At present, the precise neurophysiologic basis of this sensation cannot be stated with any confidence. Campbell and Howell have expanded the basis of their theory and suggest that dyspnea may be experienced (1) if the neurochemical demand for breathing is *inappropriate* to the apparent needs (as at altitude), (2) if the neuromuscular effort of breathing is *inappropriate* to the breathing that is achieved (as in asthma), (3) if the neural effort is *inappropriate* to the muscular act that is achieved (as in muscular paralysis). These relations are sensed unconsciously; when there is a certain level of inappropriateness, the sensation reaches consciousness, and when this level is excessive, it causes distress.

There are several ways to gain more information to test theories of the origin of dyspnea, but because only conscious man can complain of dyspnea, he must be the subject of the study. For example, anesthetists can inject a local anesthetic agent to block his vagus nerves; if he can still experience dyspnea, obviously mechanisms must be involved other than (or in addition to) those requiring the lungs. Guz and associates found that bilateral vagal block permitted longer periods of breath holding and lessened distress from it; it also abolished the unpleasant sensation ("can't get enough air") associated with inhalation of increased concentration of CO_2. However, it did not change the perception of increased airway resistance or decreased compliance. In patients with dyspnea associated with different types of cardiopulmonary disease, bilateral vagal block had no effect on some (patients with chronic bronchitis and emphysema or with a rigid chest wall) but slowed the frequency of breathing and decreased dyspnea in others (including patients with pulmonary fibrosis, left ventricular failure, pulmonary vascular obstruction and asthma). In some patients in whom bilateral temporary block decreased dyspnea, surgical section of one vagus nerve produced similar effects for longer periods. Relief from unilateral section could be explained by the fact that it eliminates spatial summation or potentiation of afferent impulses; it is well known that simultaneous stimulation of two afferent nerves whose impulses impinge on the same central neurons may produce a response even though stimulation of each singly produces none. From his studies on the role of the vagi in transmitting the sensation of dyspnea, Guz concluded that dyspnea can be experienced in the absence of vagal impulses but that impulses in some fibers (possibly small, nonmyelinated afferents) do contribute to this distressing symptom.

Investigators have also examined the role of afferent impulses from the chest wall and diaphragm. These travel upward in the spinal cord and can be blocked by spinal anesthesia. Such impulses are of course also prevented from reaching the brain in patients unfortunate enough to have a complete transection of the cervical spinal cord. If the block or transection is below the fourth or fifth cervical segment, none of the respiratory muscles except the diaphragm receives motor impulses; if above the fourth segment, no motor impulses can reach either the intercostal muscles or the diaphragm, and the patient requires artificial ventilation. Physicians have also studied patients whose respiratory muscles are completely paralyzed as a result of poliomyelitis and volunteers paralyzed by injections of neuromuscular blocking agents; neither of these conditions blocks ordinary sensation. Finally, both phrenic nerves have been blocked to paralyze the diaphragm without affecting movements of the thoracic cage or blocking afferent impulses from respiratory muscles or lungs.

The results of these studies suggest that (1) sensations that permit detection of abnormal resistance and compliance are still present after any one or several of these blocks and these probably arise from unblocked regions, i.e., the upper respiratory tract, (2) the unpleasant sensations of prolonged breath holding are lessened or abolished by respiratory muscle block (phrenic nerve block, poliomyelitis, neuromuscular blocking agents and transection of the spinal cord high enough to paralyze all respiratory muscles including the diaphragm), and these must arise at least in large part from respiratory muscles, and (3) the sensations associated with the hyperpnea of CO_2 inhalation are abolished by vagal block alone (and not by sensory block of the chest wall alone), and therefore depend on impulses traveling up the vagi during the hyperpnea.

COUGH

This is discussed on page 230.

CLUBBING OF THE FINGERS

A clublike enlargement of the ends of the fingers and toes accompanies some types of chronic pulmonary disease. It may occur in patients with pulmonary infection (lung abscess, infected bronchiectasis and tuberculosis), with bronchogenic cancer or with pulmonary arteriovenous anastomoses. Blood flow increases to the affected fingers and toes, and the soft tissues swell with an increase in the amount of connective tissues. Pulmonary disease may also be accompanied by hypertrophic osteoarthropathy: the wrists and ankles become red, swollen and painful; the periosteum of the distal ends of the long bones of the forearms and legs (less often of the metacarpals and phalanges) is thickened, and new bone is laid down. Patients with pulmonary disease may have clubbed fingers and toes or pulmonary osteoarthropathy or both.

The origin of these manifestations is a mystery. Clubbing is not necessarily related to pulmonary insufficiency (hypoxemia or hypercapnia or both), to the presence of venous-to-arterial shunts or to pulmonary infections, because it can occur in bronchogenic cancer when none of these is present. Flavell reported in 1956 that cutting all of the pulmonary branches of the vagus nerves on the side of unilateral carcinoma in 5 patients led promptly to cessation of the joint pain and to disappearance of joint swelling and clubbing of the fingertips. Presumably, receptors in the lung, activated by unknown stimuli, sent afferent impulses over the vagi, which by unknown paths and mechanisms produced changes in the extremities. The "purpose" of this is not clear, but a solution of the problem may reveal unknown facets of the functions of the lungs. Others have suggested that normal lungs remove vasodilator materials from mixed venous blood and that pulmonary artery-to-vein shunts exist in abnormal lungs that permit these substances to enter the systemic arterial blood; why these, if present, should lead to clubbing or to osteoarthropathy is uncertain.

PAIN

Mechanical or chemical stimulation of the tracheobronchial tree causes a sensation of irritation and cough. Greatly increased or hindered breathing causes dyspnea. When does *pain* result from the lung? The lung has a rich supply of nerve endings—many of them sensory—but few of these cause pain when stimulated. The lung tissue itself and its outer lining (the visceral pleura) are insensitive to stimuli that, applied to the skin, cause pain. The parietal pleura (the lining of the thoracic cage) is richly supplied with pain fibers; that lining the bony cage is supplied by the intercostal nerves, and that covering the upper surface of the diaphragm receives pain fibers from the phrenic nerve and the lower six pairs of intercostal nerves. Chemical or mechanical irritation of the parietal pleura lining the bony cage produces pain that is sharply localized to the area affected; this is the typical pain of pleurisy that becomes severe with deep breathing and leads to voluntary or involuntary limitation of breathing. Stimulation of the pain receptors of the diaphragm does not cause pain localized to the diaphragm; instead pain is referred to cutaneous areas supplied by the spinal cord segment into which sensory impulses flow from the diaphragm. Irritation of the dome and central portion of the diaphragm sends impulses up the phrenic nerves, and pain is referred to the neck and shoulder. Irritation of the outer portions of the diaphragm causes impulses to flow into the lower intercostal nerves, and pain is referred to the skin of the abdominal wall or lower thorax.

Electrical stimulation of the posterior wall of the lower trachea produces pain that is referred to the front of the chest in the midline (substernal). Stimulation of the posterior wall of a right or left main bronchus produces pain in the homolateral anterior chest within 2–4 cm of the midline or in the anterior neck within 2 cm of the midline. Impulses are usually carried in afferent vagal fibers on the side stimulated; occasionally they flow into the other vagus nerve.

These observations suggest that disease of the lung and respiratory tract produces localized or referred pain only when receptors in the parietal pleura or tracheobronchial tree are stimulated. However, they do not explain pain observed in some patients with pulmonary hypertension (without coronary insufficiency) or pulmonary embolism or following injections of chemicals (such as lobeline) into the pulmonary circulation; clearly, we need more information on the various sensory nerve endings in the lungs and pulmonary circulation.

POLYCYTHEMIA

This is discussed on page 251.

BLEEDING (HEMOPTYSIS)

Not all blood coughed up by a patient comes from the lungs; it may have originated in the mouth, nose, pharynx or even the esophagus or stomach. Bleeding definitely of pulmonary origin may be due to disease of the heart or lungs. Narrowing of the mitral valve (mitral stenosis) may so increase resistance to flow of blood into the left ventricle that blood pressure rises in the left atrium, pulmonary veins and pulmonary venules; it may also rise in bronchial veins that drain into the pulmonary veins. Any of these small vessels may rupture and lead to hemoptysis. Occlusion of a pulmonary artery may lead to ischemia of the pulmonary capillary walls, leakage of blood and hemoptysis. A high pressure in pulmonary veins due to direct artery-to-vein communications may also lead to rupture. Sometimes infectious processes or tumors of the lung or airway erode through the walls of pulmonary or bronchial arteries, arterioles or venules and cause hemorrhage and hemoptysis.

Physiologic Diagnosis

PULMONARY PHYSIOLOGISTS have developed a large number of tests to aid them in better understanding of the functions of the lungs and to aid physicians in the qualitative and quantitative evaluation of function in patients with suspected abnormalities of the heart, lungs and respiration. As a result, hospital "cardiac catheterization" laboratories have changed in name and purpose to become "cardiopulmonary function" laboratories, a large number of separate pulmonary function laboratories have sprung up, and many physicians now use some of the simpler tests in their own offices. This is a remarkable illustration of how new physiologic knowledge has been applied almost immediately to clinical medicine. In many cases this has led to earlier and more precise diagnosis, more objective evaluation of therapy and better guides to prognosis. The new tests have also led to a better understanding of the pathologic physiology and natural course of pulmonary disease. They have aided in the early detection of pulmonary dysfunction in some patients considered to be normal on the basis of clinical and radiologic examination and have assisted in differential diagnosis in patients with known disease in whom a specific diagnosis could not be made with certainty by other methods. They have been invaluable in securing physical, measurable data in patients who may or may not have pulmonary disability, and in determining, during the life of the patient, the specific func-

tion of the lung that has been impaired.

The introduction of physiologic tests does not mean that these have supplanted other diagnostic procedures. Physiologic tests indicate only how disease has altered *function*; they cannot make an anatomic, a bacteriologic or a pathologic diagnosis. For example, function tests may reveal the existence of a right-to-left shunt but, except for a few very elaborate tests, cannot locate it anatomically as being intracardiac or intrapulmonic. Again, physiologic tests may indicate that there is impairment of diffusion across the alveolocapillary membranes but cannot differentiate interstitial edema from intra-alveolar edema or determine whether the intra-alveolar fluid is exudate or transudate. Furthermore, they do not reveal alterations in all types of pulmonary disease but only in those that disturb function and disturb it sufficiently that present tests can recognize with certainty the deviation from normal values. In general, present tests cannot detect slight reduction in functioning pulmonary tissue or the presence of small regions in the lungs that have neither ventilation nor blood flow. Results of physiologic tests will be normal in the presence of lesions such as fibrotic tuberculous cavities, cysts or carcinomatous nodules, unless these lesions occupy so much space that they reduce the lung volume well below normal limits or are located so strategically that they disturb pulmonary function. Pulmonary function studies will not tell *where* the lesion is, *what* the lesion is or even that a lesion exists, if it does not interfere with the function of the lung. Therefore, they supplement and do not replace a good history and physical examination or radiologic, bacteriologic, bronchoscopic and pathologic studies.

A number of monographs have been written recently on the technics of using these tests and interpretation of the data obtained. In this chapter, I shall mention only general principles. First, there are many tests and many variations of each (some of these are discussed in Chapters 2 and 10 to 14). One cannot say that one variant is superior to another. It *is* important to be able, when necessary, to measure each of the components of pulmonary function by some reasonably reliable test. Table 21-1 shows that many tests are available to measure (1) lung volumes, (2) volume and distribution of pulmonary ventilation, (3) pressure, flow, and resistance in the pulmonary circulation and the uniformity of distribution of blood flow, (4) alveolocapillary diffusion, (5) the end results of pulmonary gas exchange—i.e., arterial O_2, CO_2 and pH, and (6) the overall mechanical properties of the lungs and thorax and each individual component. Sometimes the physician can obtain all of the information needed from simple tests that can be used in his own office or small clinic (column A); sometimes he must refer his patient to a cardiopulmonary laboratory for the tests listed in column B, and when the problem is very difficult, new research procedures (column C) will be required for a well-documented diagnosis. It is best to start with the simple tests, which, as a rule, are also the least expensive.

Second, normal typical values have been established; some are given in Table 21-2. However, these values do not apply to the newborn (Table 21-3), to children or older patients, to smaller or larger men or to women; special formulas or tables should be consulted for these. Further, values often differ considerably in individual members even of a homogeneous group of healthy men or women (by as much as $\pm 20\%$ of the mean).

Third, an abnormality in a single test rarely points with certainty to a specific disease. Physiologic tests do not really diagnose *diseases;* they diagnose abnormalities in *function*. They can place the disorder in one of a number of patterns, and the physician can then determine the specific disease. Some of the patterns that have been described are: (1) aging, (2) hypoventilation, (3) diffuse obstruction of small airways, (4) impaired diffusion, (5) restriction, (6) left-to-right shunt, (7) uneven pulmonary capillary blood flow, (8) pulmonary vascular congestion, (9) precapillary obstruction in pulmonary circulation.

If, for example, the pattern is that of diffuse obstruction of small airways, the physician knows that his patient probably has bronchial asthma, emphysema or bronchitis. He can then make a specific diagnosis of asthma if the pattern returns to normal after he has given the patient thorough antiasthmatic, bronchodilator therapy. But, to give a second example, if the pattern is that of hypoventilation, it may be due to (1) depression of respiratory centers by general anesthesia, excessive doses of morphine or barbiturates, cerebral trauma, increased intracranial pressure, prolonged hypoxia or cerebral ischemia, high concentration of CO_2 or electric shock, (2) interference with neural conduction or with neuromuscular transmission to the respiratory muscles by traumatic spinal cord lesions, infections such as poliomyelitis, peripheral neuritis, or neuromuscular block produced by curare, decamethonium, succinylcholine, nerve gases, myasthenia gravis, botulinus or nicotine poisoning, (3) diseases of respiratory muscles, (4) limitation of movement of thorax by arthritis, scleroderma, emphysema, thoracic deformity or elevation of the diaphragm, (5) limitation of movement of lungs by pleural effusion or pneumothorax, or (6) pulmonary diseases associated with decrease in functioning lung tissue caused by disorders such as atelectasis, tumor or pneumonia; de-

TABLE 21-1.—CLASSIFICATION OF TESTS OF PULMONARY FUNCTION*,†

For Measurement of	Procedures Used in:		
	A. Office, Clinic or Small Hospital	B. Cardiopulmonary Laboratory in Medical Center	C. Research Cardiopulmonary Laboratory
1. Lung volumes	Vital capacity, inspiratory capacity, expiratory reserve volume	Residual volume, functional residual capacity, total lung capacity, RV/TLC ratio. Thoracic gas volume (body plethysmograph)	X-ray planimetry
2. Pulmonary ventilation *a)* Volume	Clinical and fluoroscopic analysis of physical basis for hypoventilation. Spirometric measurement of rate, tidal volume and minute volume; calculation of alveolar ventilation based on above measurements and estimated anatomic dead space	Alveolar or arterial blood P_{CO_2}. Ventilatory response to inhaled $5-10\%$ CO_2 in air	Alveolar ventilation calculated from *measured* anatomic dead space. Low O_2 response curve. CO_2 response curve. pH and $[HCO_3^-]$ of spinal fluid. Alveolar P_{O_2}, using rapid O_2 electrode. Response to exercise (breathing air vs. O_2)
b) Distribution	Clinical and radiologic examination for uneven expansion of lungs and uneven air flow (uneven breath sounds, percussion notes, chest expansion; uneven radiolucence seen fluoroscopically)	Single-breath N_2 meter test. Pulmonary N_2 elimination rate. Volume of trapped gas (body plethysmograph)	Inhalation of radioactive xenon to determine regional pattern. Measurement of "closing volume"; bolus method using ^{85}Kr or SF_6. FEV_1 roentgenograms
3. Pulmonary circulation *a)* Changes in pressure, flow, resistance or volume	Clinical, ECG and radiologic examination for evidence of pulmonary hypertension or congestion; circulation times (?)	Cardiac catheterization and measurement of pressure, flow, resistance and O_2 content at selected points between venae cavae and pulmonary artery. Injection of acetylcholine or similar vasodilator drug to determine reversibility of increased vascular resistance	Pulmonary capillary blood volume (CO method). Pulmonary capillary blood flow (N_2O uptake) at rest and during exercise. Magnification angiography. Pulmonary artery pressure during exercise or during unilateral pulmonary artery occlusion

FOR MEASUREMENT OF	A. OFFICE, CLINIC OR SMALL HOSPITAL	PROCEDURES USED IN: B. CARDIOPULMONARY LABORATORY IN MEDICAL CENTER	C. RESEARCH CARDIO-PULMONARY LABORATORY
b) Distribution	Radiologic examination for evidence of nonuniform pulmonary vascular markings; listening for bruits	Lung scanning after injection of ^{131}I macro-aggregated albumin. Selective pulmonary angiography. Broncho-spirometry (O_2 consumption of right vs. left lung). Arterial blood – mixed expired alveolar gas CO_2 tension difference. Arterial O_2 tension during inhalation of O_2	Location of ^{133}Xe (by scintillation camera) after intravenous injection. "Alveolar" dead space. Measurement of shunts using H_2, He or ^{85}Kr. Bronchial arterial angiogram. Bronchial arterial blood flow
4. Alveolocapillary diffusion	No specific test, but can suspect diagnosis on clinical and radiologic evidence	Diffusing capacity (CO). Arterial O_2 saturation during exercise and during inhalation of O_2 (not specific)	Membrane-diffusing capacity (CO). Erythrocyte "resistance" (CO). Maximal diffusing capacity (exercise). Pulmonary diffusing capacity for O_2
5. Arterial O_2, CO_2 and pH	Look for cyanosis. Packed cell volume and RBC/mm^3 (not specific). Measure change in respiration and pulse rate during inhalation of O_2	Arterial P_{O_2} and P_{CO_2} using electrodes. Arterial O_2 content, capacity and saturation; arterial CO_2 content and tension; pH. Base excess	Spectrophotometric analysis for abnormal Hb. P_{50} for Hb + O_2. Complete Hb + O_2 association curve. Concentration of 2-3 diphosphoglycerate in erythrocytes
6. Mechanical factors in breathing	Maximal expiratory flow rates; spirogram; FEV_1 (all tests performed before and after administration of bronchodilator drugs)	Pulmonary compliance. Total pulmonary resistance. Maximal inspiratory and expiratory pressures (oral and esophageal). Flow-volume curve. Airway resistance (body plethysmograph)	Pressure-volume, resistance-volume. resistance-pressure, and flow-pressure curves. Airway resistance by forced oscillation technic. "Dynamic compliance." Pulmonary tissue resistance. Compliance of thoracic cage. Fiberoptic bronchoscopy. Tantalum bronchoscopy

*Modified from Comroe, J. H., Jr., *et al.*: *The Lung* (2d ed.; Chicago: Year Book Medical Publishers, Inc., 1962).

†Clinical history, physical findings and radiologic evidence are only mentioned here; they may be of considerable importance in identifying physiologic disturbances, but have been described in great detail in many other books and monographs.

TABLE 21-2.—TYPICAL VALUES FOR PULMONARY FUNCTION TESTS*

These are values for a healthy, resting, recumbent young male (1.7 m² surface area) breathing air at sea level, unless other conditions are specified. They are presented merely to give approximate figures. These values may change with position, age, size, sex and altitude; there is variability among members of a homogeneous group under standard conditions.

LUNG VOLUMES

Inspiratory capacity, ml	3,600
Expiratory reserve volume, ml	1,200
Vital capacity, ml	4,800
Residual volume (RV), ml	1,200
Functional residual capacity, ml	2,400
Thoracic gas volume, ml	2,400
Total lung capacity (TLC), ml	6,000
$RV/TLC \times 100$, %	20

VENTILATION

Tidal volume, ml	500
Frequency, respirations/min	12
Minute volume, ml/min	6,000
Respiratory dead space, ml	150
Alveolar ventilation, ml/min	4,200

DISTRIBUTION OF INSPIRED GAS

Single-breath test (% increase N_2 for 500 ml expired alveolar gas), % N_2	< 1.5
Pulmonary nitrogen emptying rate (7 min test), % N_2	< 2.5
Helium closed-circuit (mixing efficiency related to perfect mixing), %	76

ALVEOLAR VENTILATION/PULMONARY CAPILLARY BLOOD FLOW

Alveolar ventilation (L/min)/blood flow, (L/min)	0.8
(Physiologic shunt/cardiac output) $\times$ 100, %	< 7
(Physiologic dead space/tidal volume) $\times$ 100, %	<30

PULMONARY CIRCULATION

Pulmonary capillary blood flow, ml/min	5,400
Pulmonary artery pressure, mm Hg	24/9
Pulmonary capillary blood volume, ml	75 – 100
Pulmonary "capillary" blood pressure (wedge), mm Hg	8

ALVEOLAR GAS

Oxygen partial pressure, torr	104
CO_2 partial pressure, torr	40

DIFFUSION AND GAS EXCHANGE

O_2 consumption (STPD), ml/min	240
CO_2 output (STPD), ml/min	192
Respiratory exchange ratio, R (CO_2 output/O_2 uptake)	0.8
Diffusing capacity, O_2 (STPD) resting, ml O_2/min/torr	>15
Diffusing capacity, CO (steady state) (STPD) resting, ml CO/min/torr	17
Diffusing capacity, CO (single-breath) (STPD) resting, ml CO/min/torr	25
Diffusing capacity, CO (rebreathing) (STPD) resting, ml CO/min/torr	25

ARTERIAL BLOOD

O_2 saturation (% saturation of Hb with O_2), %	97.1
O_2 tension, torr	100
CO_2 tension, torr	40
Alveolar-arterial P_{O_2} difference (100% O_2), torr	33
O_2 saturation (100% O_2), %	100
O_2 tension (100% O_2), torr	640
pH	7.4

MECHANICS OF BREATHING

Maximal voluntary ventilation, L/min	125 – 170
Forced expiratory volume, % in 1 sec	83
% in 3 sec	97
Maximal expiratory flow rate (for 1 L), L/min	400
Maximal inspiratory flow rate (for 1 L), L/min	300
Compliance of lungs and thoracic cage, L/cm H_2O	0.1
Compliance of lungs, L/cm H_2O	0.2
Airway resistance, cm H_2O/L/sec	1.6
Work of quiet breathing, kgM/min	0.5
Maximal work of breathing, kgM/breath	10
Maximal inspiratory and expiratory pressures, mm Hg	60 – 100

*From Comroe, J. H., Jr., et al.: The Lung (2d ed.; Chicago: Year Book Medical Publishers, Inc., 1962).

TABLE 21-3.— APPROXIMATE VALUES FOR
PULMONARY FUNCTION IN A 3-KG
NEWBORN BABY

Vital capacity (vigorous cry)	120 ml
Functional residual capacity	80 ml
Total lung capacity	160 ml
Residual volume	40 ml
Tidal volume	16 ml
Anatomic dead space	7 ml
Frequency of breathing	40/min
Minute volume of breathing	640 ml/min
Alveolar ventilation	360 ml/min
Pulmonary compliance	0.006 L/cm H_2O
Pulmonary compliance/FRC	0.07 L/cm H_2O/L
Airway resistance	18 cm H_2O/L/sec
*Arterial O_2 saturation	88 – 100%
*Arterial Pco_2	34 – 40 torr
*Arterial pH	7.30 – 7.40 units
Arterial hemoglobin	17.6 gm/100 ml

*Varies during the first day of life, depending on time and completeness of closure of venous-to-arterial shunts (foramen ovale and ductus arteriosus) and opening of all alveoli.

creased distensibility of lung tissue as in restrictive disease and congestion, or obstruction lesions in the upper or lower respiratory tract.

Fourth, it is now obvious that only certain patients have a single, "pure" pattern. For example, one hypoventilating patient may have a depressed medullary respiratory center and nothing else, but a second patient may be hypoventilating because his airways are severely obstructed. Again, impaired diffusion may rarely be the sole abnormality but more often is part of severe emphysema that has disrupted the normal alveolar structure and decreased the alveolar surface area in contact with blood flowing through alveolar capillaries.

Artificial Respiration and Inhalation Therapy

ARTIFICIAL RESPIRATION

WHEN A PATIENT stops breathing or is breathing inadequately, the physician must do many things almost at once. He must ventilate the patient's lungs by emergency methods (and place a call for special apparatus in the event that a long period of artificial or assisted ventilation is needed). He must be sure the air reaches the alveoli and that blood is flowing through the alveolar capillaries. And he must determine the cause of the apnea or hypoventilation and correct it as soon and as completely as he can. Apnea or severe hypoventilation may occur when the respiratory muscles fail to receive the proper signals from the brain, when they do not respond to these or when they are not powerful enough to achieve adequate ventilation because of increased resistance or decreased compliance of the lungs or thorax.

Recently, a term "respiratory failure" has been used widely to designate any condition in which a patient is not breathing enough, no matter what the cause. For several decades a more definitive term "pulmonary insufficiency" (or "pulmonary failure") has been used specifically to describe the condition of patients whose *diseased lungs or thorax, or both*, prevented adequate ventilation despite normal neuromuscular mechanisms, and the definitive term "respiratory failure" has been reserved spe-

cifically for patients whose lungs and thorax were normal (at least initially) but suffered primarily from *depression or disorders of central or peripheral neuromuscular structures*. It seems preferable to retain the more precise and definitive older terms since specific, precise labels are more apt to lead to precise treatment.

When there is complete respiratory or pulmonary failure and complete asphyxia, irreversible brain damage usually occurs after 5 minutes except in the newborn. Therefore, in treating apnea the method that can provide ventilation immediately is the method of choice. Speed is also essential in starting a stopped heart or correcting serious hypotension if there are cardiovascular as well as respiratory problems. Well-oxygenated blood sitting in the pulmonary capillaries does not help the patient; the blood must be moved to the left ventricle and through the coronary and cerebral capillary beds to be effective in resuscitation. Closed-chest cardiac massage can move blood around the circulation until electrical defibrillation or pacing can re-establish cardiac contractions.

All methods of resuscitation fail if the airway is obstructed. Immediate attention should be given to relieving the obstruction. Airway obstruction is common in the unconscious apneic patient because of relaxation of soft tissues of the pharynx, falling back of the tongue or blocking of airways by mucus or vomitus. When respiratory obstruction is complete or almost complete, the physician must be prepared to institute adequate therapy, no matter how drastic it may seem. A plastic oropharyngeal airway may be all that is needed, but if the obstruction is in the larynx, tracheotomy is necessary. In addition to its usefulness for bypassing laryngeal obstruction, tracheotomy permits frequent and efficient aspiration of the airway. For example, a patient who is unconscious or whose respiratory muscles are paralyzed cannot cough, but his glands may continue to secrete mucus so that obstruction and infection are likely; if such a patient cannot swallow properly, tracheotomy may prevent fatal inhalation of food.

A tracheotomy does pose new problems: it is harder for the patient to cough effectively, and the tube bypasses normal mechanisms for warming, filtering and humidifying inspired air. But the air can be passed through humidifiers, and an attendant can aspirate secretions regularly from the bronchial tree while the tracheotomy tube is in place.

The opening in the skin and trachea heals promptly when the tube is removed.

Manual Methods

Two methods require little or no apparatus and can be started at once; these are the manual methods and mouth-to-mouth ventilation. Most manual methods can produce adequate pulmonary ventilation in a healthy subject who has voluntarily suspended his breathing, but some are totally inadequate in apneic patients in actual need of artificial respiration. Most of these patients have mechanical problems in breathing and require an additional inflating force to produce adequate tidal volume; in addition, they are unconscious and may have upper airway obstruction. The Schafer method has now been abandoned for several reasons. (1) The patient is prone. (Many students cannot remember which is the *prone* and which the *supine* position; the patient is *supine* when he lies on his *s(u)pine.*) The operator first pushes air out of the lungs by pressure on the rib cage; when he releases this pressure, the thorax and lungs recoil to their original resting volume. The maximal tidal volume obtainable with this technic is the expiratory reserve volume; this is much smaller, even in normal persons, than the inspiratory capacity. (2) The expiratory reserve volume in the prone position is smaller than normal because the weight of the body forces the diaphragm up and compresses the rib cage; it may be even less because of pre-existing disease or obstruction of some of the air passages. (3) The pressure-volume curve of the lungs and thorax is such that more pressure is required to move 500 ml of the expiratory reserve volume than 500 ml of the inspiratory capacity.

The arm-lift back-pressure (Holger-Nielsen) and the Silvester methods (Fig. 22-1) provide better ventilation because they include a phase in which the thorax is expanded actively ("pulled") into the inspira-

Fig. 22-1.—Respiratory level and tidal volume during artificial ventilation by different methods. The tracing at the *left* shows normal tidal volume, vital capacity, inspiratory capacity and expiratory reserve volume; the *horizontal line* represents the normal resting expiratory level.

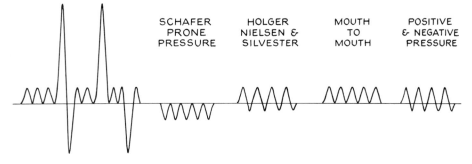

SCHAFER
PRONE
PRESSURE

HOLGER
NIELSEN &
SILVESTER

MOUTH
TO
MOUTH

POSITIVE
& NEGATIVE
PRESSURE

tory capacity range as well as compressed by manual pressure; they are "push-pull" methods instead of just "push" (Fig. 22-1). The Silvester method has the disadvantage that the patient is supine, and this position favors airway obstruction; however, there may also be serious mechanical obstruction of the airway when the Holger-Nielsen prone method is used, because of the position of the head.

Mouth-to-Mouth Method

The mouth-to-mouth method (Table 22-1) is now the method of choice for immediate, short-term artificial ventilation because: (1)

TABLE 22-1.— INSTRUCTIONS FOR MOUTH-TO-MOUTH (MOUTH-TO-NOSE) METHOD OF ARTIFICIAL RESPIRATION*

If foreign matter is visible in the mouth, wipe it out quickly with your fingers or a cloth wrapped around them.

1. Tilt the patient's head back so the chin is pointing upward. Pull or push the jaw into a jutting-out position. These maneuvers should relieve obstruction of the airway by moving the base of the tongue away from the back of the throat.
2. Open your mouth wide and place it tightly over the victim's mouth. At the same time pinch the victim's nostrils shut or close the nostrils with your cheek. Or close the victim's mouth and place your mouth over the nose. Blow into the victim's mouth or nose. (Air may be blown through the victim's teeth, even though they may be clenched.) The first blowing efforts should determine whether or not obstruction exists.
3. Remove your mouth, turn your head to the side, and listen for the return rush of air that indicates air movement. Repeat the blowing effort.
   For an adult, blow vigorously at the rate of about 12 breaths/minute. For a child, use relatively shallow breaths appropriate for the child's size, at the rate of about 20/minute.
4. If you are not getting air movement, check the head and jaw position. If you still do not get air movement, quickly turn the victim on his side and administer several sharp blows between the shoulder blades in the hope of dislodging foreign matter. Again sweep your fingers through the victim's mouth to remove foreign matter.

If you do not wish to come in contact with the patient, you may hold a cloth over the victim's mouth or nose and breathe through it. The cloth does not greatly affect the exchange of air.

---

*These instructions are condensed from those given by the American Red Cross.

---

no equipment is required, though it is better to insert a plastic airway (if one is immediately available) because it improves the effectiveness of the method, provides an airway and a breathing tube and makes the method esthetically more acceptable. (2) The operator can see the degree of inflation of the chest. (3) He can sense obstruction of the airway. (4) He will probably stay within safe inflating pressures, since he provides his own force. Most persons, by their expiratory muscle effort, can develop an air pressure equal to or greater than the pressure that mechanical respirators are now permitted to provide. (5) The composition of the gas delivered is adequate for emergency use; for a 500 ml tidal volume, the first 150 ml would come from the anatomic dead space of the operator and therefore would be fresh air; the next 350 ml would be alveolar gas (approximately 14% O_2 and 5.6% CO_2), but only 200 ml of this would enter the patient's lungs, the last 150 ml filling his anatomic dead space. The mean composition of the "fresh air" entering the patient's alveoli would be about 17% O_2 and 3.2% CO_2 (instead of 21% and 0%). The operator could bring the composition of this gas closer to that of air by inspiring deeply, thus raising his own alveolar P_{O_2} and lowering his alveolar P_{CO_2}, but this, carried too far, could lower the operator's arterial P_{CO_2} so much that he himself might suffer from cerebral vasoconstriction.

Mechanical Methods

These are of two general types: negative- and positive-pressure apparatus.

NEGATIVE-PRESSURE RESPIRATORS. The body respirator (Drinker respirator; tank respirator; "iron lung") was conceived as a method that would mimic natural "negative-pressure" breathing. The patient is supine and all but his head is enclosed in a rigid tank; a rubber diaphragm around his neck seals the tank (Fig. 10-39, p. 141). The pressure around the body is cycled. First, it is lowered below atmospheric; this enlarges the thorax, lowers intrathoracic and intra-alveolar pressure and causes ambient air to flow into the lungs. Then the pressure returns to atmospheric, and this permits the lungs and thorax to return by elastic recoil to the resting position; this causes expiratory flow. The cycle is then repeated at the desired frequency.

POSITIVE-PRESSURE APPARATUS. A tightly fitting mask is placed over the patient's face or a connection is made with a cuffed endotracheal tube if one is in place. Positive pressure can then be used to inflate the lungs; it can be pressure applied by hand to a rubber anesthesia bag or a bellows attached to the mask or tube, or pressure generated by automatic cycling machines. The latter are powered by compressed gases, usually O_2. They are often set so that they inflate the lungs to a maximal pressure, and this pressure then automatically cycles the valve to the expiratory line; expiration is either to the functional residual capacity because of the natural recoil of the lungs-thorax system or below that if the respirator is one with a subatmospheric phase (negative-pressure phase). Positive-pressure apparatus might, on the other hand, be set to deliver a specific volume or continue to a predetermined maximal flow rate rather than to deliver gas until a specific pressure is reached.

POSITIVE VS. NEGATIVE PRESSURE. Is there a decided advantage to using negative pressure around the thorax to achieve inflation of the lungs instead of applying positive pressure to the nose, mouth or trachea? The lungs cannot be inflated unless the gas pressure at the mouth is greater than that in the alveoli. The amount of this difference in pressure (the transairway pressure) determines the tidal volume for a given compliance of the lungs and thorax. The flow of air will be the same when mouth pressure is 760 and alveolar pressure 755 mm Hg (natural-, negative- or subatmospheric-pressure breathing) as when they are 765 and 760 mm Hg (positive-pressure breathing); in

each case, the pressure difference is 5 mm Hg. As far as ventilation is concerned, there is no difference between the methods; all that matters to the lungs is that a proper transairway pressure is created, by either "pushing" or "pulling." However, natural breathing, acting as a thoracic pump, favors return of venous blood to the right side of the heart. This is evident if we consider the pressure difference responsible for returning blood to the right atrium. If the pressure in the venules in the legs is +10 mm Hg (relative to atmospheric pressure) and the pressure in the great veins in the thorax is −3 mm Hg, the pressure difference for venous blood flow is 13 mm Hg. If the peripheral venular pressure +10 mm Hg and the intrathoracic pressure is +3 mm Hg, the "pushing pressure" is only 7 mm Hg. During positive-pressure breathing, the mean intrathoracic pressure during each respiratory cycle is increased; this decreases the pressure difference and reduces venous return to the right heart. Patients with good circulatory responses react to positive-pressure breathing by increasing their peripheral venous blood pressure. This restores the driving pressure for venous flow, and the cardiac output returns to previous values. This response requires an active sympathetic nervous system and is absent or reduced when spinal anesthesia or ganglionic or peripheral sympathetic blocking agents have been used or when deep narcosis is present. Therefore, positive-pressure breathing may cause or aggravate hypotension in specific circumstances.

Whittenberger has pointed out that the body respirator really has the same effects on the circulation as positive-pressure breathing. The respirator encloses the body from the neck down, and its negative-pressure cycle lowers the pressure not only in the great veins of the thorax but all over the body, except in the head. Therefore, the effect of a tank respirator on the circulation is approximately the same as that of positive-pressure breathing; the effects would be identical if only the patient's face protruded from the respirator instead of his whole head. In the body respirator, the head and neck are at atmospheric pressure when the body is at subatmospheric; with a positive-pressure device, the face is at a pressure greater than atmospheric and the body is at atmospheric. However, the body respirator, like positive-pressure devices, does not ordinarily decrease the patient's cardiac ouput and systemic blood pressure, particularly if he is not narcotized and has active cardiovascular reflexes.

PROBLEMS IN USING MECHANICAL RESPIRATORS. Certain problems and misunderstandings deserve discussion.

1. Machines, even at maximal pressure, may not produce adequate ventilation if the compliance of the patient's lungs and thoracic cage is very low. Exceeding the "safe" pressures for inflation (20–30 mm Hg) may produce more ventilation but may rupture alveoli. Alveoli rupture when distended to a certain volume and the latter is determined by their compliance and transpulmonary pressure. This critical volume may be exceeded for a few alveoli if airways to them are open and others are not, so that they preferentially receive a large volume of air despite a "safe" overall tidal volume. This volume may also be exceeded even at a "safe" pressure if some alveoli have weak walls. Clearly we need more information about the bursting pressure and volume of the weakest alveoli in infants and adults with many kinds of pulmonary disorders.

2. Machines, set to inflate lungs to a certain pressure and then reverse to permit expiration, cycle back and forth rapidly when the airway is obstructed. This is because the volume required to raise pressure in the trachea or upper airway alone is very small. This "chattering" is a signal to find and relieve obstruction.

3. One cannot depend on a "setting" to decide whether the ventilation is adequate. When artificial respiration is to be continued for more than a few minutes, arterial, alveolar or end-tidal P_{CO_2} serves as a better guide than a measurement of the volume of gas breathed.

4. When a patient is still breathing, there are technical problems not encountered in a completely apneic patient. A breathing patient may be breathing rapidly or irregularly, and the cycle provided by the apparatus may not be synchronous with his cycle. If the patient is breathing *in* when the machine is breathing *out* and vice versa, the alveolar ventilation may be less when the breathing machine is used than when the patient breathes on his own. Devices in which the inspiratory phase is triggered by the patient's own inspiratory effort may avoid his asynchrony.

5. Some physicians believe that positive pressure applied during inspiration (intermittent positive-pressure breathing—IPPB) actually forces the airways open during inspiration. Positive inspiratory pressure does, of course, provide a pressure across the bronchial wall that tends to widen the airways, but so does natural inspiration. Pressure breathing does not cause greater widening of intrathoracic airways than the forces exerted in natural breathing for the same tidal volume. A transbronchial pressure of 10 torr achieved by *in*creasing pressure *within the airway* (by positive-pressure breathing) is not different from that achieved by *de*creasing the pressure *around the airway* (by natural, negative intrathoracic pressure). Thus, inspiratory positive-pressure breathing causes bronchial dilation only if it causes breathing to be deeper than natural breathing. The increased transmural pressure in extrathoracic airways during positive pressure ventilation has no known effect on the lungs or respiration.

6. There is a difference between intermittent positive-pressure breathing and continuous positive-pressure breathing. In the former alveolar pressure decreases to atmospheric pressure at end-expiration; in the latter an added positive pressure is maintained throughout the respiratory cycle, including expiration. As mentioned earlier in discussing physiologic treatment of respiratory dis-

tress syndrome of newborn and "shock lung" of adults, continuous pressure helps to prevent alveolar collapse when there is a deficiency of pulmonary surfactant.

INDICATIONS FOR MECHANICAL VENTILATION. The main indication of course is hypoventilation, with resulting hypoxemia, CO_2 retention and respiratory acidosis. Inhalation of O_2-rich gas can correct the hypoxemia due to hypoventilation but cannot correct the CO_2 retention; increased alveolar ventilation is necessary to eliminate excess CO_2. Is it always necessary to correct hypoventilation? If it occurs in an ambulatory patient, is mild and has developed gradually, permitting time for adequate compensation for acidosis, mechanical ventilation is scarcely indicated. However, if the same degree of hypoventilation occurs abruptly in a critically ill patient (e.g., with coronary occlusion), mechanical ventilation *is* indicated. And when severe hypoventilation occurs in a patient with narcotic poisoning (by morphine, heroin or barbiturates), mechanical ventilation is lifesaving.

Mechanical ventilation is sometimes needed even when the volume of a patient's alveolar ventilation is normal, e.g., when the patient is exhausting his respiratory muscles to maintain his alveolar ventilation. This can occur when there is unusually great resistance or low compliance in the respiratory system. And sometimes continuous positive airway pressure is needed to keep alveoli from collapsing during expiration; this is an instance when mechanical ventilation of a special type is more effective than O_2 inhalation in oxygenating the blood.

THE INTENSIVE-RESPIRATORY-CARE UNIT

The best management of patients with apnea, with depressed breathing or with serious mechanical problems and pulmonary insufficiency requires expensive equipment, round-the-clock recording or monitoring of critical cardiovascular and pulmonary functions and a team of highly trained and knowledgeable physicians and assistants who have the capacity to respond immediately. The best setting for achieving this is a hospital's intensive-respiratory-care unit (which may be an integral part of an overall intensive-care unit). It contains equipment for maintaining an open airway, for delivering different patterns of assisted or complete mechanical ventilation, for continuous measurement of ventilation, expired alveolar CO_2, arterial blood pressure and heart rate, for frequent measurements of the P_{O_2} and P_{CO_2} of systemic arterial blood and for continuous display of these variables and alarm systems that alert nearby staff when a critical change has occurred. The team responsible for such care must be physiologists (in addition to being physicians or physicians' assistants), for no two patients are alike and decisions must be based on sound physiologic knowledge. Although physicians in charge of these units are essentially clinical physiologists, they have elected to call themselves "intensivists" (a dreadful name that they may abandon if their colleagues decide to call them "expensivists").

INHALATION THERAPY

Oxygen

The inspired gas may be enriched with O_2 by adding it to inspired air in a tent surrounding the patient or in a hood surrounding his head or by passing it into his nasopharynx through a nasal tube; these methods increase the inspired O_2 from 20.93% to between 30 and 80%. The inspired gas may be 100% O_2 if a well-fitted face mask is used.

The effects of inhaling 100% O_2 at sea level on gas tensions in the lungs and blood are shown in Table 22-2. First let us consider the effects on body N_2. When inspired P_{O_2} is 760 torr, inspired P_{N_2} is zero. The inspired O_2 dilutes alveolar N_2 and washes it out, breath by breath (see Fig 2-9, p. 18). As alveolar P_{N_2} decreases, N_2 passes from the mixed venous blood into the alveolar gas so that it is eventually eliminated from blood; this cre-

TABLE 22-2.—EFFECTS OF INHALATION OF AIR VS. OXYGEN ON COMPOSITION OF ALVEOLAR GAS AND BLOOD*

	INSPIRED GAS (DRY)		ALVEOLAR GAS		END-PULMONARY CAPILLARY BLOOD		ARTERIAL BLOOD		END-SYSTEMIC CAPILLARY BLOOD	
	Air	O_2	Air	O_2	Air	O_2	Air‡	O_2‡	Air	O_2
P_{O_2}, torr	159.1	760	104	673	104	673	100	640	40	53.5
P_{CO_2}, torr	0.3	0	40	40	40	40	40	40	46	46
P_{H_2O}, torr	0.0	0	47	47	47	47	47	47	47	47
P_{N_2}, torr	600.6	0	569	0	569	0	573†·	0	573†	0
P total, torr	760.0	760	760	760	760	760	760	727	706	146.5
O_2 saturation, %					98	100	97	100	75	85.5
Dissolved O_2, ml/100 ml					0.31	2.02	0.30	1.92	0.12	0.16
O_2 combined with Hb, ml/100 ml					19.70	20.10	19.50	20.10	15.07	17.19
Total O_2 content, ml/100 ml					20.01	22.12	19.80	22.02	15.19	17.35

*These values apply to man at sea level with Hb concentration of 15 gm/100 ml, alveolar ventilation of 4.27 L/min, O_2 consumption of 250 ml/min and R values of 0.8. The O_2 consumption and A-V O_2 difference (4.6 ml O_2/100 ml) are assumed to be the same during inhalation of O_2 and air.

†Blood P_{N_2} is higher than that of mixed alveolar gas because of differences in the ratio of ventilation to blood flow that occur in different alveoli, even of healthy lungs (see p. 181).

‡Values for arterial P_{O_2} are based on assumed pulmonary artery-to-vein shunt of 2%.

ates a difference in partial pressure between tissue and capillary blood N_2, and N_2 is washed out of tissues. If a man is surrounded by O_2 (so that no N_2 enters the body through skin or mucous membranes) and breathes O_2, all of his tissue, blood and pulmonary N_2 will eventually be eliminated. The rate of the elimination is slower if there are many poorly ventilated regions of the lung or many body tissues with relatively slow circulation (e.g., fat pads).

This process of *nitrogen* elimination has led some to believe that inhalation of O_2 also leads to elimination of CO_2 from the lungs, blood and tissues. It does not. This is because N_2 originates in the air we breathe, but CO_2 is derived from the metabolic activity of our tissues. Inhalation of O_2 can, of course, affect P_{CO_2} if it causes hypo- or hyperventilation. Theoretically, inhalation of O_2 can also interfere with CO_2 transport if HbO_2 is not dissociated to Hb and O_2 in tissue capillaries (see Chapter 16).

What happens to *total* gas tensions when man breathes pure O_2? The total gas tension of alveolar gas must remain at 760 torr at end-inspiration and end-expiration at sea level if all of the airways are open to the atmosphere. Many students believe that total blood and tissue gas tensions must also remain at 760 torr if man is at sea level, but this is not true. Because of the shapes of the O_2

and CO_2 dissociation curves (Fig 14-6), even when man breathes air his total tissue and end-systemic capillary blood have a total tension of 706, or 54 torr less than atmospheric; the transfer of 5 ml of O_2 from 100 ml of blood is associated with a decrease of 60 torr P_{O_2}, while the transfer of 4 ml of CO_2, in the opposite direcion, is associated with a rise of only 6 torr P_{CO_2}. When man breathes O_2, since the transfer of O_2 from capillary blood to tissues calls on dissolved O_2 first, blood P_{O_2} decreases from 640 to 53.5 torr while blood is passing through an ordinary capillary bed; since blood P_{CO_2} rises only 6 torr and P_{N_2} is now zero the *total* of the gas tensions in venous blood falls to 146.5.

ABSORPTION OF GASES FROM CLOSED SPACES. This change in *total* tissue and end-capillary gas tension explains why gas is absorbed from any closed space (such as subcutaneous spaces, the gastrointestinal tract, cerebral ventricles, peritoneal cavity, pleural cavity, paranasal sinuses and alveoli not in free communication with their airway) when the patient breathes air and why absorption is far more rapid when he breathes O_2.

Let us take a subcutaneous gas pocket as an example. The sum of the partial pressures of gases in the pocket must equal 760 torr (at sea level) because the total barometric pressure is transmitted directly to this pocket and maintains its pressure at 760 torr until the last molecules of gas are absorbed into the blood. The subcutaneous gas is in contact with tissues and tissue capillaries and will be absorbed into the capillary blood because the sum of the partial pressures there is less than in the pocket. No matter what the initial composition of gas in the subcutaneous pocket is, the gas will be absorbed more rapidly if O_2 is inhaled, because total gas pressure is 760 torr in the pocket in either case, but only 146.5 in the tissue when O_2 is inhaled vs. 706 when air is inhaled. It is difficult for some physicians to grasp the concept that body tissues and capillary or venous blood have gas tensions which add up to less than the total atmospheric pressure. It may help if one remembers that gas tensions decrease in the Van Slyke manometric apparatus when O_2 absorbent is added and soaks up the O_2 molecules, or if one realizes that boiling drives all dissolved gases from water, leaving its $Po_2 + Pn_2 + Pco_2 = 0$ until it is again equilibrated with air, slowly by diffusion from the air-water interface or rapidly by shaking.

Sometimes more rapid absorption brought about by inhalation of O_2 is desirable and sometimes undesirable. In the middle ear, if the eustachian tube is blocked, gas absorption causes the drum to be drawn in. In the paranasal sinuses, if the ostia are blocked, it leads to congestion and pain. Postoperative atelectasis is more apt to occur if alveoli contain gas rich in O_2; its incidence can be decreased by making sure that the alveoli contain 80% N_2 and that the patient is breathing air in the recovery room. Atelectasis is more apt to occur if the subject is breathing O_2 at less than 1 atmosphere of pressure (as in aircraft or spaceships). For example, if a pilot breathes pure O_2 at 760 torr total pressure, his alveolar Po_2 is $760 - 47$ torr $Ph_2o - 40$ torr Pco_2, or 673, but if he breathes pure O_2 at 200 torr total pressure, his alveolar $Po_2 = 200 - 47 - 40 = 113$ torr; in the first case, his alveoli contain 6 times as many molecules as in the second case, and, if O_2 uptake is the same in each case, it will take 6 times as long to empty the O_2 from any blocked alveoli that still have pulmonary capillary blood flow.

Oxygen is sometimes used to hasten the elimination of gases in closed intestinal loops or from cavities that contain gas either accidentally (subcutaneous emphysema) or as a result of diagnostic or therapeutic procedures (pneumoencephalogram or pneumothorax). Its main use, however, is in the correction or prevention of hypoxemia.

CORRECTION OF HYPOXEMIA AND HYPOXIA. In Table 22-3 a classification of hypoxemia and hypoxia is presented. In *1a*, the lungs are normal but the Po_2 in inspired air is low, either because the percent of O_2 in air is decreased below 20.93 by the presence of other gases or because the *total* barometric pressure is low; inhalation of O_2 will correct this type of hypoxemia by bringing inspired and alveolar Po_2 up to normal values. However, when the total barometric pressure is very low (as at a very high altitude), hypoxemia will occur even if 100% O_2 is inspired; at a total barometric pressure of $\frac{1}{5}$ atmosphere (152 torr), alveolar Po_2 may be only 65 torr because alveolar gas is always moist ($Ph_2o = 47$ torr) and contains CO_2 ($Pco_2 = 40$ torr unless there is hyperventilation).

TABLE 22-3.—CAUSES OF HYPOXEMIA OR HYPOXIA

1. Inadequate oxygenation of normal lung
    a) Deficiency of O_2 in atmosphere
    b) Airway obstruction; neuromuscular disorders
2. Inadequate oxygenation of abnormal lung
    a) Hypoventilation
    b) Uneven alveolar ventilation/pulmonary capillary blood flow
    c) Impaired diffusion
3. Venous-to-arterial shunts
4. Inadequate circulatory transport of O_2
    a) Anemia; abnormal hemoglobin
    b) General circulatory deficiency
    c) Localized circulatory deficiency
5. Inadequate tissue oxygenation
    a) Inadequate release of O_2 from HbO_2
    b) Tissue edema
    c) Abnormal tissue demand for O_2
    d) Poisoning of cellular enzymes

In *1b* and *2a*, in which there is hypoventilation, inhalation of O_2 corrects the hypoxemia because it brings more O_2 molecules to the alveoli each minute than are removed by the mixed venous blood, but it does not correct the hypoventilation and associated CO_2 retention and respiratory acidosis; only an adequate volume of alveolar ventilation/minute will do this, with or without O_2.

In *2b*, inhalation of O_2 corrects the hypoxemia because it brings many more O_2 molecules to poorly ventilated areas, but again it does not correct CO_2 retention if present and may make it worse by depressing chemoreceptor drive and decreasing ventilation. When there is hypoxemia due to impaired diffusion (*2c*), as in alveolocapillary block, inhalation of O_2 corrects it by raising alveolar Po_2 and creating a very large initial Po_2 difference between alveolar Po_2 and the Po_2 of mixed venous blood entering the alveolar capillaries; impaired diffusion rarely results in CO_2 retention, so that additional volume of ventilation is unnecessary. If a patient's dyspnea is due to hyperventilation caused by hypoxemia, O_2 inhalation, by relieving hypoxemia, will also relieve the dyspnea; in most cases, O_2 inhalation does not relieve dyspnea, meaning that dyspnea in most cases is caused by other factors.

In absolute shunts of systemic venous to arterial blood, O_2 inhalation can never bring arterial blood to *maximal* values for O_2 content (O_2 combined with Hb plus dissolved O_2) and the failure to do so is an infallible indication that such a shunt exists (see p. 175). When the shunt is small and the hypoxemia mild (93–94% saturation), O_2 inhalation may restore O_2 *saturation* to normal (but not the maximal O_2 content). When the shunt is large, O_2 inhalation cannot correct the hypoxemia because only the mixed venous blood that flows through capillary beds of ventilated alveoli is exposed to the high alveolar Po_2.

In patients whose inspired gas and lungs are normal, hypoxia may occur because of inadequate transport of oxygenated blood (Table 22-3, *4*). If systemic and local blood flow are normal and only the amount of hemoglobin is deficient (anemia due to hemorrhage, hemolysis or decreased formation of red cells), inhalation of O_2 can compensate wholly or in part for the lack of O_2-carrying pigment, but correction of the anemia is a better way of treating the anemic patient than is inhalation of O_2. When the problem is too little blood flow to a part (peripheral vascular obstruction, coronary artery occlusion or cerebral thrombosis), hypoxemia is only part of the problem; for their survival, tissues require many things in blood in addition to O_2, and inhalation of O_2 is only a partial or temporary measure. The same is true when the circulatory deficiency is widespread, as in hemorrhage, hypotension and circulatory shock. Inhalation of O_2 does no harm in these circumstances unless the physician who employs it believes that it alone has the power to cure a complex situation.

In Table 22-3, *5*, arterial blood is normal in its O_2 content, O_2 tension and volume flow, but there is too little O_2 available in relation to the metabolic needs of tissues. If there is an unusually great tissue demand for O_2 (*5c*), there will certainly also be a great demand for substances in blood that yield energy, and O_2 inhalation will supply only the O_2 and not the glucose or free fatty acids needed. Tissue edema (*5b*) is similar at the cellular level to alveolocapillary block in the lung; a high arterial Po_2, created by O_2 inhalation, will drive the O_2 over the longer path to the cells, but will not help the delivery of substrates. In *5d*, if the cytochrome oxidase system is inactivated by cyanide, the cells will not take up O_2, even at higher pressure, and the venous blood returns to the heart fully saturated.

HYPERBARIC OXYGENATION. Oxygen can be administered at more than 1 atmosphere of pressure if the patient is placed in a rigid chamber capable of withstanding 2, 3 and 4 atmospheres. Since hemoglobin is fully saturated when patients breathe O_2 at 1 atmosphere (except for those with large venous-to-arterial shunts), how can inhalation of O_2

at 2, 3 or 4 atmospheres provide more O_2? Oxygen dissolves in the blood in direct proportion to the partial pressure: when man inhales O_2 at 1 atmosphere, 100 ml of his blood contains $[(760 - 40 - 47) \times 0.003]$, or 2 ml of dissolved O_2; when he breathes O_2 at 2 atmospheres, it contains $[(1520 - 40 - 47) \times 0.003]$, or 4.3 ml; when he breathes O_2 at 4 atmospheres, it contains $[(3040 - 40 - 47) \times 0.003]$, or 8.8 ml of dissolved O_2 (Fig. 22-2). One can increase the dissolved O_2 without limit by increasing the O_2 pressure without limit. However, remember two important points.

1. One cannot inhale O_2 at high pressures without developing rather alarming signs, such as convulsions (see p. 282); one must never exceed specified periods of inhalation of O_2 at 1, 2, 3 or 4 atmospheres.

2. Maintaining an optimal environment for the cells in the body requires removing CO_2, H^+ and lactate and supplying O_2, substrates of energy (glucose, fatty acids) and components needed for proper function,

growth and repair of cells. For this there must be adequate blood flow *and* O_2; neither blood flow without O_2 nor O_2 without blood flow can maintain mammalian cell function for long.

The main source of energy in the body is the hydrolysis of adenosine triphosphate (ATP). A little ATP can be synthesized from glucose without O_2 (anaerobic glycolysis); much more can be synthesized from glucose, fatty acids or amino acids in the presence of O_2 (oxidative phosphorylation). Oxygen is neither energy nor a source of energy. It *is* required as the terminal electron acceptor in a complex mitochondrial electron transport system that generates ATP; this system functions well at very low intracellular O_2 tension (~ 1 torr) and no better at very high tensions. Increasing intracellular oxygen tension above normal does not improve cell function, does not accelerate metabolism, does not increase cardiac output or tissue blood flow, does not supply the cells with more glucose, free fatty acids or hor-

Fig. 22-2.—Total O_2 in blood when man breathes O_2 at high pressures. **A,** standard HbO_2 dissociation curve (0–100 torr Po_2). **B,** dissolved O_2 and O_2 combined with Hb when oxygen pressures increase to 3,000 torr (approximately 4 atmospheres). When Po_2 exceeds 200–300 torr, hemoglobin is fully saturated but O_2 continues to dissolve in blood as Po_2 increases. The horizontal arrow indicates the Po_2 0 to 100 torr portion of each curve.

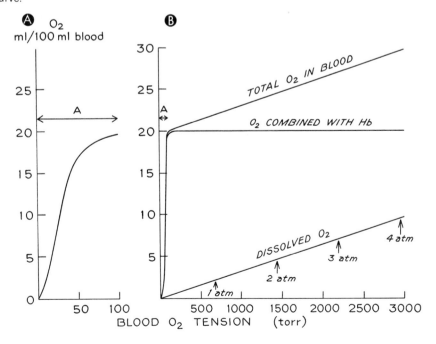

mones, does not remove more metabolites from the cells and does not buffer more effectively the hydrogen ions liberated intracellularly during metabolism.

Hyperbaric oxygenation is at its best in specific clinical conditions in which there is no deficiency in blood flow and only a need for more O_2 than can be supplied by breathing O_2 at 1 atmosphere. This may be infection with anaerobic organisms that cannot live in a high Po_2, carbon monoxide poisoning or possibly crises of sickle cell anemia. Hyperbaric O_2 has been used for short periods to restore arterial oxygen saturation and tension to normal in hypoxemic patients with large vein-to-artery shunts across the lungs or across the heart and to prolong the safe period of total cardiac arrest when cardiac surgeons must electively stop the heart long enough to correct defects of the heart valves or interatrial or interventricular septa.

Hyperbaric O_2 has also been used in patients whose arterial blood O_2 is normal but who suffer from restricted blood flow to a part. This use, within safe limits, is rational because tissue cells, with the exception of muscle, have no oxygen stores to match their intracellular stores of glycogen and fat. If O_2 can diffuse into ischemic cells and act intracellularly to accept electrons, the cells may remain alive until their intracellular materials required for generation of ATP are exhausted. But this period of grace, for most mammalian cells, is a short one. After a period of hyperbaric oxygenation (2 atmospheres), the hearts of animals can be safely stopped for 8 minutes as compared to 5 minutes (if the body temperature has first been lowered to 28 C). When extra dissolved O_2 is made available, utilization of tissue substrates can continue for only a few more minutes; irreversible cell death then occurs.

After cells have utilized their stores of glycogen or fat, they break down structural proteins, and this means cell death. Further, when blood flow is insufficient to carry away metabolites formed in aerobic or anaerobic metabolism, the metabolites accumulate and injure cells. When blood is exposed to 3 atmospheres of pressure, so much O_2 is dissolved in blood that Hb (fully saturated with O_2) never gives up any O_2 (Fig 22-3), and can no longer play its important role in CO_2 transport from tissues to pulmonary capillaries; acidosis results.

POSSIBLE HARM FROM OXYGEN INHALATION.

1. Cessation of respiration. This is the most dramatic side effect following inhalation of O_2. It is rare, however, and occurs only when O_2 is given to a severely hypoxic patient whose respiratory center is not responsive to CO_2 and whose only important drive to maintain respiration is the chemoreceptor reflex. The cells of the carotid and aortic bodies, their pathways and central synapses appear to resist depression by narcotics, hypoxia, etc., more than do central chemoreceptors and other reflex paths. When a patient is severely hypoxic and the Po_2 in arterial blood is 30–60 torr, practically all of his carotid and aortic chemoreceptors are maximally stimulated. His ventilation may stop when he inhales O_2, and his arterial blood Po_2 increases suddenly from 40 to more than 600 torr.

2. Depression of ventilation. Depression of breathing after inhalation of O_2 is more common than apnea and may be even more serious because it is more likely to be overlooked. In some patients with chronic pulmonary disease and respiratory acidosis, inhalation of O_2 is followed by depression of breathing and somnolence, or even coma. This is uncommon; in our experience, among 66 patients with mild to severe chronic hypoxemia who were treated with O_2 therapy, this reaction developed in nine, one of whom died as a result. No patient given O_2 to breathe become comatose unless (1) initial arterial Pco_2 was 50 torr or more, (2) arterial O_2 saturation was below 90% and (3) the O_2 therapy relieved hypoxemia. Because

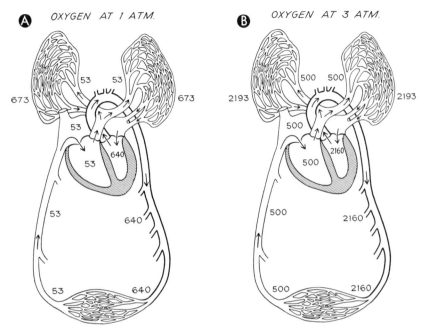

Fig. 22-3. — O_2 tensions in blood in arteries, capillaries and veins when man breathes oxygen at 1 atmosphere (**A**) and at 3 atmospheres (**B**). Note that venous blood in **B** has a Po_2 of 500 torr. Hemoglobin must therefore still be fully saturated; this interferes with the normal blood buffering mechanism that depends on conversion of HbO_2 to deoxygenated Hb in tissue capillaries.

coma is an uncommon reaction and the prompt use of mechanical ventilators can correct hypoventilation when it occurs, patients with hypoxemia should not be denied the possible benefits of O_2 therapy.

However, since there is no way of predicting whether coma will develop, it appears best to begin O_2 therapy with 30–40% O_2 and to watch patients for the first few hours of therapy. If true coma occurs, the physician should increase the patient's ventilation mechanically to insure elimination of CO_2; he should provide extra O_2 if needed to correct hypoxemia.

The somnolence and coma are usually attributed to the depression of breathing and consequent increase in arterial Pco_2. Normal men given 10% CO_2 to breathe may become unresponsive; inhalation of 30% CO_2 causes surgical anesthesia. There is, however, no knowledge of the level of CO_2 or the amount of change required to produce this effect in healthy persons or in patients with respiratory acidosis.

Possible mechanisms for "oxygen coma" other than "carbon dioxide narcosis" should be mentioned:

a) By relieving hypoxemia, inhalation of pure O_2 might lead to spasm of cerebral blood vessels and thus precipitate coma.

b) Hypoxemia reflexly stimulates the cerebral cortex as well as the respiratory and vasomotor centers. The restlessness and delirium associated with hypoxemia are probably manifestations of this effect. Inhalation of high concentrations of O_2 may result in sudden withdrawal of this cortical stimulation and so lead to coma.

c) Patients with chronic pulmonary insufficiency may have high cerebrospinal fluid pressure, presumably because of the marked vasodilation of cerebral vessels by low Po_2 and high Pco_2. Some investigators have noted that cerebrospinal fluid pressure rises even higher in these patients when they inhale O_2.

d) Patients with chronic hypoxemia may have compensatory alterations in cerebral metabolism. Sudden removal of these may lead to inability to utilize O_2 at normal or even high pressures, and coma results.

3. *Pulmonary irritation.* Animals exposed continuously to 80–100% O_2 die of pulmonary congestion, exudation and edema. Normal men breathing 100% O_2 continuously for 24 hours may experience substernal distress that is aggravated by deep breathing; their vital capacity may decrease by 500–800 ml. Symptoms disappear after a few hours of breathing air. Inhalation of 50% O_2 for long periods does not result in this syndrome, nor does breathing of 100% O_2 at 18,000 ft (0.5 atmosphere).

4. *Retrolental fibroplasia.* Inhalation of 100% O_2 is the cause of retrolental fibroplasia and blindness of premature infants, presumably because of local vasoconstriction caused by the high Po_2. Inhalation of 40% O_2 appears to be safe.

5. *Atelectasis and absorption of gases from closed spaces (see p. 276).*

6. *Convulsions.* These occur only when O_2 is breathed at more than 1 atmosphere of pressure. This can occur in therapeutic hyperbaric oxygenation. It can also occur in a diver breathing O_2 (p. 250). The symptoms often begin with twitching of the lips, eyelids or hands, ringing in the ears and dizziness. Convulsions may come on suddenly and be very severe. The toxicity is a function of Po_2, the duration of exposure and the amount of exercise. At 6 atmospheres of O_2, convulsions develop in resting subjects in a few minutes; at 4 atmospheres, symptoms may appear in less than 15 minutes. The safe time is less during exercise—such as in a diver breathing O_2. Safe periods during which no symptoms occur in divers, are 45 minutes at 30 feet, 75 minutes at 25 feet and 110 minutes at 20 feet; every 33 feet below the surface of salt water is the equivalent of one atmosphere of gas pressure. Safe limits for high pressures of O_2 have not yet been determined for unconscious or anesthetized patients undergoing treatment in high pressure chambers.

The central nervous system effects are believed to be due to inactivation of certain enzymes (especially dehydrogenases in which sulfhydryl groups are essential for activity) as a direct result of the high Po_2.

Carbon Dioxide

The only centrally acting, specific respiratory stimulant is CO_2. However, inhalation of air or O_2, enriched with CO_2 is rarely advisable in the treatment of central respiratory depression. Whenever there is apnea or severe depression of breathing, there must be an increase in arterial Pco_2 (unless metabolism is decreased). Adding 3, 5 or 7% CO_2 to the inspired air will increase blood and tissue Pco_2 further and aggravate the respiratory acidosis. Further, CO_2 in high concentration is a narcotic. Although inhalation of 10% CO_2 tremendously stimulates breathing in healthy persons, it may produce some stupor even in them. As noted before, inhalation of 25–30% CO_2 produces complete narcosis; inhalation of less than 10% CO_2 may depress the brain of a patient suffering from chronic hypoxia and CO_2 retention.

Inhalation of 7–10% CO_2 in air for a few minutes may be a useful test to gauge the severity of narcotic depression of the respiratory center in cases of poisoning by morphine, heroin or barbiturates; if respiratory depth increases noticeably, narcosis is not excessive and the patient will recover if given good nursing and medical care. Inhalation of 5–10% CO_2 in air for 1–3 minutes intermittently is also useful to prevent atelectasis in patients who are hypoventilating postoperatively.

There is a rationale for the use of CO_2 in combating the action of gaseous poisons, notably CO: if inhalation of 7–10% CO_2 in O_2 increases the depth of breathing, it should hasten elimination of CO from the lungs and blood. From the practical point of view, inhalation of pure O_2 is recommended because of its ready availability.

DRUGS STIMULATING RESPIRATION. *Aminophylline* can also produce central stimulation of respiration, probably as part of its excitatory effect on the central nervous system. The subjective improvement described by patients after the use of aminophylline may be partly due to such stimulation. The side effects of adequate doses of aminophylline taken orally (gastrointestinal irritation) usually prevent its administration over long periods.

Large doses of *salicylates* stimulate respiration and increase respiratory minute volume, probably by direct stimulation of the medullary respiratory centers. The hyperventilation that results in healthy men from toxic doses of salicylates may be severe enough to cause marked lowering of alveolar and arterial Pco_2 and tetany. In patients with pulmonary insufficiency, such hyperventilation is impossible, owing to mechanical difficulties, but salicylates may cause some increase in breathing. The dose required to do this is large and may cause petechial hemorrhages in the brain.

Analeptics such as pentylenetetrazol, nikethamide, ethamivan and doxapram are occasionally used to overcome depression of breathing in patients with barbiturate or heroin overdoses and less often as respiratory stimulants in patients with chronic pulmonary insufficiency. However, these drugs are not *specific* respiratory stimulants, and the dose required to increase breathing is very close to the amount that produces widespread central nervous system stimulation, twitching and convulsions.

Helium-Oxygen Therapy

Helium-oxygen therapy was proposed some years ago as physiologic therapy for obstructed breathing, because the *density* of 80% He-20% O_2 is much less than that of air or O_2. Its viscosity, however, is actually greater than that of air. Inhalation of 80% He-20% O_2 should be useful only in those conditions in which a decrease in gas *density* might be beneficial; such a decrease permits greater flow for the same driving pressure when air flow is turbulent. This occurs only where flow is most rapid or where irregularities in the lumen of air passages cause eddy currents (e.g., glottic narrowing, foreign bodies); inhalation of He-O_2 mixtures may permit increased ventilation for the same effort in such cases. A general increase in air velocities, as during an MVV test, increases the degree of turbulence in the air passages; for this reason the MVV is greater while the patient is breathing He-O_2.

Because the trachea subdivides terminally into hundreds of thousands of fine air passages with a large total cross-sectional area, the velocity of flow through any one small airway is extremely low. Therefore, flow is streamlined in smaller tubes unless unusual obstructions exist. Inhalation of He-O_2 might actually be disadvantageous because its greater viscosity compared to air should require more driving pressure (and hence more effort) to achieve streamlined flow through the small airways.

Aerosol Therapy

Many chemicals have been introduced locally into the respiratory tract in the form of aerosols. These include bronchodilators, antibiotic agents, adrenal cortical hormones, proteolytic or mucolytic enzymes, detergents and components of pulmonary surfactant (dipalmitoyl lecithin). Aerosols are droplets or solids suspended in air. They can be generated manually by squeezing a bulb or by the use of compressed air or O_2. By employing suitable nebulizers and baffles, droplets of the desired size (within limits) can be propelled into the respiratory tract in the hope that they settle at the desired location. The most widely used aerosols are bronchodilator agents.

Bronchodilator drugs are generally sympathomimetic agents that actively enlarge the lumen of bronchioles by effects on bronchiolar smooth muscle. They may be given locally or systemically. Aerosol administration achieves a high concentration of the drug locally, with minimal systemic absorption and few undesired effects. The aerosol, however, goes only where the inspired gas goes and does not reach completely blocked areas of the lung; therefore it goes preferentially where it is needed least. On the other hand, a bronchodilator drug given systemically reaches all bronchioles through the systemic bronchial circulation and reaches alveolar ducts through the pulmonary circulation, whether the corresponding airways are occluded or not.

Where droplets settle in the respiratory tract depends largely on their size. If deposition on bronchiolar mucosa is desired, the particle size should be $1-3$ μ, and a nebulizer certified to deliver in this range should be used. (It is difficult to produce an aerosol in which all particles are of identical size and all settle in one anatomic region; some will be larger and settle in the upper airways.) The bronchodilator most widely used in aerosol form is isoproterenol (isopropyl norepinephrine), which stimulates β receptors in bronchi; drugs such as propranolol that block β receptors may induce asthmatic attacks or make them more severe.

Not all inhaled particles or droplets dilate. Dusts, smokes, fumes and irritating vapors usually constrict bronchioles, and patients with obstructive airway disease should avoid inhaling these.

Positive-pressure breathing, without aerosols, has been used to dilate bronchioles. Probably its value lies in inducing increased tidal volume. Increase in depth of breathing normally widens the bronchioles. A deep breath may be helpful in relieving bronchial obstruction in several ways: (1) A maximal inspiration can temporarily overcome bronchoconstriction such as that induced experimentally by inhalation of smoke or aerosols of histamine. (2) A deep inspiration can aid in clearing the lumen of mucus. If the bronchiolar lumen is bridged by mucus, the air trapped behind the obstruction is absorbed; the breaking of fluid bridges by bronchodilation permits air to pass the obstruction and provides the alveolar gas necessary for effective coughing.

For a discussion of mucolytic aerosols, see page 224.

23

Nonrespiratory Functions of the Lungs and Pulmonary Circulation

THE RESPIRATORY FUNCTIONS of the lungs and pulmonary circulation have been discussed in Chapters 2 and 11–16, and some of the defense functions of the lungs have been discussed in Chapter 17. Here we consider some additional functions of the lungs that are concerned neither with gas exchange nor with defense of the upper and lower respiratory tracts.

RESERVOIR FOR LEFT VENTRICLE

The pulmonary vessels normally contain about 600 ml of blood; most of this is in readily distensible vessels. This blood and that in the left atrium together serve as a reservoir that supplies blood to fill the left ventricle and maintains its output, even when the right ventricular output falls behind for a few beats. Guz and associates have demonstrated this nicely; they placed one electromagnetic flowmeter on a pulmonary trunk and another on the ascending aorta so that they could simultaneously measure pulmonary arterial blood flow (the inflow to the pulmonary circulation) and aortic blood flow (which in a steady state is the output from the pulmonary circulation). In this way they could calculate the beat-by-beat change in pulmonary blood volume. Figure 23-1 shows the response to blocking completely the inflow to the pulmonary circulation. The stroke volume of the left ventricle continued unchanged for two beats and then gradually declined. In another experiment, when the pulmonary circulation was congested and its blood volume considerably increased, left ventricular output was maintained even long-

Fig. 23-1.—Aortic blood flow after complete occlusion of the main pulmonary artery. Left ventricular output (aortic flow) remains unchanged for 2 beats and then gradually decreases. ⊢—⊣ = 1 second. (Courtesy of J. Hoffman, A. Guz, A. Charlier and D. Wilcken.)

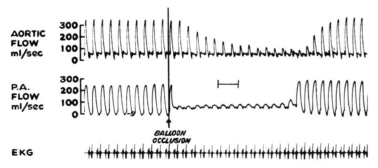

er even though no blood flowed into the pulmonary circulation.

FILTER TO PROTECT
SYSTEMIC CIRCULATION

The pulmonary circulation, strategically located between the mixed venous blood and the systemic arterial blood, serves the important function of retaining fine particles present in mixed venous blood so that these do not enter the systemic circulation and lodge in end arteries in other, potentially more troublesome, sites such as the coronary or cerebral circulation. There are many more pulmonary capillaries than are needed for effective gas exchange in resting man, and some of these can be sacrificed to protect other vascular beds. Indeed, in one diagnostic test for patency of pulmonary vessels, the physician injects macroaggregates of serum albumin intravenously with the deliberate plan of plugging some previously open pulmonary arterioles, to map regions of the lung with and without blood flow (see p. 146). If he injects about 70,000 such emboli (average diameter 30 μ), these occlude only about 5% of the pulmonary precapillary vessels (assuming that each embolus plugs a different precapillary vessel); this has no noticeable effect on the patient and produces no measurable change in his diffusing capacity for carbon monoxide (a sensitive test of the size of his functioning pulmonary capillary bed).

Small pulmonary vessels can therefore trap particles that find their way into mixed venous blood as the result of natural processes, trauma or therapeutic measures. These particles include small fibrin or blood clots, fat cells, bone marrow, detached cancer cells, gas bubbles, tangled sickle cells, agglutinated red blood cells, masses of platelets or white blood cells, debris in stored blood and particles in intravenous solutions. Some of these simply block mechanically; some produce local or systemic responses (see p. 89).

Although the pulmonary circulation can accept a modest number of particles once or twice, obviously it cannot tolerate even a smaller number day by day unless it also has mechanisms for ridding itself of plugs promptly and reopening closed channels. Gold and associates found that an iodized oil used by radiologists to outline lymph channels in patients blocked enough pulmonary vessels to decrease the pulmonary diffusing capacity for carbon monoxide (Dco) by 32%, but the Dco returned to normal values in these patients in four days. This means that the pulmonary circulation does possess mechanisms for passing or disposing of macro- or microemboli and re-establishing the full number of open capillaries — ready for the next emergency. These mechanisms may include an abundance of special lytic enzymes, of competent macrophages and of ready lymph channels. They deserve more study because their proper functioning may insure health and their failure to function may lead to ischemia of pulmonary tissues and cell damage.

This function of the pulmonary circulation — to act as a filter and protect the systemic circulation from emboli — is diminished when some precapillary vessels or capillaries are greatly widened by disease and whenever there are shunts that permit entry of mixed venous blood directly into the systemic arterial circulation. This function is lost completely when the lungs are bypassed by a pump oxygenator during operations on the open heart; special devices must then be used to filter blood passing through the pump and precautions taken to prevent air bubbles from entering the patient's circulation.

A special type of filtering is sequestering altered white blood cells. Although normal, intact white cells pass through pulmonary capillaries without trapping, those that have been manipulated, even gently (to permit their separation from blood, tagging and intravenous reinjection), seem then to be selectively removed during their passage through the pulmonary circulation. This observation has led some to suggest that the lungs play a role in regulating the level of circulating white cells, by storage and release mechanisms.

FLUID EXCHANGE

Water introduced into alveoli passes rapidly into pulmonary capillary blood. This is because the pulmonary capillary pressure of a healthy man (8 – 10 mm Hg), which tends to filter fluid from the blood into the alveoli, is always far below the colloidal osmotic pressure of the plasma proteins (25 – 30 mm Hg), which tends to pull fluid from the alveoli into the blood. In 1873 Colin introduced 25 L of water into the trachea of a horse over a 6-hour period, and noted that the respiratory tract absorbed the whole quantity without causing any apparent discomfort to the animal; he introduced a solution of potassium ferricyanide into the trachea and noted its appearance $3\frac{1}{2}$ minutes later in blood drawn from the jugular vein and 8 minutes later in urine collected from a ureter.

The low capillary pressure provides an elegant mechanism for preventing transudation of fluid from blood to alveoli and for speeding absorption of any fluid in alveoli into blood. However, rapid absorption of fluid can be a hazard. For example, aerosols of drugs such as isoproterenol or procaine, intended for airways only, will enter blood almost as rapidly as if injected intravenously if the drugs reach the alveolar surface. Again, inhalation and rapid absorption of large quantities of water in fresh-water drowning can cause hemolysis of red blood cells, large increases in plasma volume and overload of the heart.

Molecules that do not pass readily through capillary walls are not absorbed so quickly. Some plasma protein placed in alveoli may enter capillaries rapidly, but most of it stays there several days; it is removed slowly by lymphatics. This explains the slow return to normal of the lungs of patients with pneumonia and protein exudates in their alveoli, even after the pneumococci have been killed by antibiotics.

Some wonder how the pulmonary capillaries, with such a low filtration pressure, supply substrates and hormones to the alveolar cells. Transfer of such materials across capillary walls can occur by ultrafiltration, by diffusion, by active transport or by pinocytosis (transport through the capillary wall in vesicles). Only the mass flow of water requires a high capillary (filtration) pressure. Diffusion can move gases and small molecules rapidly over the short distances between capillaries and alveolar tissues. Further, the pulmonary blood flow is far in excess of that needed to supply metabolic needs of alveolar tissues.

METABOLIC FUNCTIONS OF THE LUNG

Most of us think of the lung as a fantastically thin membrane with a vast area designed for rapid exchange of gas. This is true. But most of us also think of the lung as an organ that does no metabolic work. The reasoning is as follows: (1) the muscles of the thoracic cage do the work of moving air through the air tubes, (2) the muscle of the right ventricle does the work of pushing blood through the pulmonary capillaries and (3) gas exchange then occurs by diffusion; since blood entering the pulmonary capillaries has a higher P_{CO_2} and lower P_{O_2} than air entering the alveoli, no active transport mechanisms and metabolic work are required.

Thinking of the lung solely as an organ of gas exchange has led to the conventional view that the lung tissues need just enough O_2 and substrates to keep the epithelial and endothelial cells alive and to enable vascular and airway smooth muscle to contract occasionally and do the small amount of work required to constrict tubes that have a very low transmural pressure. This view held until the 1960s, even though Dale had speculated in 1929 that, since the lungs of many species contain more histamine than do other organs, the lung is either an organ of internal secretion for histamine or it captures histamine that has escaped from other tissues. Dale also commented on the large amount of heparin in the lung, though only the liver (the *hepar*) was then thought to contain much heparin. We now know that pulmonary tissues *are* active metabolically and have a variety of cells that can selectively capture some materials in the mixed venous blood, concentrate and store these, and later release them in the original or in a chemically altered form. We also know now that the lungs can also synthesize new chemical substances in addition to those required by the usual processes of maintenance and repair of cells of any organ. Convincing proof of these functions is that there are nongaseous substances in pulmonary vein blood leaving the lung that were not present in pulmonary artery blood entering the lung, and there are nongaseous substances in pulmonary arterial blood that are either not present at all, or much reduced in concentration in the pulmonary vein blood.

Modern biochemical technics have been used to learn what the lung does to a number of substances passing through it in mixed venous blood. Does the lung clear the blood completely of these substances, or only partially? Does the lung store the captured materials and later release them unchanged, or does it first alter them metabolically? Does the metabolic action cause physiologically active substances to be inactive or inactive substances to become active?

It is of course not correct to attribute *specific* metabolic functions to the lung unless passage of materials through the pulmonary circulation changes their concentration or nature more than passage through another circulatory bed or than contact with blood for the same number of seconds that they are in the pulmonary vessels. Acetylcholine, for example, is rapidly changed to choline and acetate by *blood* cholinesterase; the lung has no unique role in this metabolic change. And it is possible that some of the lung's metabolic function is not specific in a qualitative sense but only appears to be so because of its vast capillary bed and consequent large number of endothelial cells.

UPTAKE BY LUNGS OF CHEMICAL SUBSTANCES IN THE MIXED VENOUS BLOOD. In 1925 Starling and Verney, perfusing the kidney with defibrinated blood, noted that the renal vessels progressively constricted unless the blood first passed through the pulmonary circulation. Their observations could have been explained if there had been inert particles in the blood that were filtered out mechanically by passing the blood first through any capillary bed. But in 1953 Gaddum showed that the lung removed a *chemical* substance from blood; it was 5-OH-tryptamine (serotonin), a naturally occurring vasoconstrictor substance released from platelets. We now know that many chemical substances in mixed venous blood are taken up in passage through the pulmonary vessels, while others pass through without any change in concentration; Table 23-1 lists some of these (many substances remain to be tested).

What purpose do the lungs serve by capturing some chemical substances as they pass through its capillary bed and storing, inactivating or detoxifying these? Even the wisest of ancient gods could not have predicted the

TABLE 23-1.—UPTAKE BY LUNGS OF CHEMICAL SUBSTANCES IN MIXED VENOUS BLOOD

SUBSTANCE IN MIXED VENOUS BLOOD ENTERING LUNG	% IN BLOOD LEAVING LUNG
Acetylcholine	5
Prostaglandins E_1, E_2, $F_{2\alpha}$	5
5HT (serotonin)	5–15
Bradykinin	5–20
Angiotensin I	30*
Imipramine; chlorpromazine	20
ATP; AMP	10–60
Norepinephrine	70
Epinephrine	95
Isoproterenol	100
Dopamine	100
Angiotensin II	100
Oxytocin	100
Vasopressin	100
Histamine	100
Prostaglandins A_1, A_2	100
Substance P	100
Gastrin	100
Eledoisin	100

*70% of the amount of angiotensin I entering the lungs leaves as angiotensin II.

present era of intravenous medication and placed a biochemical sieve in the lung to protect man from his future physicians. But millions of years ago our lungs were gills, and the gill circulation presented a huge absorbing surface through which any chemical material in the water, in addition to O_2, might enter the circulating blood. A detoxifying station in the gills would serve a useful defense mechanism for the rest of the body.

As man evolved from fish and his respiratory surfaces were enfolded within the body, what useful purpose could then be served by a biochemical sieve in the pulmonary circulation? Vane has proposed that such a sieve – between the postcapillary and precapillary beds of the systemic circulation – can be biologically useful in removing from the blood substances never intended to enter the systemic circulation. Chemicals liberated locally in organs and tissues and intended to influence only local tissue function[1] often spill into the end-capillary blood and enter mixed venous blood, though they were never meant to be distributed by systemic arterial blood to every tissue in the body. According to Vane, the lung captures these and stores or inactivates them. The lung, however, does little or nothing to true hormones released from endocrine organs into end-capillary blood; these hormones are intended for distribution through systemic arterial blood to many body tissues. Thus, substances such as acetylcholine, 5HT, some prostaglandins, norepinephrine and ATP, formed locally and intended for local action, are taken up wholly or in considerable part by lungs when mixed venous blood containing them passes through the pulmonary vascular bed; true hormones such as epinephrine, angiotensin II and pitressin, intended for fairly widespread distribution to tissues, are not removed from blood in the lungs.

---

[1]These substances are sometimes called "local hormones." All dictionaries define a *hormone* as a chemical substance formed in one organ of the body and carried by the blood to another organ or tissue where it has specific effects. This makes the term "local hormone" an impossible one; when you use it or see it, remember it as such.

This hypothesis is intriguing, but it leads one to classify isoproterenol as a hormone even though no one has yet demonstrated its natural occurrence in the body and suggests that histamine, prostaglandins A_1, A_2 and substance P are hormones, though no one has demonstrated a useful function for their widespread distribution simultaneously to all organs and tissues.

FORMATION OF CHEMICAL SUBSTANCES IN LUNGS AND RELEASE FOR LOCAL USE. Pulmonary surfactant, formed mainly in the alveolar type II cells, is one substance that is released and used locally; it coats alveolar surfaces, promotes alveolar stability and prevents collapse of alveoli (pp. 109–114).

Another example of local action is the intrapulmonary release of histamine and serotonin from mast cells in response to pulmonary embolism or anaphylaxis; after release each may cause bronchoconstriction and stimulation of certain sensory nerve endings that initiate pulmonary or cardiopulmonary reflexes. A third example is the intrapulmonary release of histamine by hypoxia; some believe that such release is responsible for hypoxic pulmonary vasoconstriction.

FORMATION OF CHEMICAL SUBSTANCES IN LUNGS FOR RELEASE INTO AIRWAYS. In the fetus, chemical substances formed in alveolar cells and released onto the surface of alveoli drift into the airways and move upward. Near the time of birth, pulmonary surfactant appears in the amniotic fluid, and its concentration there is a useful guide to determining the maturity of the lung (see p. 113).

CONVERSION OF CHEMICAL MATERIALS IN LUNG FOR RELEASE INTO BLOOD. Some substances are activated in the lungs. For example, enzymes on the luminal surface of pulmonary endothelial cells convert angiotensin I into the active form, angiotensin II, within the few seconds needed for passage of blood through the pulmonary circulation. Increase or decrease in the activity of the converting enzyme could be a mechanism for increasing or decreasing systemic arterial blood pressure by altering the level of circulating angiotensin II.

Other substances in blood captured by the lungs are *in*activated before being released into pulmonary vein blood; serotonin and ATP are handled in this way.

RELEASE INTO BLOOD OF SUBSTANCES STORED IN PULMONARY TISSUES OR CELLS. Bradykinin, stored in the lungs, is released into pulmonary blood of the newborn lamb when its lungs are initially inflated with O_2. Histamine and perhaps serotonin are released during pulmonary embolism. Prostaglandin E_2 is released during overinflation and during hyperventilation. Heparin, histamine, serotonin and prostaglandins E_2 and $F_{2\alpha}$ are released during anaphylactic shock. Imipramine, stored unchanged in the lungs, can be displaced into blood by administering chlorpromazine.

Site of Metabolic Activity

Blood flowing through the pulmonary circulation comes in contact with all cells lining arteries, arterioles, capillaries, venules and veins and, in addition, supplies cells of the alveolar walls, alveolar ducts and respiratory bronchioles. Table 23-2 lists these cells and some of their synonyms. The alveolar type I cell covers most of the alveolar surface and represents the main area for gas exchange (Fig. 12-2, p. 161). The type II cell (Fig. 10-18, p. 112) has characteristic lamellar inclusion bodies and microvilli protruding from the free edge into the alveolar space; this cell is considered to be the main source of pulmonary surfactant. Alveolar macrophages, definitely scavengers, may also have other metabolic functions (p. 225).

The endothelial cells lining the pulmonary vessels have received much attention recently. Figure 23-2 shows these cells as pictured by the scanning electron microscope. Of particular interest is the tremendous surface area of these cells, created both by projections from the capillary wall into the lumen of the vessel and by indentations into the capillary wall (caveolae or vesicles separated from the capillary lumen only by an extremely delicate membrane). There is now

TABLE 23-2.—CELLS OF THE LUNG THAT RECEIVE PULMONARY
ARTERY BLOOD

CELL	OTHER NAMES FOR SAME CELL
Alveolar type I cell	Type A cell; type I pneumonocyte; membranous cell or pneumocyte; surface epithelial cell; squamous alveolar cell; attenuated squamous cell; small alveolar cell
Alveolar type II cell	Type B cell; type II pneumonocyte; granular pneumonocyte; great, large or cuboidal alveolar cell; secretory alveolar cell; niche, septal or wall cell
Alveolar type III cell (rat)	Type III pneumonocyte; alveolar brush cell
Terminal bronchiolar cell	Clara cell; nonciliated bronchiolar cell
Alveolar macrophages	Phagocytic pneumonocyte; free alveolar cell; dust cell; heart failure cell
Vascular endothelial cells	
Mast cells	Dopamine cells (in ruminants)
Megakaryocytes	
Nerves	
Interstitial tissue, fibroblasts, elastic fibers, collagen, lymphatics and lymphoid tissue	

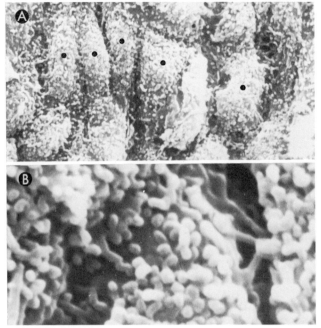

Fig. 23-2.—Scanning electron micrographs of inner surface of pulmonary artery of a dog. **A**, the endothelial cells are denoted by a •. The main body of each endothelial cell is richly covered by an array of irregular projections that thin out toward the borders of the cell (× 3,000). **B**, higher power scanning electron micrograph showing the endothelial projections in greater detail; they are 250–350 nm in diameter and 300–3000 nm in length, ×17,500. (From Smith, U., Ryan, J. W., Michie, D., and Smith, D. S.: Science 173:925, 1971.)

good evidence that serotonin, angiotensin I, bradykinin, ATP and some prostaglandins are taken up from blood by the vascular endothelial cells. Figure 23-3 shows that these cells capture radioactively labeled serotonin and concentrate it. Pulmonary endothelial cells therefore do more than separate blood and tissue cells; they are active metabolically in uptake, storage and metabolic conversion of chemical substances in pulmonary arterial blood.

Postganglionic sympathetic nerve endings elsewhere in the body take up norepinephrine and store it in granules; they also take up precursors and synthesize norepinephrine from them. When appropriate, nerve endings release norepinephrine onto or near adrenoreceptors on arterioles and other tissues; similar uptake and release undoubtedly occurs in nerve endings in the lung.

Pulmonary mast cells presumably synthesize and then store heparin and histamine (and in ruminants, large amounts of dopamine) and release these into the pulmonary capillary blood during anaphylaxis.

Learning the precise function of each cell type listed in Table 23-2 will require methods for clean separation of living cells and growing each type in pure cell culture. In general, organs, tissues and cells have more than one function; time will probably show that this is true for the cells of the lung.

Clinical Implications

What are the clinical implications of these newly discovered functions of the lungs and pulmonary circulation? (1) We formerly thought that arterial blood differed from venous blood only in that arterial blood contained more O_2, less CO_2, fewer H^+ and thinner red blood cells. We must now conclude that, normally and in pathologic states, venous and arterial blood can differ in other ways, and we can no longer use analyses of systemic arterial blood to tell us how much norepinephrine, 5HT, bradykinin or prostaglandins are present in mixed venous blood, or depend on analyses of venous blood to estimate their concentrations in arterial blood. (2) Since some tissues of the lung are supplied by pulmonary artery blood and some by bronchial artery blood, substances removed entirely by the pulmonary circula-

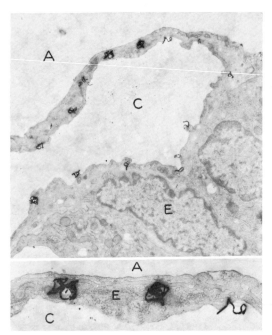

Fig. 23-3.—Electron microscope autoradiographs of a pulmonary capillary from a rat lung that has been infused with ^{3}H-5-hydroxytryptamine. **Top**, silver grains (black threads), which show the location of radioactive material, overlie only the endothelium; 5-hydroxytryptamine has been concentrated specifically in the capillary endothelial cells. $\times$ 11,800. **Bottom**, higher magnification of same capillary. The silver grains (threads) are present over only the endothelial cells. $\times$ 49,000. A = alveolus. C = capillary lumen. E = endothelial cell. (From Strum, J. M., and Junod, A.F.: J. Cell Biol. 54:460, 1972.)

substance given intra-arterially. (4) Widespread disease of pulmonary tissue may lead to systemic disturbances other than increased P_{CO_2} and decreased P_{O_2} and pH of systemic arterial blood — if the inactivation or detoxification functions of the pulmonary circulation are greatly diminished. Immaturity of biochemical process in the lungs of newborn babies can, because of lack of detoxifying or synthetic mechanisms, lead to serious problems. Large pulmonary artery to pulmonary vein shunts create a similar problem. Total bypass of the pulmonary circulation for hours or days by a pump oxygenator or artificial lung causes a complete bypass of the lung's metabolic function, and this must be taken into account in giving drugs intravenously to patients without natural lungs. Further, at the end of a long bypass procedure during which the lungs have been ischemic for several hours, lungs may extract more or less of substances or drugs in mixed venous blood now presented to them. (5) If two drugs are inactivated in the lungs by the same process, previous intravenous injection of one may prevent inactivation of the other and lead to its unexpectedly high concentration in arterial blood. (6) A second drug (e.g., chlorpromazine) might abruptly release a first drug (e.g., imipramine) presumed to be stored safely in pulmonary cells. And commonly used procedures may release stored materials; for example, hyperventilation is believed to release prostaglandin E_2 and, in newborn lambs, expansion of the lungs with O_2 leads abruptly to the appearance of free bradykinin in left atrial blood.

tion will act only on pulmonary arterioles, alveolar walls, alveolar ducts and afferent nerve endings in these, but not on the bronchi or bronchial arterioles or their afferent nerve endings. (3) Some substances given intravenously may have much less systemic action than the same amount of the same

References

Review articles on all aspects of respiratory physiology may be found in:

Fenn, W. O., and Rahn, H. (eds): *Handbook of Physiology*, Sec. 3. *Respiration*, Vol. I (Washington, D.C.: American Physiological Society, 1964), Vol. II (1965). These consist of 73 Chapters (1,696 pages); with few exceptions, these chapters are not listed separately in the references in this text.

Annual Review of Physiology. Each volume since 1939 (with the exception of 1942) contains a critical review of respiratory physiology or selected aspects of it; each contains excellent bibliographies.

Selected references to each chapter of this text follow.

Chapter 1. Introduction

Altman, P. L., and Dittmer, D. S. (eds.): *Respiration and Circulation* (Bethesda, Md.: Federation of American Societies for Experimental Biology, 1971).

Bartels, H., Dejours, P., Kellogg, R. H., and Mead, J.: Glossary on respiration and gas exchange, J. Appl. Physiol. 34:549, 1973.

Bates, D. V., Macklem, P. T., and Christie, R. V.: *Respiratory Function in Disease* (2d ed.; Philadelphia: W. B. Saunders Company, 1971).

Caro, C. G. (ed.): *Advances in Respiratory Physiology* (London: Edward Arnold & Co., 1966).

Ciba Foundation Symposium on Development of the Lung, de Reuck, A. V. S., and Porter, R. (eds.) (Boston: Little, Brown & Company, 1967).

Ciba Foundation Symposium on Pulmonary Structure and Function, de Reuck, A. V. S., and O'Conner, M. (eds.) (London: J. & A. Churchill, Ltd., 1961).

Cole, R. B.: *Essentials of Respiratory Disease* (New York: Pitman Publishing Corporation, 1971).

Comroe, J. H., Jr.: The functions of the lung, Harvey Lect. 48:110, 1952–53.

Cumming, G., and Semple, S. J.: *Disorders of the Respiratory System* (Oxford: Blackwell Scientific Publications, 1973).

Cunningham, D. J. C., and Lloyd, B. B. (eds.): *The Regulation of Human Respiration* (J. S. Haldane Centenary Symposium) (Oxford: Blackwell Scientific Publications, 1963).

Dejours, P.: *Respiration* (transl. by Farhi, L. E.) (New York: Oxford University Press, 1966).

Engel, S.: *Lung Structure* (Springfield, Ill.: Charles C Thomas, Publisher, 1962).

Haldane, J. S., and Priestley, J. G.: *Respiration* (London: Oxford University Press, 1935).

Hayek, H. von: *The Human Lung* (transl. by Krahl, V. E.) (New York: Hafner Publishing Company, 1960).

Krogh, A.: *The Comparative Physiology of Respiratory Mechanisms* (Philadelphia: University of Pennsylvania Press, 1941).

Miller, W. S.: *The Lung*, (2d ed.; Springfield, Ill.: Charles C Thomas, Publisher, 1947).

Nagaishi, Chūzō: *Functional Anatomy and Histology of the Lung* (Baltimore: University Park Press, 1972).

Nahas, G. G. (ed.): *Regulation of Respiration*, Ann. N.Y. Acad. Sci. 109:411, 1963.

Pappenheimer, J., *et al.*: Standardization of definitions and symbols in respiratory physiology, Fed. Proc. 9:602, 1950.

Rossier, P. H., Bühlmann, A. A., and Wiesinger, K.: *Respiration: Physiologic Principles and Their Clinical Applications* (transl. by Luchsinger, P. C., and Moser, K. M.) (St. Louis: C. V. Mosby Company, 1960).

Schulz, H.: *The Submicroscopic Anatomy and Pathology of the Lung* (Berlin: Springer-Verlag, 1959).

Staub, N. C.: The interdependence of pulmonary structure and function, Anesthesiology 24:831, 1963.

Chapter 2. Alveolar Ventilation

Comroe, J. H., Jr., Forster, R. E., II, DuBois, A. B., Briscoe, W. A., and Carlsen, E.: *The Lung: Clinical Physiology and Pulmonary Function Tests* (2d ed.; Chicago: Year Book Medical Publishers, Inc., 1962).

Davy, H.: *Researches, Chemical and Philosophical, Chiefly Concerning Nitrous Oxide or Dephlogisticated Air and Its Respiration* (2d ed.; London: 1839).

DuBois, A. B., Botelho, S. Y., Bedell, G. N., Marshall, R., and Comroe, J. H., Jr.: A rapid plethysmographic method for measuring thoracic gas volume: A comparison with a nitrogen washout method for measuring functional residual capacity in normal subjects, J. Clin. Invest. 35:322, 1956.

Fowler, W. S.: Lung function studies: II. The respiratory dead space, Am. J. Physiol. 154:405, 1948.

Hogg, W., Brunton, J., Kryger, M., Brown, R., and Macklem, P. T.: Gas diffusion across collateral channels, J. Appl. Physiol. 33:568, 1972.

Hutchinson, J.: Lecture on vital statistics, embracing an account of a new instrument for detecting the presence of disease in the system, Lancet 1:567, 594, 1844.

Kory, R. C.: Routine measurement of respiratory rate: An expensive tribute to tradition, J.A.M.A. 165:448, 1958.

Kory, R. C., Callahan, R., Boren, H. G., and Syner, J. C.: Clinical spirometry in normal men, Am. J. Med. 30:243, 1961.

Macklem, P. T.: Airway obstruction and collateral ventilation, Physiol. Rev. 51:368, 1971.

Radford, E. P., Jr.: The Physics of Gases, in Fenn, W. O., and Rahn, H. (eds.): *Handbook of Physiology*, Sec. 3. *Respiration*, Vol. I (Washington, D.C.: American Physiological Society, 1964), p. 125.

Rossier, P. H., and Bühlmann, A.: The respiratory dead space, Physiol. Rev. 35:860, 1955.

Salvatore, A. J., Sullivan, S. F., and Papper, E. M.: Postoperative hypoventilation and hypoxemia in man after hyperventilation, N. Engl. J. Med. 280:467, 1969.

Storey, W. F., and Staub, N. C.: Ventilation of terminal air units, J. Appl. Physiol. 17:391, 1962.

West, J. B.: Gas exchange when one lung region inspires from another, J. Appl. Physiol. 30:479, 1971.

Chapter 3. Regulation of Respiration — The Respiratory Centers

Brown, H. W., and Plum, F.: The neurologic basis of Cheyne-Stokes respiration, Am. J. Med. 30:849, 1961.

Cherniack, N. S., and Longobardo, G. S.: Cheyne-Stokes breathing: An instability in physiologic control, N. Engl. J. Med. 288:952, 1973.

Cohen, M. I.: How Respiratory Rhythm Originates: Evidence from Discharge Patterns of Brainstem Respiratory Neurones, in Porter, R. (ed.): *Breathing: Hering-Breuer Centenary Symposium* (London: J. & A. Churchill, Ltd., 1970), p. 125.

Guilleminault, C., Eldridge, F. L., and Dement, W. C.: Insomnia with sleep apnea: A new syndrome, Science 181:856, 1973.

Guyton, A. C., Crowell, J. W., and Moore, J. W.: Basic oscillating mechanism of Cheyne-Stokes breathing, Am. J. Physiol. 187:395, 1956.

Kaada, B. R.: Angulate, Posterior Orbital, Anterior Insular and Temporal Pole Cortex, in Magoun, H. W. (ed.): *Handbook of Physiology*, Sec. 1. *Neurophysiology*, Vol. II (Washington, D.C.: American Physiological Society, 1960), p. 1345.

Lange, R. L., and Hecht, H. H.: The mechanism of Cheyne-Stokes respiration, J. Clin. Invest. 41:42, 1962.

Liljestrand, A.: Neural control of respiration, Physiol. Rev. 38:691, 1958.

Oberholzer, R. J. H., and Tofani, W. O.: The Neural Control of Respiration, in Magoun, H. W. (ed.): *Handbook of Physiology*, Sec. 1. *Neurophysiology*, Vol. II (Washington, D. C.: American Physiological Society, 1960), p. 1111.

Pitts, R. F.: Organization of the respiratory center, Physiol. Rev. 26:609, 1946.

Plum, F.: Neurological Integration of Behavioural and Metabolic Control of Breathing, in Porter, R. (ed.): *Breathing: Hering-Breuer Centenary Symposium* (London: J. & A. Churchill, Ltd., 1970), p. 159.

Wang, S. C., and Ngai, S. H.: General Organization of Central Respiratory Mechanisms, in Fenn, W. O., and Rahn, H. (eds.): *Handbook of Physiology*, Sec. 3. *Respiration*, Vol. I (Washington, D. C.: American Physiological Society, 1964), p. 487.

Chapter 4. The Response to Oxygen and Oxygen Lack

Biscoe, T. J.: Carotid body: Structure and function, Physiol. Rev. 51:437, 1971.

Chiodi, H., Dill, D. B., Consolazio, F., and Horvath, S. M.: Respiratory and circulatory responses to acute CO poisoning, Am. J. Physiol. 134:683, 1941.

Comroe, J. H., Jr.: The location and function of the chemoreceptors of the aorta, Am. J. Physiol. 127: 176, 1939.

Comroe, J. H., Jr.: The Peripheral Chemoreceptors, in Fenn, W. O., and Rahn, H. (eds.): *Handbook of Physiology*, Sec. 3. *Respiration*, Vol. I (Washington, D. C.: American Physiological Society, 1964), p. 557.

Daly, M. deB., Lambertsen, C. J., and Schweitzer, A.: Observations on the volume of blood flow and oxygen utilization of the carotid body in the cat, J. Physiol. (Lond.) 125:67, 1954.

Dripps, R. D., and Comroe, J. H., Jr.: The effect of the inhalation of high and low oxygen concentrations on respiration, pulse rate, ballistocardiogram and arterial oxygen saturation (oximeter) of normal individuals, Am. J. Physiol. 149:277, 1947.

Eyzaguirre, C., and Zapata, P.: A Discussion of Possible Transmitter or Generator Substances in Carotid Body Chemoreceptors, in Torrance, R. W. (ed.): *Arterial Chemoreceptors* (Oxford: Blackwell Scientific Publications, 1968), p. 213.

Guazzi, M., Baccelli, G., and Zanchetti, A.: Reflex chemoceptive regulation of arterial pressure during natural sleep in the cat, Am. J. Physiol. 214:969, 1968.

Guz, A., Noble, M. I. M., Widdicombe, J. G., Trenchard, D., and Mushin, W. W.: Peripheral chemoreceptor block in man, Respir. Physiol. 1:38–40, 1966.

Hatcher, J. D., and Jennings, D. B. (eds.): *International Symposium on the Cardiovascular and Respiratory Effects of Hypoxia* (New York: Hafner Publishing Company, 1966).

Heymans, C.: Action of drugs on carotid body and sinus, Pharmacol. Rev. 7:119, 1955.

Heymans, C., and Neil, E.: *Reflexogenic Areas of the Cardiovascular System* (Boston: Little, Brown & Company, 1958).

Korner, P. I.: Circulatory adaptations in hypoxia, Physiol. Rev. 39:687, 1959.

Korner, P. I.: Integrative neural cardiovascular control, Physiol. Rev. 51:312, 1971.

Landgren, S., and Neil, E.: Chemoreceptor impulse activity following haemorrhage, Acta physiol. scandinav. 23:158, 1951.

McDonald, D. M., and Mitchell, R. A.: A Quantitative Analysis of the Synaptic Connections in the Rat Carotid Body, in Purves, M. (ed.): *Chemoreceptor Mechanisms* (Cambridge, England: Cambridge University Press, 1974).

Mills, E., and Edwards, McI. W.: Stimulation of aortic and carotid chemoreceptors during carbon monoxide inhalation, J. Appl. Physiol. 25:494, 1968.

Neurophysiological and metabolic aspects of chemoreceptor function (Physiology Society Symposium), Fed. Proc. 31:1365, 1972.

Purves, M. J. (ed.): *Chemoreceptor Mechanisms* (Cambridge, England: Cambridge University Press, 1974).

Schmidt, C. F., and Comroe, J. H., Jr.: Functions of the carotid and aortic bodies, Physiol. Rev. 20:115, 1940.

Sorenson, S. C.: The chemical control of ventilation, Acta physiol. scand., Supp. 361, 1971.

Torrance, R. W.: Prolegomena, in Torrance, R. W. (ed.): *Arterial Chemoreceptors* (Oxford: Blackwell Scientific Publications, 1968), p. 1.

Chapter 5. The Response to Carbon Dioxide

Douglas, C. G., and Haldane, J. S.: The regulation of normal breathing, J. Physiol. (Lond.) 38:420, 1909.

Dripps, R. D., and Comroe, J. H., Jr.: The respiratory and circulatory response of normal man to inhalation of 7.6 and 10.4 per cent CO_2 with a comparison of the maximal ventilation produced by severe muscular exercise, inhalation of CO_2 and maximal voluntary hyperventilation, Am. J. Physiol. 149:43, 1947.

Gray J. S.: *Pulmonary Ventilation and Its Physiologic Regulation* (Springfield, Ill.: Charles C Thomas, Publisher, 1950).

Haldane, J. S.: Acclimatization to high altitudes, Physiol. Rev. 7:363, 1927.

Jacobs, M. H.: The production of intracellular acidity by neutral and alkaline solutions containing carbon dioxide, Am. J. Physiol. 53: 457, 1920.

Kellogg, R. H.: Central Chemical Regulation of Respiration, in Fenn, W. O., and Rahn, H. (eds.): *Handbook of Physiology:* Sec. 3. *Respiration*, Vol. I (Washington, D.C.: American Physiological Society, 1964), p. 507.

Leusen, I.: Regulation of cerebrospinal fluid composition with reference to breathing, Physiol. Rev. 52:1, 1972.

Lloyd, B. B., Jukes, M. G. M., and Cunningham, D. J. C.: The relation between alveolar oxygen pressure and the respiratory response to carbon dioxide in man, Q. J. Exp. Physiol. 43: 214, 1958.

Loeschke, H. H., and Gertz, K. H.: Einfluss des O_2-Druckes in der Einatmungszeit auf die Atemtätigkeit des Menschen, geprüft unter Konstanthaltung des alveolaren CO_2-Druckes, Arch. ges. Physiol. 267:460, 1958.

Mitchell, R. A., Loeschke, H. H., Severinghaus, J. W., Richardson, B. W., and Massion, W. H.: Regions of respiratory chemosensitivity on the surface of the medulla, Ann. NY Acad. Sci. 109:661, 1963.

Mitchell, R. A., and Severinghaus, J. W.: Cerebrospinal fluid and the regulation of respiration, Physiol. Physicians 3:1, 1965.

Symposium: Carbon dioxide and man, Anesthesiology 21:585, 1960.

Tschirgi, R. D.: Chemical Environment of the Central Nervous System, in Magoun, H. W. (ed.): *Handbook of Physiology*, Sec. 1. *Neurophysiology*, Vol. III (Washington, D. C.: American Physiological Society, 1960), p. 1865.

Chapter 6. The Response to Hydrogen Ions

Gesell, R.: The chemical regulation of respiration, Physiol. Rev. 5:551, 1925.

Lambertsen, C. J., Semple, S. J. G., Smyth, M. G., and Gelfand, R.: H$^+$ and Pco$_2$ as chemical factors in respiratory and cerebral circulatory control, J. Appl. Physiol. 16:473, 1961.

Leusen, I.: Regulation of cerebrospinal fluid composition with reference to breathing, Physiol. Rev. 52:1, 1972.

Mitchell, R. A.: Cerebrospinal Fluid and the Regulation of Respiration, in Caro, C. G. (ed.): *Advances in Respiratory Physiology* (London: Edward Arnold & Co., 1966), p. 1.

Severinghaus, J. W., Mitchell, R. A., Richardson, B. W., and Singer, M. M.: Respiratory control at high altitude suggesting active transport regulation of CSF pH, J. Appl. Physiol. 18: 1155, 1963.

Symposium on Cerebrospinal Fluid and the Regulation of Ventilation (Brooks, C. McC., Kao, F. F., and Lloyd, B. B., eds.): (Oxford: Blackwell Scientific Publications, 1965).

Winterstein, H.: The action of substances introduced into the cerebrospinal fluid and the problem of intracranial chemoreceptors, Pharmacol. Rev. 13:71, 1961.

Chapter 7. Cerebral Blood Flow and Respiratory Regulation

Betz, E.: Cerebral blood flow: Its measurement and regulation, Physiol. Rev. 52:595, 1972.

Defares, J. G.: Principles of Feedback Control and their Application to the Respiratory Control System, in Rahn, H., and Fenn, W. O. (eds.): *Handbook of Physiology*, Sec. 3. *Respiration*, Vol. I (Washington, D.C.: American Physiological Society, 1964), p. 649.

Lambertsen, C. J.: Chemical Factors in Respiratory Control, in Bard, P. (ed.): *Medical*

Physiology (11th ed.; St. Louis: C. V. Mosby Company, 1961), p. 633.

Purves, M. J.: *The Physiology of the Cerebral Circulation* (Cambridge, England: Cambridge University Press, 1972).

Schmidt, C. F.: The influence of cerebral bloodflow on respiration, Am. J. Physiol. 84:202, 1928.

Chapter 8. Reflexes from the Lungs

Adrian, E. D.: Afferent impulses in the vagus and their effect on respiration, J. Physiol. (Lond.) 79:332, 1933.

Bartoli, A., Bystrzycka, E., Guz, A., Jain, S. K., Noble, M. I. M., and Trenchard, D.: Studies of pulmonary vagal control of central respiratory rhythm in the absence of breathing movements, J. Physiol. 230:449, 1973.

Breuer, J.: Self-Steering of Respiration through the *Nervus Vagus* (transl. by Ullmann, E.), in Porter, R. (ed.): *Breathing: Hering-Breuer Centenary Symposium* (London: J. & A. Churchill, Ltd., 1970), p. 365.

Breuer, J., and Hering, E.: Self-Steering of Respiration through the *Nervus Vagus* (transl. by Ullmann, E.), in Porter, R. (ed.): *Breathing: Hering-Breuer Centenary Symposium* (London: J. & A. Churchill, Ltd., 1970), p. 359.

Clark, F. J., and Euler, C. von: On the regulation of depth and rate of breathing, J. Physiol. 222: 267, 1972.

Costantin, L. L.: Effect of pulmonary congestion on vagal afferent activity, Am. J. Physiol. 196: 49, 1959.

Cross, K. W.: Head's paradoxical reflex, Brain 84:529, 1961.

Davis, H. L., Fowler, W. S., and Lambert, E. H.: Effect of volume and rate of inflation and deflation on transpulmonary pressure and response of pulmonary stretch receptors, Am. J. Physiol. 187:558, 1956.

Guz, A., Noble, M. I. M., Eisele, J. H., and Trenchard, D.: The effect of lung deflation on breathing in man, Clin. Sci. 40:451, 1971.

Guz, A., Noble, M. I. M., Eisele, J. H., and Trenchard, D.: The Role of Vagal Inflation Reflexes in Man and Other Animals, in Porter, R. (ed.): *Breathing: Hering-Breuer Centenary Symposium* (London: J. & A. Churchill, Ltd., 1970), p. 17.

Guz, A., Noble, M. I. M., Widdicombe, J. G., Trenchard, D., Mushin, W. W., and Makey, A. R.: The role of vagal and glossopharyngeal afferent nerves in respiratory sensation, control of breathing and arterial pressure regulation in conscious man, Clin. Sci. 30:161, 1966.

Hung, K. S., Hertweck, M. S., Hardy, J. D., and

Loosli, C. G.: Electron microscopic observations of nerve endings in the alveolar walls of mouse lungs, Am. Rev. Respir. Dis. 108:328, 1973.

Knowlton, G. C., and Larrabee, M. G.: A unitary analysis of pulmonary volume receptors, Am. J. Physiol. 147:100–114, 1946.

Larrabee, M. G., and Knowlton, G. C.: Excitation and inhibition of phrenic mononeurones by inflation of the lungs, Am. J. Physiol. 147:90–99, 1946.

Larsell, O., and Dow, R. S.: The innervation of the human lung, Am. J. Anat. 52:125, 1933.

Mead, J.: Control of respiratory frequency, J. Appl. Physiol. 15:325–336, 1960.

Mills, J. E., Sellick, H., and Widdicombe, J. G.: Epithelial Irritant Receptors in the Lungs, in Porter, R. (ed.): *Breathing: Hering-Breuer Centenary Symposium* (London: J. & A. Churchill, Ltd., 1970), p. 77.

Paintal, A. S.: Vagal sensory receptors and their reflex effects, Physiol. Rev. 53:159, 1973.

Phillipson, E. A., Hickey, R. F., Bainton, C. R., and Nadel, J. A.: Effect of vagal blockade on regulation of breathing in conscious dogs, J. Appl. Physiol. 29:475, 1970.

Simmons, D. H., and Hemingway, A.: Acute respiratory effects of pneumothorax in normal and vagotomized dogs, Am. Rev. Tuberc. 76:195, 1957.

Whitteridge, D.: Multiple embolism of the lung and rapid shallow breathing, Physiol. Rev. 30:475, 1950.

Widdicombe, J. G.: Respiratory Reflexes, in Fenn, W. O., and Rahn, H. (eds.): *Handbook of Physiology*, Sec. 3. *Respiration*, Vol. I (Washington, D. C.: American Physiological Society, 1964), p. 585.

Chapter 9. Other Reflexes

Anderson, H. T.: Physiological adaptations in diving vertebrates, Physiol. Rev. 46:212, 1966.

Aviado, D. M., Jr., and Schmidt, C. F.: Reflexes from stretch receptors in blood vessels, heart and lungs, Physiol. Rev. 35:247, 1955.

Comroe, J. H., Jr., Van Lingen, B., Stroud, R. C., and Roncoroni, A.: Reflex and direct cardiopulmonary effects of 5-OH-tryptamine (serotonin): Their possible role in pulmonary embolism and coronary thrombosis, Am. J. Physiol. 173:379, 1953.

Dawes, G. S., and Comroe, J. H., Jr.: Chemoreflexes from the heart and lungs, Physiol. Rev. 34:167, 1954.

Fink, B. R.: Influence of cerebral activity in wakefulness on regulation of breathing, J. Appl. Physiol. 16:15, 1961.

Gray, J. S.: The multiple factor theory of the control of respiratory ventilation, Science 103:739, 1946.

Irving, L.: Respiration in diving mammals, Physiol. Rev. 19:112, 1939.

Jain, S. K., Subramanian, S., Julka, D. B., and Guz, A.: Search for evidence of lung chemoreflexes in man: Study of respiratory and circulatory effects of phenyldiguanide and lobeline, Clin. Sci. 42:163, 1972.

Nathan, P. W., and Sears, T. A.: Effects of posterior root section on the activity of some muscles in man, J. Neurol. Neurosurg. Psychiatry 23:10, 1960.

Reed, D. J., and Kellogg, R. H.: Effect of sleep on CO_2 stimulation of breathing in acute and chronic hypoxia, J. Appl. Physiol. 15:1135, 1960.

Reeve, E. B., Nanson, E. M., and Rundle, F.F.: Observations on inhibitory respiratory reflexes during abdominal surgery, Clin. Sci. 10:65, 1951.

Whitehead, R. W., and Draper, W. B.: A respiratory reflex originating from the thoracic wall of the dog, Anesthesiology 8:159, 1947.

Chapter 10. Mechanical Factors in Breathing

Agostoni, E.: Action of Respiratory Muscles, in Fenn, W. O., and Rahn, H. (eds.): *Handbook of Physiology*, Sec. 3. *Respiration*, Vol. I (Washington, D. C.: American Physiological Society, 1964), p. 377.

Agostoni, E.: Mechanics of the pleural space, Physiol. Rev. 52:58, 1972.

Avery, M. E.: The pulmonary surfactant in foetal and neonatal lungs, in *Foetal and Neonatal Physiology* (*Proceedings of Barcroft Centenary Symposium*) (Cambridge, England: Cambridge University Press, 1973).

Avery, M. E., and Mead, J.: Surface properties in relation to atelectasis and hyaline membrane disease, Am. J. Dis. Child. 97:517, 1959.

Bayliss, L. E., and Robertson, G. W.: The viscoelastic properties of the lungs, Quart. J. Exp. Physiol. 29:27, 1939.

Campbell, E. J. M.: *The Respiratory Muscles and the Mechanics of Breathing* (Chicago: Year Book Medical Publishers, Inc., 1958).

Campbell, E. J. M.: Motor Pathways, in Fenn, W. O., and Rahn, H. (eds.): *Handbook of Physiology*, Sec. 3. *Respiration*, Vol. I (Washington, D.C.: American Physiological Society, 1964), p. 535.

Campbell, E. J. M., Martin, H. B., and Riley, R. L.: Mechanisms of airway obstruction, Bull. Johns Hopkins Hosp. 101:329, 1957.

Chu, J., Clements, J. A., Cotton, E. K., Klaus, M.

H., Sweet, A. Y., and Tooley, W. H.: Neonatal pulmonary ischemia: I. Clinical and physiological studies, Pediatrics 40:709, 1967.

Clements, J. A.: Sixth Bowditch Lecture: Surface phenomena in relation to pulmonary function, Physiologist 5:11, 1962.

Clements, J. A.: Pulmonary surfactant, Am. Rev. Respir. Dis. 101:984, 1970.

Clements, J. A., et al.: Assessment of the risk of the respiratory-distress syndrome by a rapid test for surfactant in amniotic fluid, N. Engl. J. Med. 286:1077, 1972.

Dayman, H.: Mechanics of airflow in health and in emphysema, J. Clin. Invest. 30:1175, 1951.

DeGraff, A. C., and Bouhuys, A.: Mechanics of airflow in airway obstruction, Annu. Rev. Med. 24:111, 1973.

DuBois, A. B., Botelho, S. Y., and Comroe, J. H., Jr.: A new method for measuring airway resistance in man using a body plethysmograph: Values in normal subjects and in patients with respiratory disease, J. Clin. Invest. 35:327, 1956.

Fry, D. L., and Hyatt, R. E.: Pulmonary mechanics: A unified analysis of the relationship between pressure, volume and gas flow in the lungs of normal and diseased human subjects, Am. J. Med. 29:672, 1960.

Hogg, J. C., Macklem, P. T., and Thurlbeck, W. M.: Site and nature of airway obstruction in chronic obstructive lung disease, N. Engl. J. Med. 278:1355, 1968.

Horsfield, K., Dart, G., Olson, D. E., Filley, G. F., and Cumming, G.: Models of the human bronchial tree, J. Appl. Physiol. 31:207, 1971.

Hyatt, R. E., and Black, L. F.: The flow-volume curve: A current perspective, Am. Rev. Respir. Dis. 107:191, 1973.

Leuallen, E. C., and Fowler, W. S.: Maximal midexpiratory flow, Am. Rev. Tuberc. 72:783, 1955.

Macklem, P. T.: Airway obstruction and collateral ventilation, Physiol. Rev. 51:368, 1971.

Macklem, P. T., and Mead, J.: Factors determining maximum expiratory flow in dogs, J. Appl. Physiol. 25:159, 1968.

Macklin, C. C.: The musculature of the bronchi and lungs, Physiol. Rev. 9:1, 1929.

Macklin, C. C.: The pulmonary alveolar mucoid film and the pneumonocytes, Lancet 1:1099, 1954.

Marshall, R., and DuBois, A. B.: Measurement of the viscous resistance of the lung tissues in normal man, Clin. Sci. 15:161, 1956.

Mead, J.: Mechanical properties of lungs, Physiol. Rev. 41:281, 1961.

Mead, J., Takishima, T., and Leith, D.: Stress distribution in lungs: A model of pulmonary elasticity, J. Appl. Physiol. 28:596, 1970.

Mead, J., Turner, J. M., Macklem, P. T., and Lit-tle, J. B.: Significance of the relationship between lung recoil and maximum expiratory flow, J. Appl. Physiol. 22:95, 1967.

Murray, J. F., Greenspan, R. H., Gold, W. M., and Cohen, A. B.: Early diagnosis of chronic obstructive lung disease, Calif. Med. 116:37, 1972.

Nadel, J. A., Colebatch, H. J. H., and Olsen, C. R.: Location and mechanism of airway constriction after barium sulfate microembolism, J. Appl. Physiol. 19:387, 1964.

Neergaard, K., and Wirz, K.: Über eine Methode zur Messung der Lungenelastizität am lebenden Menschen, insbesondere beim Emphysem, Z. klin. Med. 105:35, 1927.

Otis, A. B.: The work of breathing, Physiol. Rev. 34:449, 1954.

Otis, A. B.: The Work of Breathing, in Fenn, W. O., and Rahn, H. (eds.): Handbook of Physiology, Sec. 3. Respiration, Vol. I (Washington, D.C.: American Physiological Society, 1964), p. 463.

Otis, A. B., McKerrow, C. B., Bartlett, R. A., Mead, J., McIlroy, M. B., Selverstone, N. J., and Radford, E. P.: Mechanical factors in distribution of pulmonary ventilation, J. Appl. Physiol. 8:427, 1956.

Pattle, R. E.: Lining layer of alveoli, Br. Med. Bull. 19:41, 1963.

Pattle, R. E.: Surface lining of lung alveoli, Physiol. Rev. 45:48, 1965.

Petty, T. L., and Ashbaugh, D. G.: The adult respiratory distress syndrome, Chest 60:233, 1971.

Pride, N. B., Permutt, S., Riley, R. L., and Bromberger-Barnea, B.: Determinants of maximal expiratory flow from the lungs, J. Appl. Physiol. 23:646, 1967.

Radford, E. P., Jr.: Static Mechanical Properties of Mammalian Lungs, in Fenn, W. O., and Rahn, H. (eds.): Handbook of Physiology, Sec. 3. Respiration, Vol. I (Washington, D.C.: American Physiological Society, 1964), p. 429.

Rahn, H., et al.: The pressure-volume diagram of the lung and thorax, Am. J. Physiol. 146:161, 1946.

Widdicombe, J. G.: Regulation of tracheobronchial smooth muscle, Physiol. Rev. 43:1–37, 1963.

Widdicombe, J. G.: The Regulation of Bronchial Calibre, in Caro, C. G. (ed.): Advances in Respiratory Physiology (London: Edward Arnold & Company, 1966), p. 48.

Chapter 11. The Pulmonary Circulation

Adams, W. R., and Veith, I. (eds.): Pulmonary Circulation (New York: Grune & Stratton, Inc., 1959).

Anthonisen, N. R., and Milic-Emili, J.: Distribution of pulmonary perfusion in erect man, J. Appl. Physiol. 21:760, 1966.

Aviado, D. M.: The pharmacology of the pulmonary circulation, Pharmacol. Rev. 12:159, 1960.

Carlens, E., Hanson, H. E., and Nordenström, B.: Temporary unilateral occlusion of the pulmonary artery, J. Thoracic Surg. 22:527, 1951.

Cournand, A.: Pulmonary circulation: Its control in man, with some remarks on methodology, Science 125:1231, 1957, p. 1667.

Fishman, A. P.: Dynamics of the Pulmonary Circulation, in Hamilton, W. F. (ed.): *Handbook of Physiology*, Sec. 2. *Circulation*, Vol. II (Washington, D. C.: American Physiological Society, 1963), p. 1667.

Fishman, A. P.: Respiratory gases in the regulation of the pulmonary circulation, Physiol. Rev. 41:214, 1961.

Forster, R. E.: The Pulmonary Capillary Bed: Volume, Area and Diffusing Characteristics, in *Pulmonary Circulation* (New York: Grune & Stratton, Inc., 1959), p. 45.

Harris, P., and Heath, D.: *The Human Pulmonary Circulation* (Edinburgh and London: E. & S. Livingstone, Ltd., 1962).

Hellems, H. K., Haynes, F. W., and Dexter, L.: Pulmonary "capillary" pressure in man, J. Appl. Physiol. 2:24, 1949.

Lee, G. de J., and DuBois, A. B.: Pulmonary capillary blood flow in man, J. Clin. Invest. 34: 1380, 1955.

Liljestrand, G.: Chemical control of the distribution of the pulmonary blood flow, Acta physiol. scandinav. 44:216, 1958.

Milnor, W. R.: Pulsatile blood flow, N. Engl. J. Med. 287:27, 1972.

Richards, D. W.: Right heart catheterization: Its contributions to physiology and medicine, Science 125:1181, 1957.

Roughton, F. J. W.: The average time spent by the blood in the human lung capillary, Am. J. Physiol. 143:621, 1945.

Singhal, S., Henderson, R., Horsfield, K., Harding, K., and Cumming, G.: Morphometry of the human pulmonary arterial tree, Circ. Res. 33:190, 1973.

West, J. B.: *Ventilation/Blood Flow and Gas Exchange* (2d ed.; Oxford: Blackwell Scientific Publications, 1970).

Chapter 12. Pulmonary Gas Diffusion

Barcroft, J.: *The Respiratory Function of the Blood:* Part I. *The Diffusion of O_2 through Pulmonary Epithelium*, Vol. I (Cambridge, England: Cambridge University Press, 1925), p. 63.

Forster, R. E.: Exchange of gases between alveolar air and pulmonary capillary blood: Pulmonary diffusing capacity, Physiol. Rev. 37:391, 1957.

Forster, R. E.: Rate of Gas Uptake by Red Cells, in Fenn, W. O., and Rahn, H. (eds.): *Handbook of Physiology*, Sec. 3. *Respiration*, Vol. I (Washington, D.C.: American Physiological Society, 1964), p. 827.

Forster, R. E.: Diffusion of Gases, in Fenn, W. O., and Rahn, H. (eds.): *Handbook of Physiology*, Sec. 3. *Respiration*, Vol. I (Washington, D.C.: American Physiological Society, 1964), p. 839.

Gold, W. M., Youker, J., Anderson, S., and Nadel, J. A.: Pulmonary function abnormalities following lymphangiography, N. Engl. J. Med. 273:519, 1965.

Hogg, W., Brunton, J., Kryger, M., Brown, R., and Macklem, P.: Gas diffusion across collateral channels, J. Appl. Physiol. 33:568, 1972.

Krogh, M.: Diffusion of gases through the lungs of man, J. Physiol. (Lond.) 49:271, 1914–15.

Lilienthal, J. L., Jr., Riley, R. L., Proemmel, D. D., and Franke, R. E.: An experimental analysis in man of the oxygen pressure gradient from alveolar air to arterial blood during rest and exercise at sea level and at altitude, Am. J. Physiol. 147:199, 1946.

McNeill, R. S., Rankin, J., and Forster, R. E.: The diffusing capacity of the pulmonary membrane and the pulmonary capillary blood volume in cardiopulmonary disease, Clin. Sci. 17: 465, 1958.

Ogilvie, C. M., et al.: A standardized breath holding technique for the clinical measurement of the diffusing capacity of the lung for carbon monoxide, J. Clin. Invest. 36:1, 1957.

Weibel, E. R.: Morphological basis of alveolar-capillary gas exchange, Physiol. Rev. 53:419, 1973.

Chapter 13. Matching of Gas and Blood

Ball, W. C., Stewart, P. B., Newsham, L. G. S., and Bates, D. V.: Regional pulmonary function studied with xenon[133], J. Clin. Invest. 41:519, 1962.

Bouhuys, A., and Lundin, G.: Distribution of inspired gas in lungs, Physiol. Rev. 39:731, 1959.

Canfield, R. E., and Rahn, H.: Arterial-alveolar N_2 gas pressure differences due to ventilation-perfusion variations, J. Appl. Physiol. 10:165, 1957.

Comroe, J. H., Jr., and Fowler, W. S.: Detection of uneven ventilation during a single breath of O_2, Am. J. Med. 10:408, 1951.

Dolfuss, R. E., Milic-Emili, J., and Bates, D. V.: Regional ventilation of the lung, studied with boluses of [133]xenon, Respir. Physiol. 2:234, 1967.

Dollery, C. T., and Hugh-Jones, P.: Distribution of gas and blood in the lungs in disease, Br. Med. Bull. 19:59, 1963.

Fowler, W. S.: Intrapulmonary distribution of inspired gas, Physiol. Rev. 32:1, 1952.

Lilly, J. C.: Mixing of gases within respiratory system with a new type nitrogen meter, Am. J. Physiol. 161:342, 1950.

Milic-Emili, J., Henderson, J. A. M., Dolovich, M. B., Trop, D., and Kaneko, K.: Regional distribution of inspired gas in the lung, J. Appl. Physiol. 21:749, 1966.

Olszowska, A. J., Rahn, H., and Farhi, L. E.: *Blood gases: Hemoglobin, Base-Excess and Maldistribution* (Philadelphia: Lea & Febiger, 1973).

Rahn, H.: A concept of mean alveolar air and the ventilation−bloodflow relationships during pulmonary gas exchange, Am. J. Physiol. 158: 21, 1949, p. 735.

Rahn, H., and Farhi, L. E.: Ventilation, Perfusion, and Gas Exchange−the $\dot{V}A/\dot{Q}$ concept, in Fenn, W. O., and Rahn, H. (eds.): *Handbook of Physiology*, Sec. 3. *Respiration*, Vol. I (Washington, D.C.: American Physiological Society, 1964), p. 737.

Riley, R. L., and Cournand, A.: Analysis of factors affecting partial pressures of O_2 and CO_2 in gas and blood of lungs: Theory, J. Appl. Physiol. 4:77, 1951.

Riley, R. L., Cournand, A., and Donald, K. W.: Analysis of factors affecting partial pressures of O_2 and CO_2 in gas and blood of lungs: Methods, J. Appl. Physiol. 4:102, 1951.

Severinghaus, J. W., and Stupfel, M.: Alveolar dead space as an index of distribution of blood flow in pulmonary capillaries, J. Appl. Physiol. 10:335, 1957.

Severinghaus, J. W., Swenson, E. W., Finley, T. N., Lategola, M. T., and Williams, J.: Unilateral hypoventilation produced in dogs by occluding one pulmonary artery, J. Appl. Physiol. 16: 53, 1961.

West, J. B.: Causes of carbon dioxide retention in lung disease, N. Engl. J. Med. 284:1232, 1971.

West, J. B.: *Ventilation/Blood Flow and Gas Exchange* (2d ed.; Oxford: Blackwell Scientific Publications, 1970).

Chapter 14. The Transport of Oxygen by Blood

Benesch, R. E., and Benesch, R.: The reaction between diphosphoglycerate and hemoglobin, Fed. Proc. 29:1101, 1970.

Bunn, H. F., and Jandl, J. J.: Control of hemoglobin function within the red cell, N. Engl. J.

Med. 282:1414, 1970.

Chanutin, A., and Curnish, R. R.: Effect of organic and inorganic phosphates on the oxygen equilibrium of human erythrocytes, Arch. Biochem. Biophys. 121:96, 1967.

Cherniack, N. S., and Longobardo, G. S.: Oxygen and carbon dioxide gas stores of the body, Physiol. Rev. 50:196, 1970.

Dickens, F., and Neil, E. (eds.): *Oxygen in the Animal Organism* (Oxford: Pergamon Press, 1964).

Finch, C. A., and Lenfant, C.: Oxygen transport in man, N. Engl. J. Med. 286:407, 1972.

Hershey, D. (ed.): *Blood Oxygenation* (New York: Plenum Press, 1970).

Kilmartin, J. V., and Rossi-Bernardi, L.: Interaction of hemoglobin with hydrogen ions, carbon dioxide and organic phosphates, Physiol. Rev. 53:836, 1973.

Lübbers, D. W., Luft, U. C., Thews, G., and Witzleb, E.: *Oxygen Transport in Blood and Tissue* (Stuttgart: Georg Thieme Verlag, 1968).

Peters, J. P., and Van Slyke, D. D.: *Hemoglobin and Oxygen: Carbonic Acid and Acid Base Balance* (Reprinted from *Quantitative Clinical Chemistry*, Vol. I, ch. XII and XVIII) (Baltimore: Williams & Wilkins Company, 1931).

Rahn, H., and Fenn, W. O.: *A Graphical Analysis of the Respiratory Gas Exchange: The O_2-CO_2 Diagram* (Washington, D.C.: American Physiological Society, 1955).

Roughton, F. J. W.: Transport of Oxygen and Carbon Dioxide, in Fenn, W. O., and Rahn, H. (eds.): *Handbook of Physiology*, Sec. 3. *Respiration*, Vol. I (Washington, D.C.: American Physiological Society, 1964), p. 767.

Roughton, F. J. W., and Darling, R. C.: The effect of carbon monoxide on the oxyhemoglobin dissociation curve, Am. J. Physiol. 141:17, 1944.

Severinghaus, J. W.: Blood gas calculator, J. Appl. Physiol. 21:1108, 1966.

Stamatoyannopoulos, G., Bellingham, A. J., Lenfant, C., and Finch, C. A.: Abnormal hemoglobins with high and low oxygen affinity, Annu. Rev. Med. 22:221, 1971.

Chapter 15. Blood-Tissue Gas Exchange

American Physiological Society: Symposium on tissue oxygen tension, Fed. Proc. 16:665, 1957.

Bircher, H. I., and Bruley, D. R. (eds.): *Oxygen Transport to Tissue* (New York: Plenum Press, 1974).

Farhi, L. E.: Atmospheric nitrogen and its role in modern medicine, J.A.M.A. 188:152, 1964.

Farhi, L. E.: Gas Stores of the Body, in Fenn, W. O., and Rahn, H. (eds.): *Handbook of Physiol-*

ogy, Sec. 3. *Respiration*, Vol. I (Washington, D. C.: American Physiological Society, 1964), p. 873.

Kessler, M., Bruley, D. F., Clark, L. C., Lübbers, D. W., Silver, I. A., and Strauss, J. (eds.): *Oxygen Supply* (Baltimore: University Park Press, 1973).

Kety, S. S.: The theory and applications of the exchange of inert gas at the lungs and tissues, Pharmacol. Rev. 3:1–41, 1951.

Wittenberg, J. B.: Myoglobin-facilitated oxygen diffusion: Role of myoglobin in oxygen entry into muscle, Physiol. Rev. 50:559, 1970.

Chapter 16. Transport and Elimination of Carbon Dioxide

Astrup, P., Jørgensen, K., Siggaard-Andersen, O., and Engel, K.: The acid-base metabolism: A new approach, Lancet 1:1035, 1960.

Berliner, R. W., and Orloff, J.: Carbonic anhydrase inhibitors, Pharmacol. Rev. 8:137, 1956.

Campbell, E. J. M.: RIpH, Lancet 1:681, 1962.

Christiansen, H. N.: *Body Fluids and Their Neutrality* (New York: Oxford University Press, 1963).

Davenport, H.: *The ABC of Acid Base Chemistry* (5th ed.; Chicago: University of Chicago Press, 1969).

Dorman, P. J., Sullivan, W. J., and Pitts, R. F.: The renal response to acute respiratory acidosis, J. Clin. Invest. 33:82, 1954.

Elkinton, J. R.: Hydrogen ion turnover in health and in renal disease, Ann. Intern. Med. 57:660, 1962.

Filley, G. F.: Acid-base regulation: Classical concepts and modern measurements, Johns Hopkins Med. J. 120:355, 1967.

Gilman, A., and Brazeau, P.: The role of the kidney in the regulation of acid-base metabolism, Am. J. Med. 15:765, 1953.

Henderson, L. J.: *Blood: A Study in General Physiology* (New Haven: Yale University Press, 1928).

Peters, J. P., and Van Slyke, D. D.: Hemoglobin and Oxygen: Carbonic Acid and Acid Base Balance (reprinted from *Quantitative Clinical Chemistry*, Vol. I, ch. XII and XVIII) (Baltimore: Williams & Wilkins Company, 1931).

Pitts, R. F.: *Physiology of the Kidney and Body Fluids* (3d ed.: Chicago: Year Book Medical Publishers, Inc., 1974).

Pitts, R. F.: The role of ammonia production and excretion in regulation of acid-base balance (Physiology in Medicine), N. Engl. J. Med. 284: 32, 1971.

Roughton, F. J. W.: Kinetics of gas transport in blood, Brit. Med. Bull. 19:80, 1963.

Schwartz, W. B., and Relman, A. S.: A critique of the parameters used in the evaluation of acid-base disorders, N. Engl. J. Med. 268:1382, 1963.

Singer, R. B.: A new diagram for the visualization and interpretation of acid-base changes, Am. J. Med. Sci. 221:199, 1951.

Van Slyke, D. D., and Sendroy, J., Jr.: Line charts for graphic calculations by Henderson-Hasselbalch equation and for calculating plasma CO_2 content from whole blood content, J. Biol. Chem. 79:781, 1928.

Chapter 17. Defense Mechanisms of the Lungs

Angell James, J. E., and Daly, M. deB.: Reflex respiratory and cardiovascular effects of stimulation of receptors in the nose of dog, J. Physiol. 220:673, 1972.

Boyd, E. M.: Expectorants and respiratory tract fluid, Pharmacol. Rev. 6:521, 1954.

Brain, J. D.: Free cells in the lungs, Arch. Intern. Med. 126:477, 1970.

Dalhamm, T.: Mucous flow and ciliary activity in the trachea of healthy rats and rats exposed to respiratory irritant gases, Acta physiol. scandinav. vol. 36, supp. 123, 1956.

Gee, J. B. L.: The alveolar macrophage: Pulmonary frontiersman, Am. J. Med. Sci. 260:195, 1970.

Green, G.: In defense of the lung, Am. Rev. Respir. Dis. 102:691, 1970.

Greenwood, M. F., and Holland, P.: The mammalian respiratory tract surface, Lab. Investig. 27:296, 1972.

Grimstone, A. V.: Cilia and flagella, Br. Med. Bull. 18:238, 1962.

Hilding, A. C.: Production of negative pressure in the trachea of the hen by ciliary action, Am. J. Physiol. 167:108, 1951.

Jakowska, S. (ed.): *Mucous Secretions*, Ann. NY Acad. Sci. 106:157, 1963.

Johnson, P., Robinson, J. S., and Salisbury, D.: The Onset and Control of Breathing After Birth, in *Foetal and Neonatal Physiology (Proceedings of Barcroft Centenary Symposium)* (Cambridge, England: Cambridge University Press, 1973), p. 217.

Kratschmer, F.: Ueber Reflexe von der Nasenschleimhaut auf Athmung und Kreislauf, Wien. Akad. Sitzungsb. 62:147, 1870.

Moritz, A. R., Henriques, F. C., Jr., and McLean, R.: The effects of inhaled heat on the air passages and lungs: An experimental investigation, Am. J. Pathol. 21:311, 1945.

Nadel, J. A., Wolfe, W. G., and Graf, P. D.: Powdered tantalum as a medium for bronchography in canine and human lungs, Invest. Radiol. 3:229, 1968.

Negus, V.: The air-conditioning mechanism of the nose, Br. Med. J. 1:367, 1956.

Sorokin, S. P.: Properties of alveolar cells and tissues that strengthen alveolar defenses, Arch. Intern. Med. 126:450, 1970.

Walker, J. E. C., and Wells, R. E., Jr.: Heat and water exchange in the respiratory tract, Am. J. Med. 30:259, 1961.

Wright, G. W.: Structure and function of respiratory tract in relation to infection, Bacteriol. Rev. 25:219, 1961.

Yeager, H.: Tracheobronchial secretions, Am. J. Med. 50:493, 1971.

Chapter 18. Special Acts Involving Breathing

Borison, H. L., and Wang, S. C.: Physiology and pharmacology of vomiting, Pharmacol. Rev. 5: 193, 1953.

Faulkner, M., and Sharpey-Schafer, E. P.: Circulatory effects of trumpet playing, Br. Med. J. 1: 685, 1959.

Fowler, W. S.: Breaking point of breath-holding, J. Appl. Physiol. 6:539, 1954.

Godfrey, S., and Campbell, E. J. M.: Mechanical and chemical control of breath holding, Q. J. Exp. Physiol. 54:117, 1969.

Hall, F. G., Black, J. W., Neely, K. K., and Hall, K.: Influence of loud speaking on pulmonary gas exchange, J. Aviation Med. 23:211, 1952.

Heusner, A. P.: Yawning and associated phenomena, Physiol. Rev. 26:156, 1946.

Mithofer, J. C.: Breath Holding, in Fenn, W. O., and Rahn, H. (eds.): Handbook of Physiology, Sec. 3. Respiration. Vol. II (Washington, D.C.: American Physiological Society, 1965)., p. 1011.

Ross, B. B., Gramiak, R., and Rahn, H.: Physiological dynamics of the cough mechanism, J. Appl. Physiol. 8:264, 1955.

Stevens, K. N.: Acoustical Aspects of Speech Production, in Fenn, W. O., and Rahn, H. (eds.): Handbook of Physiology, Sec. 3. Respiration, Vol. I (Washington, D.C.: American Physiological Society, 1964)., p. 347.

Chapter 19. Respiratory Adjustments in Health

Asmussen, E., and Nielsen, M.: Studies on the initial changes in respiration at the transition from rest to work and from work to rest, Acta physiol. scandinav. 16:270, 1948.

Avery, M. E.: In pursuit of understanding the first breath, Am. Rev. Respir. Dis. 100:295, 1969.

Avery, M. E.: The Lung and its Disorders in the Newborn Infant (Philadelphia: W. B. Saunders Company, 1964).

Bainton, C. R.: Effect of speed vs. grade and shivering on ventilation in dogs during active exercise, J. Appl. Physiol 33:778, 1972.

Bean, J. W.: Effects of oxygen at increased pressure, Physiol. Rev. 25:1, 1945.

Beaver, W. L., and Wasserman, K.: Tidal volume and respiratory rate changes at start and end of exercise, J. Appl. Physiol. 29:872, 1970.

Bert, P.: Barometric Pressure: Researches in Experimental Physiology (transl. by Hitchcock, M. A. and F. A.) (Columbus, Ohio: College Book Company, 1943).

Bullard, R. W.: Physiological problems of space travel, Annu. Rev. Physiol. 34:205, 1972.

Campiche, M. A., Gautier, A., Hernandez, E. I., and Reymond, A.: An electron microscope study of the fetal development of human lung, Pediatrics 32:976, 1963.

Chiodi, H.: Respiratory adaptations to chronic high altitude hypoxia, J. Appl. Physiol. 10:81, 1957.

Comroe, J. H., Jr.: The hyperpnea of muscular exercise, Physiol. Rev. 24:319, 1944.

Cross, K. W.: Respiration in the new-born baby, Br. Med. Bull. 17:160, 1961.

Dawes, G. S.: Changes in the circulation at birth, Br. Med. Bull. 17:148, 1961.

Dawes, G. S.: Foetal and Neonatal Physiology (Chicago: Year Book Medical Publishers, Inc., 1968).

Dawes, G. S., Fox, H. E., Leduc, B. M., Liggins, G. C., and Richards, R. T.: Respiratory movements and rapid eye movement sleep in the foetal lamb, J. Physiol. 220:119, 1972.

Dejours, P.: Control of Respiration in Muscular Exercise, in Fenn, W. O., and Rahn, H. (eds.): Handbook of Physiology, Sec. 3. Respiration, Vol. I (Washington, D.C.: American Physiological Society, 1964), p. 631.

Dejours, P.: Chemoreflexes in breathing, Physiol. Rev. 42:335, 1962.

Dripps, R. D., and Severinghaus, J. W.: General anesthesia and respiration, Physiol. Rev. 35: 741, 1955.

Dunnill, M. S.: Postnatal growth of the lung, Thorax 17:329, 1962.

Foetal and Neonatal Physiology (Proceedings of Barcroft Centenary Symposium) (Cambridge, England: Cambridge University Press, 1973).

Forbes, W. H., Sargent, F., and Roughton, F. J. W.: The rate of carbon monoxide uptake by normal men, Am. J. Physiol. 143:594, 1945.

Kao, F. F.: An Experimental Study of the Pathways Involved in Exercise Hyperpnoea Employing Cross-Circulation Techniques, in

Cunningham, D. J. C., and Lloyd, B. B. (eds.): *The Regulation of Human Respiration* (Oxford: Blackwell Scientific Publications, 1963), p. 461.

Krogh, A., and Lindhard, J.: The regulation of respiration and circulation during the initial stages of muscular work, J. Physiol. (Lond.) 47:112, 1913.

Lambertsen, C. J., Bond, G., and Jacobson, J. H. (eds.): Hyperbaric oxygenation, Ann. NY Acad. Sci. 117:647, 1965.

Lanphier, E. H.: Medical progress; Diving medicine, N. Engl. J. Med. 256:120, 1957.

Lenfant, C., and Sullivan, K.: Adaptation to high altitude, N. Engl. J. Med. 284:1298, 1971.

Lugliani, R., Whipp, B. J., Seard, C., and Wasserman, K.: Effect of bilateral carotid-body resection on ventilatory control at rest and during exercise in man, N. Engl. J. Med. 285:1105, 1971.

Olver, R. E., Reynolds, O. E. R., and Strang, L. B.: Foetal Lung Fluid, in *Foetal and Neonatal Physiology (Proceedings of Barcroft Centenary Symposium)* Cambridge, England: Cambridge University Press, 1973), p. 186.

Phillipson, E. A., Hickey, R. F., Bainton, C. R., and Nadel, J. A.: Effect of vagal blockade on regulation of breathing in conscious dogs, J. Appl. Physiol. 29:475, 1970.

Physiology Symposium: Respiratory physiology in manned spacecraft, Fed. Proc. 22:1022, 1963.

Porter, R., and Knight, J. (eds.): *High Altitude Physiology: Cardiac and Respiratory Effects* (London: Churchill Livingstone, 1971).

Roth, E. M.: Gas physiology in space operations, N. Engl. J. Med. 275:196, 255, 1966.

Rudolph, A. M.: *Congenital Diseases of the Heart* (Chicago: Year Book Medical Publishers, Inc., 1974).

Severinghaus, J. W.: Hypoxic respiratory drive and its loss during chronic hypoxia, Clin. Physiol. 2:57, 1972.

Severinghaus, J. W., Bainton, C. R., and Carcelen, A.: Respiratory insensitivity to hypoxia in chronically hypoxic man, Respir. Physiol. 1: 308, 1966.

Severinghaus, J. W., and Larson, C. P.: Respiration in Anesthesia, in Fenn, W. O., and Rahn, H. (eds.): *Handbook of Physiology*. Sec. 3, *Respiration*, Vol. II (Washington, D.C.: American Physiological Society, 1965), p. 1221.

Smith, C. A.: The first breath, Sci. Am. 209:27, 1963.

Weil, J. V., Byrne-Quinn, E., Sodal, I. E., Filley, G. F., and Grover, R. F.: Acquired attenuation of chemoreceptor function in chronically hy-poxic man at high altitude, J. Clin. Invest. 50: 186, 1971.

Whitteridge, D.: Effect of anesthetics on mechanical receptors, Br. Med. Bull. 14:5, 1958.

Chapter 20. Manifestations of Pulmonary Disease

Brown, E. B., Jr.: Physiological effects of hyperventilation, Physiol. Rev. 33:445, 1953.

Bucher, K.: Pathophysiology and pharmacology of cough, Pharmacol. Rev. 10:43, 1958.

Campbell, E. J. M., and Howell, J. B. L.: Sensation of breathlessness, Br. Med. Bull. 19: 36, 1963.

Comroe, J. H., Jr.: Dyspnea, Mod. Concepts Cardiovasc. Dis. 25:347, 1956.

Comroe, J. H., Jr., and Botelho, S.: The unreliability of cyanosis in the recognition of arterial anoxemia, Am. J. Med. Sci. 214: 1, 1947.

Gardner, F. H.: *Polycythemia, Disease-a-Month* (Chicago: Year Book Medical Publishers, Inc., June, 1962).

Guz, A., Noble, M. I. M., Eisele, J. H., and Trenchard, D.: Experimental Results of Vagal Block in Cardiopulmonary Disease, in Porter, R. (ed.): *Breathing: Hering-Breuer Centenary Symposium* (London: J. & A. Churchill, Ltd., 1970), p. 315.

Hamilton, W. F., Woodbury, R. A., and Harper, H. T., Jr.: Arterial, cerebrospinal and venous pressures in man during cough and strain, Am. J. Physiol. 141:42, 1944.

Howell, J. B. L., and Campbell, E. J. M. (eds.): *Breathlessness* (Oxford: Blackwell Scientific Publications, 1966).

Hurtado, A., Merino, C., and Delgado, E.: Influence of anoxemia on the hemopoietic activity, Arch. Intern. Med. 75:284, 1945.

McIlroy, M. B.: Dyspnea and the work of breathing in diseases of the heart and lungs, Prog. Cardiovasc. Dis. 1:284, 1959.

Morton, D. R., Klassen, K. P., and Curtis, G. M.: The clinical physiology of the human bronchi: I. Pain of tracheobronchial origin, Surgery 28: 699, 1950.

Noble, M. I. M., Eisele, J. H., Trenchard, D., and Guz, A.: Effect of Selective Nerve Block on Respiratory Sensations, in Porter, R. (ed.): *Breathing:* Hering-Breuer Centenary Symposium (London: J. & A. Churchill, Ltd., 1970), p. 233.

Porter, R. (ed.): *Breathing: Hering-Breuer Centenary Symposium* (London: J. & A. Churchill, Ltd., 1970).

Ratto, O., Briscoe, W. A., Morton, J. W., and Comroe, J. H., Jr.: Anoxemia secondary to polycythemia and polycythemia secondary to anoxemia, Am. J. Med. 19:958, 1955.

Sharpey-Schafer, E. P.: The mechanism of syncope after coughing, Br. Med. J. 2:860, 1953.

Stead E. A., Jr.: *Hyperventilation, Disease-a-Month* (Chicago: Year Book Medical Publishers, Inc., February, 1960).

Wright, G. W., and Branscomb, D. V.: The origin of the sensations of dyspnea, Trans. Am. Clin. Climatol. Assoc. 66:116, 1954.

10:77, 210, 356, 375, 481, 642, and 719, 1951.

Severinghaus, J. W., and Bradley, A. F.: Electrodes for blood P_{O_2} and P_{CO_2} determination, J. Appl. Physiol. 13:515, 1958.

Severinghaus, J. W.: Respiratory System: Methods; Gas Analysis, in Glasser, O. (ed.): *Medical Physics* (Chicago: Year Book Medical Publishers, Inc., 1960), Vol. III, p. 550.

Wright, G. W.: Disability evaluation in industrial pulmonary disease, J.A.M.A. 141:1218, 1949.

Chapter 21. Physiologic Diagnosis

Arcangeli, P., *et al.* (eds.): *Introduction to the Definition of Normal Values for Respiratory Function in Man* (Torino, Italy: Panminerva Medica, 1970).

Bartels, H., Bucheri, E., Hertz, C. W., Rodewald, G., and Schwab, M.: *Methods in Pulmonary Physiology* (transl. by Workman, J. M.) (New York: Hafner Publishing Company, 1963).

Bates, D. V., and Christie, R. V.: *Respiratory Function in Disease* (2d ed.; Philadelphia: W. B. Saunders Company, 1971).

Cander, L., and Moyer, J. H. (eds.): *Aging of the Lung* (New York: Grune & Stratton, Inc., 1964).

Comroe, J. H., Jr. (ed.): Pulmonary Function Tests, in *Methods in Medical Research* (Chicago: Year Book Medical Publishers, Inc., 1950), Vol. 2, p. 74.

Comroe, J. H., Jr., Forster, R. E., II, DuBois, A. B., Briscoe, W. A., and Carlsen, E.: *The Lung: Clinical Physiology and Pulmonary Function Tests* (2d ed.; Chicago: Year Book Medical Publishers, Inc., 1962).

Denolin, H., Sadoul, P., and Orie, N. G. M.: *L'Exploration Fonctionnelle Pulmonaire: Techniques d'Études et Applications Cliniques* (Paris: Editions Médicales Flammarion, 1964).

Dittmer, D. S., and Grebe, R. M. (eds.): *Handbook of Respiration* (Proj. 7158, Task 71801) (WADC TR 58-532) (ASTIA Document No. AD-155823) (Aero Medical Laboratory, 1958).

Gaensler, E. A., *et al.*: Bronchospirometry I-VI, J. Lab. & Clin. Med. 39:917, 935; 40:223, 410 and 558, 1952; 41:436, 1953.

McIlroy, M. B.: The clinical uses of oximetry, Br. Heart J. 21:293, 1959.

McNeill, R. S., Malcolm, G. D., and Brown, W. R.: A comparison of expiratory and inspiratory flow rates in health and in chronic pulmonary disease, Thorax 14:225, 1959.

Seminars in pulmonary physiology, Am. J. Med.

Chapter 22. Artificial Respiration and Inhalation Therapy

Behnke, A., and Saltzman, H. A.: Hyperbaric oxygenation, N. Engl. J. Med. 276:1423, 1478, 1967.

Carbon Dioxide and Man (Symposium), Anesthesiology 21:585, 1960.

Clark, J. M., and Lambertsen, C. J.: Pulmonary oxygen toxicity: A review, Pharmacol. Rev. 23:37, 1971.

Comroe, J. H., Jr., and Dripps, R. D.: *The Physiological Basis for Oxygen Therapy* (Springfield, Ill.: Charles C Thomas, Publisher, 1950).

Comroe, J. H., Jr., Dripps, R. D., Dumke, P. R., and Deming, M.: Oxygen toxicity; The effect of inhalation of high concentrations of oxygen for twenty-four hours on normal men at sea level and at a simulated altitude of 18,000 feet, J.A.M.A. 128:710, 1945.

Dautrebande, L.: Physiological and pharmacological characteristics of liquid aerosols, Physiol. Rev. 32:214, 1952.

Dickens, F., and Neil, E. (eds.): *Oxygen in the Animal Organism* (Oxford: Pergamon Press, 1964).

Filley, G. F.: *Pulmonary Insufficiency and Respiratory Failure* (Philadelphia: Lea & Febiger, 1967).

Nahas, G. G., and Bates, D. V. (eds.): Respiratory failure, Ann. NY Acad. Sci. 121: 651, 1965.

Pontoppidan, H., Geffin, B., and Lowenstein, E.: Acute respiratory failure in the adult, N. Engl. J. Med. 287:690, 743, 799, 1972.

Radford, E. P., Jr., Ferris, B. G., Jr., and Kriete, B. C.: Clinical use of a nomogram to estimate proper ventilation during artificial respiration, N. Engl. J. Med. 251:877, 1954.

Safar, P. (ed.): *Respiratory Therapy* (Philadelphia: F. A. Davis Company, 1965).

Sieker, H. O., and Hickam, J. B.: Carbon dioxide intoxication: The clinical syndrome, its etiology and management with particular reference to the use of mechanical respirators, Medicine 35:389, 1956.

Symposium on mouth-to-mouth resuscitation (expired air inflation), J.A.M.A. 167:317, 1958.

Symposium on inhalational therapy, Anesthesiology 23:407, 1962.

Whittenberger, J. L.: Artificial respiration, Physiol. Rev. 35:611, 1955.

Whittenberger, J. L. (ed.): *Artificial Respiration: Theory and Applications* (New York: Paul B. Hoeber, Inc., 1962).

Chapter 23. Nonrespiratory Functions of the Lungs and Pulmonary Circulation

Boileau, J. C., Compeau, L., and Biron, P.: Pulmonary fate of histamine, isoproterenol, physalaemin and substance P, Can. J. Physiol. Pharmacol. 48:681, 1970.

Comroe, J. H., Jr.: The functions of the lungs, Harvey Lect. 48:110, 1952–53.

Comroe, J. H., Jr.: The main functions of the pulmonary circulation, Circulation 33:146, 1966.

Eiseman, B., Bryant, L., and Waltuch, T.: Metabolism of vasomotor agents by the isolated perfused lung, J. Thorac. Cardiovasc. Surg. 48:798, 1964.

Gaddum, J. H., Hebb, C. O., Silver, A., and Swan, A. A. B.: 5-Hydroxytryptamine: Pharmacological action and destruction in perfused lungs, Q. J. Exp. Physiol. 38:255-262, 1953.

Hall, G. H., and Sackner, M. A.: Inactivation of endogenous vasodilator material: A detoxification process of the lung, J. Appl. Physiol. 21:923, 1966.

Heinemann, H. O., and Fishman, A. P.: Nonrespiratory functions of mammalian lung, Physiol. Rev. 49:1, 1969.

Metabolism of the Lung (American Physiological Society Symposium), Fed. Proc. 32:1955, 1973.

Meyrick, B., and Reid, L.: The alveolar wall, Br. J. Dis. Chest 64:121, 1970.

Smith, U., and Ryan, J. W.: Pinocytotic vesicles of the pulmonary endothelial cell, Chest 59:12, 1971.

Smith, U., and Ryan, J. W.: Substructural features of pulmonary endothelial caveolae, Tissue and Cell 4:49, 1972.

Smith, U., Ryan, J. W., Michie, D. D., and Smith, D. S.: Endothelial projections as revealed by scanning electron microscopy, Science 173:925, 1971.

Strum, J. M., and Junod, A. F.: Radioautographic demonstration of 5-hydroxytryptamine-^{3}H uptake by pulmonary endothelial cells, J. Cell Biol. 54:456, 1972.

Thomas, D. P., and Vane, J. R.: 5-Hydroxytryptamine in the circulation of the dog, Nature 216:335, 1967.

Tierney, D. F.: Lung metabolism and biochemistry, Annu. Rev. Physiol. 36:209, 1974.

Vane, J. R.: The release and fate of vaso-active hormones in the circulation, Br. J. Pharmacol. 35:209, 1969.

Index